Basic Skills and Professional Issues in Clinical Psychology

Janet R. Matthews
Loyola University—New Orleans

C. Eugene Walker
University of Oklahoma Medical School

Allyn and Bacon
Boston • London • Toronto • Sydney • Tokyo • Singapore

*We dedicate this book to our parents, Eugene T. and Louise B.
Rogers, Lewis G. Walker and Olga T. Brioli, the first three of
whom passed away during the work on this volume. This book is
also dedicated to Lee H. Matthews, spouse of the first editor and
former student of the second editor, whose support helped make
this project a reality.*

Library of Congress Cataloging-in-Publication Data

Basic Skills and Professional Issues in Clinical Psychology / Janet R.
 Matthews, C. Eugene Walker, editors.
   p.   cm.
 Includes bibliographical references and index.
 ISBN 0-205-16970-8
 1. Clinical psychology—Practice. 2. Clinical psychology-
-Vocational guidance. 3. Clinical psychology. I. Matthews, Janet
R. II. Walker, C. Eugene (Clarence Eugene), (date)–   .
 [DNLM: 1. Psychology, Clinical.   WM 105 B311 1997]
RC467.95.B37   1997
616.89´023—dc20
DNLM/DLC
for Library of Congress   96-38506
                                                             CIP

Printed in the United States of America

10 9 8 7 6 5 4 3 2 1   01 00 99 98 97

Contents

PART II   Professional Topics

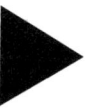 # About the Authors

Bruce Bongar, Ph.D., received his doctorate from the University of Southern California in 1977. He is Professor of Psychology at the Pacific Graduate School of Psychology and Consulting Professor, Department of Psychiatry and Behavioral Sciences, Stanford University School of Medicine. His major professional and research interests are in suicidal and life-threatening behaviors and ethical and professional practice issues.

Sheila Coonerty, Ph.D., received her doctorate in clinical psychology from Adelphi University in 1983. She is in private practice and educational consulting in Santa Cruz, California. Her major professional and research interests are in the psychology of women and gender issues in psychotherapy, projective assessment of developmental psychopathology, and psychological aspects of post-polio syndrome.

Patrick H. DeLeon, Ph.D., MPH, JD, received his doctorate from Purdue University in 1969. He is Administrative Assistant to U.S. Senator Daniel K. Inouye, the Secretary of the Board of Directors of the American Psychological Association (APA), former chair of the APA Board of Professional Affairs, and, for a decade, chair of the APA Committee on Legal Issues. His prime interests are in public service and the interface between psychology and law.

Donald K. Freedheim, Ph.D., received his doctorate in clinical psychology from Duke University in 1960. He is currently Associate Professor at Case Western Reserve University, where he coordinates graduate student practicum placements. He has written, edited, and recently developed teaching videotapes in the field of psychotherapy. He is a member of the Board of Directors of the American Psychological Association.

Peter J. Giordano, Ph.D., received his doctorate in clinical psychology from the University of North Carolina at Chapel Hill in 1989. He is Associate Professor of Psychology at Belmont University in Nashville, Tennessee. He is licensed in Tennessee as a clinical psychologist/health service provider. He is a former regional vice-president of Psi Chi. His major professional and research interests are in understanding ambivalence in the context of father–son relationships.

Jerold R. Gold, Ph.D., received his doctorate in clinical psychology from Adelphi University in 1980. He is currently Professor of Psychology at Long Island University and Clinical Professor, Postdoctoral Program in Psychoanalysis and Psychotherapy at Adelphi University. His professional and research interests are in psychotherapy integration, interpersonal approaches to assessment and treatment, and the application of narrative theories to psychotherapy.

Peggy Greco, Ph.D., received her doctorate in clinical psychology from the University of Miami, in 1993. She is a staff psychologist in Nemours Children's Clinic in Jacksonville, Florida. Her major professional and research interests are in the area of pediatric psychology.

Samuel J. Knapp, Ed.D., received his doctorate in counseling and guidance from Lehigh University in 1982. He is the Professional Affairs Officer of the Pennsylvania Psychological Association. His major professional and research interests include ethics and the regulation of professional psychology.

Kevin R. Krull, Ph.D., received his doctorate in clinical psychology from Florida State University in 1991. He is Assistant Professor of Psychology at the University of Houston. His major professional and research interests are in the abnormal development of attention and behavior control, the acute and long-term effects of exposure to neurotoxic substances from early childhood through adolescence, neuropsychological measures and electroencephalographic recordings of acquired and developmental deficits of attention and impulsivity, and behavioral and medicinal treatment of attention deficits and impulsivity.

Bob Landry, M.A., received his master's degree in clinical psychology from Pepperdine University and is currently a doctoral candidate at the Pacific Graduate School of Psychology. He will do his pre-doctoral internship at the California State University at Sacramento. His major areas of research interest are the client–therapist alliance formation and therapist training.

Janet R. Matthews, Ph.D., received her doctorate in clinical psychology from the University of Mississippi in 1976. She is Professor of Psychology at Loyola University and also maintains a private practice. She is an at-large member of the Board of Directors of the American Psychological Association (APA), former chair of the APA Policy and Planning Board, and has a long history of governance service with psychological associations. Her major professional interests are in training issues in psychology and women's issues.

Lee H. Matthews, Ph.D., received his doctorate in clinical psychology from the University of Mississippi in 1978. He is Director of Psychology at DePaul Hospital and Adjunct Associate Professor of Psychology at Loyola University. He teaches an annual assessment seminar to pre-doctoral interns in clinical psychology. Among his professional interests are clinical and neuropsychological assessment and training issues in clinical psychology.

Larry L. Mullins, Ph.D., received his doctorate from the University of Missouri–Columbia in 1983. He is Associate Professor of Psychology at Oklahoma State University. His major professional and research interests are in the areas of chronic illness in children and adults, systems consultation, and rehabilitation psychology.

Sandra K. Netherton, Ph.D., received her doctorate in counseling psychology from Texas Tech University in 1990. She is Clinical Assistant Professor, Department of Psychiatry and Behavioral Sciences at the University of Oklahoma Health Sciences Center and Director, Consultation and Liaison, Children's Hospital of Oklahoma. Her major professional and research interests are in consultation and liaison services for children and adolescents, adjustment to chronic illness, and death and bereavement.

James C. Overholser, Ph.D., received his doctorate in clinical psychology from Ohio State University. He is Associate Professor of Psychology at Case Western Reserve University. His major professional and research interests are in cognitive-behavioral approaches to the treatment of depression, suicide, and personality disorders.

Antonio E. Puente, Ph.D., received his doctorate in biological psychology from the University of Georgia in 1978. He is Professor of Psychology at the University of North Carolina at Wilmington. His major professional and research interests are in the assessment of non–English-speaking clients and reimbursement for neuropsychological services.

Robert J. Resnick, Ph.D., ABPP, received his doctorate from the University of Tennessee in 1968. He has recently retired as Professor of Psychiatry and Pediatrics. He is currently Professor of Psychology at Randolph—Macon College, Ashland, Virginia. Dr. Resnick has published extensively in the areas of public policy and attention-deficit hyperactivity disorder (ADHD) and recently coedited a comprehensive bibliography on ADHD. He was the 1995 president of the American Psychological Association.

Donald K. Routh, Ph.D., received his doctorate in clinical psychology from the University of Pittsburgh in 1967. He is Professor of Psychology at the University of Miami. His major professional and research interests are in pediatric psychology.

Randy A. Sansone, M.D., received his medical degree in 1978 from the Ohio State University. His residency in psychiatry was also from the Ohio State University. He is Associate Professor of Psychiatry and Medical Director of the Psychiatry Outpatient Clinic at the University of Oklahoma College of Medicine—Tulsa. His major professional and research interests are in eating disorders, borderline personality, and psychiatric issues in primary care.

Blaine Shaffer, M.D., received his medical degree from the University of Oklahoma Medical School in 1976. His residency in psychiatry was also from the University of Oklahoma Medical School. He is Professor of Psychiatry and Director of the Division of Adult Psychiatry at Creighton-Nebraska Department of Psychiatry. His major professional and research interests are in cultural psychiatry, psychiatric education, and anxiety and mood disorders.

Julia Shiang, Ed.D., Ph.D., received her Ed.D. in human development from Harvard University in 1984 and her Ph.D. in clinical psychology from the Pacific Graduate School of Psychology in 1992. She is Assistant Professor at Pacific Graduate School of Psychology and Lecturer at Stanford University School of Medicine. Her major professional and research interests are in psychotherapy and supervision research and in the study of culture, depression, and suicide with special interests in Chinese and Chinese American issues.

George Stricker, Ph.D., received his doctorate from the University of Rochester in 1960. He is Distinguished Research Professor at Adelphi University. His major professional and research interests are in psychotherapy integration, clinical training, ethics, and grandparenting.

Leon VandeCreek, Ph.D., received his doctorate in clinical psychology from the University of South Dakota in 1972. He is Professor and Dean, School of Professional Psychology, at Wright State University in Dayton, Ohio. His major professional and research interests include professional training and ethics and program administration. He has published widely on topics in professional issues and ethics.

Gary R. VandenBos, Ph.D., received his doctorate in clinical psychology from the University of Detroit in 1973. He is the Executive Director, Publications and Communications of the American Psychological Association, associate editor of the *American Psychologist,* and a columnist for *Psychiatric Services.* Among his major professional interests are facilitating the translation of psychological research into clinical practice and policy formation.

C. Eugene Walker, Ph.D., received his doctorate in clinical psychology from Purdue University in 1965. He is Professor Emeritus at the University of Oklahoma Medical School as well as teaching psychology courses at several universities. He is the author or editor of over fifteen books and has written or co-written over twenty-five book chapters and over fifty journal articles. Among his professional interests are general clinical and pediatric psychology and training issues.

Theresa A. Wozencraft, Ph.D., received her Ph.D. in counseling psychology from the University of Southern Mississippi in 1991. She is Associate Professor of Psychology at Midwestern State University in Wichita Falls, Texas. Her major professional interests are in training/supervision, ethics, mentoring, and teaching. Her research interests are in the areas of child abuse, sexual aggression, and eating-disordered behaviors in subclinical populations.

▶ Preface

When we first discussed writing this book, we realized that the initial practicum experience may occur at either the advanced undergraduate or early graduate level. These two groups of students have somewhat different levels of preparation as well as different responsibilities at their placements. Regardless of the educational level of the students, however, they have a need for information in similar domains. We therefore decided to develop a book that could be used by practicum students at varying levels of educational preparation.

Mental health practicum experiences are provided in several applied specialties within psychology. Rather than making repeated references to such specialties as Clinical psychology, Counseling psychology, Community psychology, and so on, we have adopted the use of the term "clinical psychology" in a generic sense (and with a lowercase "c") throughout this book. We understand that there is some controversy in the profession regarding this use of the word "clinical." Some professionals prefer to limit the use of this term to individuals who have obtained their doctoral degrees in the specialty of Clinical Psychology and use the more general term "health service provider" to refer to clinical practitioners. Other professionals make a distinction between the use of the lower- and uppercase spelling of "clinical," reserving the former for the general activity and the latter for the specialty. This is the approach we have adopted.

Traditionally, no textbook is used in the practicum course. The material that is addressed in this book typically has been taught by class discussion, individual assigned readings, or is assumed to be learned through practical experience. Our observation over many years of work with practicum students is that the experience is presented unevenly and that some students miss entire domains of exposure due to variability in placement sites and supervisor interests.

Our general goal for this book is to provide the reader with basic information about practical aspects of psychology service activities, current professional issues that are relevant to that experience, and the role of organized psychological associations in one's professional development. The book is subdivided into two broad sections. The first section covers practical issues faced by practicum students. It begins with the process of finding an appropriate placement site and progresses through issues of working with supervisors, the establishment of rapport and interviewing issues, and basic information about psychotherapy. Because psychological testing is such a major activity of many psychologists, we have devoted two chapters to this activity. The first chapter addresses screening tests and batteries. Especially in inpatient facilities, such approaches are becoming more popular as hospital stays are shorter and third-party payers are placing strict limits on services covered. The second testing chapter provides an overview of traditional psychological testing and is intended as a refresher for students who have had a strong background in tests and measurements and as a means of filling gaps for students without such a history. The record keeping chapter provides information on both the content of records and professional issues related to record keeping. Although many special populations could have been addressed in individual chapters, we chose only children for such coverage. In our experience, beginning and early practicum experiences often include work with children. Since early campus experiences are often with young adults, further coverage of children is needed before students begin placements in which they are more likely to encounter this population. Two other topics have complete chapters in this section because students often have minimal prior training in these domains. The authors of the chapter on psychotropic medication have given the reader a thorough review of this area. It is intended as a reference for students who are reading patient charts and attending interdisciplinary staffings at which such topics are often included without much explanation. It is also a foundation chapter for the later discussion about prescriptive privileges for psychologists. The final chapter in this section provides a basic introduction to clinical neuropsychology. This chapter should allow students to have a basic understanding of neuropsychological reports they may encounter even if they have not had specific course work on this topic.

The other major segment of the book has four chapters on professional issues. These chapters are designed to assist in the process of socializing the practicum student into the profession of psychology. One chapter addresses training issues including models and level of training. This chapter illustrates the professional importance of some of the topics covered in the practical issues section of the book. An appendix shows a sample vita. The chapter on professional issues discusses licensure, credentialing, continuing education, and malpractice. This chapter is followed by one on legislative concerns and the debate over prescriptive privileges for psychologists. The final chapter provides detailed information about a range of professional organizations with which both students and professionals may choose to affiliate, as well as some of the reasons for doing so.

In order to provide this range of information, we chose to have individual chapters written by carefully selected experts on each topic. Like a lecture series, the chapters of this book adopt slightly different styles depending on the preference of the author and the nature of the material. Due to the differing nature of the material, some chapters are longer than others. Some chapters have more information than may be of interest to a particular reader. We chose to include more rather than less information believing that readers who did not have that interest level could omit sections of those chapters. Some chapters are more relevant to the graduate student than to the undergraduate. Others are more crucial for the undergraduate. As editors, we have tried to maintain a reasonable degree of comparibility across chapters, including cross-referencing of related material that may be found elsewhere in the book while providing latitude to the authors to present material as they might if they were working individually with practicum students. Thus, some chapters provide more research foundations for the topic while others use an anecdotal style of addressing the specific topic. Since practicum students have theoretical course foundations for their applied experiences, we did not include much information on such topics as reliability and validity or the extensive research base for such psychotherapy variables as therapist and client characteristics. These topics are typically addressed in foundation courses. Although this style is somewhat unusual for a textbook, we feel it serves the purpose for the unique nature of the practicum course.

We thank each of the contributors to this volume as well as the editors at Allyn and Bacon for their assistance in the development of this project. We also wish to thank Daniel Houlihan, Mankato State University, and Susan Lonborg, Central Washington University, for reviewing the manuscript during its formative stage.

Janet R. Matthews, Ph.D.
C. Eugene Walker, Ph.D.

► 1

Introduction

First Steps in Professional Psychology

C. EUGENE WALKER   JANET R. MATTHEWS

This book is intended for students who are about to have their first experience in the care of clients or patients in agencies that offer mental health services to the public. Up to now you will have learned much about emotional problems and their treatment from classroom presentations and textbooks. The purpose of the present volume is to help you make the transition from what you have learned in the classroom to application with real individuals who are in need of help or service.

As you will discover, there is a great deal of difference between an academic setting and a clinical setting. In an academic setting you interact with peers and with professors in an effort to learn basic information and principles of your future profession. In this setting you are the client or consumer and the situation is structured to benefit you. However, when you enter the clinical arena, you change roles and become the provider of service or care for another person who is the consumer. This important shift in roles and function must be kept in mind. The chapters in this book will help you understand your new role and give you much useful guidance on how to function effectively in that role. Information about issues to be addressed in your continued training and your integration into the profession of psychology is also included. In the present chapter we will make some general comments regarding principles that will help you orient yourself to the new task you will be facing.

PROFESSIONAL APPEARANCE

In your new role, one of the first considerations has to do with how you present yourself, which may be more complicated than you might think at first. It is important to realize that you will be representing the agency or clinic as well as the mental health profession to the clients and patients with whom you come in contact. The exact details may vary from one setting to another, but the underlying principle to be observed is one of *professionalism*. You are becoming a mental health professional, and to be maximally effective, it is important that you maintain appropriate demeanor. One important dimension of this has to do with dress and grooming. While a t-shirt, jeans, and tennis shoes might be appropriate attire for campus life, they generally are not acceptable in a mental health agency. Dress requirements vary depending on the agency and the clients served. However, both men and women are expected to project the image of a competent and serious professional. This image involves clothing, make-up, hair styles and so forth. The main point is to communicate to your clients that you think they are important and that you are very serious in your intent to be of help to them. When clients arrive at a mental health facility, they are generally in considerable distress, somewhat confused, upset, and anxious. Your appearance and dress should reassure them and put them at ease. You can take a cue from others in the facility by noting how they dress. It is also good to discuss this topic with the site supervisor.

A second very important factor of professional appearance is one's verbal behavior as it reflects a level of closeness. Our observation of trainees over the years indicates that they tend to go to one extreme or the other. In the one extreme, trainees attempt to be overly friendly and familiar with clients. This approach often is overwhelming and upsetting to clients. It also tends to undermine their confidence in the therapist's competence. At the other extreme, some trainees adopt a severely aloof, austere, even arrogant approach in an attempt to project a very "professional" image. This often puts patients off because they feel demeaned and as though the person confronting them is not really interested in them. The best approach is the middle road in which one has a serious and businesslike approach tempered with warmth, goodwill, and sincere interest in the client.

One's appearance and verbal behavior toward the client are essential in what may well be the key to all clinical interactions, the establishment of rapport with the patient. The dictionary definition of *rapport* indicates that it means to be in agreement or in harmony with another individual. In a clinical or counseling situation it means that and much more. When one has rapport with a client or patient, there is a feeling of oneness, connectedness, and understanding as well as goodwill and sincere liking for each other. It is this contact and relationship with the patient that underlie what is often referred to as the *therapeutic alliance* and which is crucial to all interactions that will occur between the therapist and client throughout the treatment process. In the absence of rapport, very little good can come out of counseling. With rapport, tactical errors or "mistakes" can be openly discussed and dealt with so they do not impede the therapeutic process. (This topic will be covered in greater detail with examples from a professional career in Chapter 11.)

CHARACTERISTICS OF SUCCESSFUL THERAPISTS

There has been a good deal of research over the years on the characteristics of successful therapists and therapeutic relationships. Although it is difficult to summarize such a massive amount of research in a few words, some generalizations are possible. First, the characteristics of a good therapist are very similar to the characteristics of a good friend, provided that the friend remains objective and maintains a sense of personal integrity. (Some years ago William Schofield (1964) discussed this concept in a book entitled *Psychotherapy: The Purchase of Friendship.*)

More specifically, helpful therapeutic relationships involve several concepts. Among these are unconditional positive regard, warmth, empathy, and emotional congruence. Unconditional positive regard may not be totally possible and there may be times when that concept would have to be qualified. Nevertheless, it is essential that the therapist believe the patient has intrinsic worth and approach the patient with strong feelings of positive regard and respect that remain unshakable regardless of what occurs. This is an extremely important concept. Most emotionally disturbed people feel that they have been mistreated by others, rejected, let down, abandoned, and that others don't care about them, a feeling that generally stems from some truth and some misperception. The successful therapist is careful to approach the patient with the utmost respect and with a great deal of goodwill.

Second is warmth, or a sincere liking for the patient. This is obviously closely related to positive regard and implies a desire to be nurturing toward the person, to support him or her, and to be helpful. Regardless of what the patient reports having done in the past or feeling at present, the therapist must attempt to nurture the good in the patient and foster positive growth.

The third concept is empathy. It is possible for a therapist to have positive regard and warmth toward a patient but yet be misguided and misdirected. Warmth and positive feelings require the direction of empathy. One who has empathy for another is able to understand and appreciate how the other person feels and why the person might feel that way. At the same time, the individual maintains objectivity and is, therefore, in a position to be of help in resolving the problem. This differs from sympathy, in which one has the same feeling as the other person and becomes enmeshed in the sympathy-provoking situation, which prevents either party being objective and working successfully toward a solution. The origin of the word *sympathy* is from the Greek word *patheim* (to feel or suffer) and *syn* (with). Obviously, the successful therapist will have a great deal of empathy but will not be caught in sympathy. It is empathic understanding that enables a therapist to provide direction, guidance, and help.

Emotional congruence is a two edged sword. The therapist must have congruence between his or her emotions and behaviors so that he or she can be genuine in interpersonal relationships. Likewise, one of the goals of treatment is to help the patient develop congruence between feelings or emotions and behavior in order to be effective in coping with life situations.

The goal of a therapist is to have the personal characteristics and to create relationships with others that are *health-engendering*. A health engendering relationship is one that enables the patient to grow in strength, maturity, coping ability and self-esteem. Unfortunately, not all therapeutic relationships fit this model. Some therapists are noteworthy for their ability to weaken patients, undermining their self-esteem and making them unable to cope without the support of the therapist. While patients of such therapists often have high praise for them, the treatment in reality does more harm than good.

It is in the context of rapport and a helpful, health engendering relationship that therapeutic progress can be made via specific interventions and techniques. Further explanation of this process, with case examples, is found in Chapter 5.

NORMATIVE VERSUS IDIOGRAPHIC APPROACHES

One final and related point should be made regarding orientation to patients. As the foregoing discussion implies, the successful therapist must approach the client or patient with full recognition of the uniqueness and individuality of the person. It is particularly important to keep individuality in mind as one makes the transition from the classroom to the clinic because most of the information presented in the classroom is presented in terms of *group* data. However, many clients seen in counseling and treatment centers represent the extremes or the unusual cases as opposed to the ones that fit the central tendency. This is often discussed in the literature as the difference between *idiographic* and *normative* approaches to understanding behavior. In normative approaches the mean and central tendency for groups of subjects is what is of interest. All sorts of statistical tests can be performed on such data, and presence or absence of differences can be established. In the idiographic approach to human behavior one is concerned about the specific variability of the behavior of one person. Group data are useful, but only as a context. The group or central tendency information may not apply to the individual at all. And there are relatively few statistical analyses that can be performed on the limited amount of information available from one individual. For example, the first author recalls an instance some years ago in which he had just completed a course on intelligence testing. In this course he learned that IQs do not vary from one testing to another by more than 3 to 5 points. This led to a minor argument with a supervisor who stated that a patient in the clinic needed to be retested and that a significantly higher score on the second testing might be anticipated because of a traumatic experience that had occurred just before the first testing. The answer, of course, is inherent in the idiographic versus normative use of data. It is true that *on the average*, IQ scores will not vary more than 3 to 5 points from one occasion to another. However, if an individual is tested in an unfamiliar setting following a highly traumatic event, that person may do very poorly on an intelligence test. A later testing sometime following the traumatic event might yield an IQ score of as much as 10 or 20 points higher. In working with individual patients, it is important to know norms and ranges for various behaviors, but it is also important to keep in mind that for a given individual the central tendency data may not apply. It is the extreme scorers who more often show up in the clinic.

ETHICS

The following chapters in this text will discuss, in much more detail, the specifics of relating to clients and providing for their care. Legal and ethical considerations will be discussed in each of these chapters also. The complete ethical guidelines adopted by the American Psychological Association appear in Appendix A at the end of this book. These should be read carefully and questions should be discussed with your supervisor. By way of introduction, it is good to note a few frequently applicable ethical principles that are sometimes not fully appreciated by therapists who are beginning their clinical work.

Confidentiality

First is the issue of confidentiality. Statements made by a patient to a therapist are considered to be confidential. However, this principle is not adhered to in an absolute sense. It is important that the client understand the limits of confidentiality from the beginning of treatment. Many agencies have a written statement about confidentiality that is given to the patient and must be signed. This is certainly an excellent procedure. If such a written document does not exist, the therapist must make clear to the client the exact nature of their relationship and the limits of confidentiality. Since this varies from state to state and with different circumstances, it is important to discuss this topic with your supervisor before you begin to see clients. However, the following guidelines may be helpful. First, and foremost, one must explicitly discuss the limits of confidentiality with the patient. An adult patient should be told that what is discussed will be confidential; however, the patient must be aware that you will be discussing his or her treatment with your supervisor and that records will be maintained in the agency. The case should *not* be discussed with anyone else including the therapist's spouse or closest friend. The patient's right to confidentiality requires the utmost discretion.

Second, clients should understand that if they disclose certain information to you, you are required to take appropriate measures. For example, reports of child abuse require that the therapist notify the appropriate child protection agency in the state. If the client threatens to harm another individual, the therapist is required to notify that individual and the proper authorities to provide for the safety of that individual. If the client becomes at risk to harm himself or herself, such as through suicide, the therapist may need to inform family members or other individuals who can intervene in the interest of safety for the client. These issues should be explained to the client, and questions answered, before treatment begins.

In the case of a minor the therapist has to be aware of the fact that, in most states, minors are not permitted confidentiality with respect to their parent or guardian. That is, the parent or guardian has a right to request information regarding the treatment of that minor. Most professionals who work with minors have a written or verbal agreement with the parent or guardian to the effect that they will not disclose what is discussed in therapy routinely but will inform the parent or guardian if there is a danger or risk of harm to the client or any other individual. This is also explained to the young person in treatment. Generally, explaining to the parent or guardian that it would virtually make treatment impossible if the young person thought that everything said would be relayed to the parent or guardian is sufficient to obtain cooperation. However, it is important that there be an explicit understanding.

When treating young people, an issue that frequently arises has to do with noncustodial parents following a divorce. Each clinic and agency has its own policy regarding such instances. A conservative approach that is taken in pediatric psychology at the University of Oklahoma Health Sciences Center is that information regarding treatment of a young person is provided only to the legal guardian of the child. This policy has been established because the treatment contract is with the legal guardian and the child, who are thus entitled to the normal confidentiality. Further, noncustodial parents are sometimes seeking information that can be used in court to remove custody from the parent who is the guardian. It of course, would be very unfortunate if custodial parents failed to obtain treatment for a young person experiencing emotional difficulties for fear that seeking treatment might result in their losing custody of their child. Legally, noncustodial parents have a right to certain information about their child. However, we do not routinely make it available because of confidentiality. They can, however, obtain a court order and obtain the information through appropriate channels if they desire.

Confidentiality needs to be understood not only narrowly as described here, but in a more general context also. For example, it is generally understood that information about a case will be made available to other professionals within the agency or those who are actively involved in the referral and treatment of the patient. Nevertheless, this should be made clear to the client and appropriate signatures obtained when required. An important point here is that this information is available only to individuals who have a legitimate reason to obtain the information in order to provide care for the patient. Professionals in the agency who are not involved in the case should not seek or be granted access to it. A simple example to make the point is that if a professional in an agency discovers that a neighbor or friend is being treated in the facility, it is inappropriate for the professional to read the file out of curiosity.

Recording (audio or video) should never be made without the explicit consent of the client. Most centers have a separate permission form that the client must sign before a recording is made. The circumstances under which the recording may be used must be explicit. In most cases, they are used only for supervision. Sometimes the permission includes use for staffing or case presentations. In some cases, permission may be granted to use the recordings for professional presentation at workshops or conferences as well as for research. However, all uses of such tapes must be clearly understood by the patient and permission granted. The tapes must be erased or destroyed when they are no longer needed. Trainees are not to take tapes with them when they leave the agency where they have been in training. Likewise, trainees are not to take any records or files with them when they leave the agency. Such materials must be maintained in a secure setting in order to protect the confidentiality of the client.

Other aspects of the principle of confidentiality involve such things as discussion of cases in the clinic or agency where treatment is being provided. It is absolutely essential that case discussion occur in the privacy of an office or conference room where individuals who have no right to the information cannot overhear. Discussion of cases in the cafeteria or in a waiting room or hallway within earshot of other individuals is clearly inappropriate. Likewise, it is absolutely inappropriate to discuss cases in a public place such as a restaurant or at a party or any similar gathering. It is inappropriate to discuss a person's symptoms and treatment at a party even if the name is not mentioned and the therapist thinks he or she is disguising the situation enough that no one would recognize the patient. This is true for two reasons. First, an astute person can often figure out who is being discussed, thus breaching confidentiality. Second, even if no one can figure out who the client being discussed is, people who might overhear mental health professionals discussing cases at a party would be likely to lose confidence in that professional and in all mental health professionals. The thought certainly might occur to them that if they go to see someone for professional help, they might become the "good story" at the next party.

Cases presented at professional meetings or written about for publication must be thoroughly disguised and/or be used only with written permission of the patient. To avoid problems, many professionals use composite or hypothetical cases for illustration rather than actual cases.

Anotherl situation with the potential to compromise confidentiality must be mentioned. Frequently a professional will receive a call from an individual who identifies himself or herself as a relative, other professional, or other interested person. The caller may indicate that he or she is aware that Mister or Miss So and So is in treatment at the center and request or offer to provide certain information. The most acceptable response to such an overture is to explain to the individual that the clinic policy is to provide or receive information only with the permission of the client. It is not even permissible to indicate whether or not the individual is in treatment at the center without permission. The individual placing the call would first have to obtain permission from the client or suggest that the client give permission at the next appointment. When appropriate permission has been obtained, the therapist can make a decision about what to discuss.

Another question is what to do when the therapist encounters a client in a public place such as a supermarket or at a party. The general rule in this situation is to not acknowledge acquaintanceship with the individual unless the person does so first. If the person wishes to acknowledge you, he or she may do so. If the person wishes to remain anonymous and not have to explain how he or she came to know you, that is the person's prerogative.

Dual Relationships

Another extremely important ethical principle has to do with professional boundaries and dual relationships. Ethical principles of the American Psychological Association (1992) make very clear that professional boundaries must be distinct and that there be no dual relationships in the context of the practice of psychology. As with confidentiality, there are many aspects and dimensions of this topic. First, it is obviously inappropriate for a therapist to have any kind of sexual or romantic involvement with a client. The therapist also should not initiate any kind of social contact or involvement with the client. This is particularly important for beginning therapists to understand because sometimes, in a desire to be of maximum help, the young therapist permits the relationship to go beyond the bounds of professionalism. For example, one might think that it would be beneficial to take a child client to a baseball game or a movie or some other activity. Some activities of this sort during treatment time are appropriate, but after hours they generally are not. It is not appropriate to take patients to church or engage them in religious activities. Likewise, a therapist might want to visit a patient's home. This can be done during working hours (preferably accompanied by another person) on a limited basis but should not be done to excess or outside of working hours. The therapist should not maintain personal correspondence with former patients outside of official business of the agency. The therapist should not buy from or sell anything to the patient (Girl Scout cookies and similar items are excepted) or enter into any joint business relationship. Therapists should not solicit the aid of patients as volunteer workers for community activities, political organizations, or membership in organizations. Limited volunteer work for the agency may be acceptable if it is mutually beneficial and not exploitative of the patient.

Basically, contact with the client should be in the clinic or agency during normal working hours and under supervision. Emergencies should be handled in an appropriate emergency room or treatment center with supporting staff available. It is not appropriate to go to patients' homes, take them on outings, or meet them at odd hours when no one else is around. Likewise, when the case is complete, there should be no further contact other than in a professional setting and during normal working hours. There may be specific instances in which an exception might be made to these guidelines, but this should be done only with approval by your supervisor and with strict boundaries.

Therapists generally do not give their home phone numbers or addresses to patients. If patients have a crisis, they should be able to contact an operator at the facility who will put them in touch with their therapist, or they may be given a beeper number to contact the therapist or an "on call" person. Since all agencies handle this their own way, you should discuss this with your supervisor and then provide the information to your patient (preferably in writing).

Therapists should not involve themselves in treatment with close friends, relatives, or other individuals (such as employees) in which proper boundaries cannot be maintained. A not uncommon situation is the therapist and the client attending the same church or belonging to the same club. This certainly is acceptable, but during the time of treatment the therapist must still attempt to maintain a professional distance and not become overly involved. The therapist should not discuss treatment in the other context and certainly would not reveal the treatment relationship to others there.

Further aspects of dual relationships are also of interest. The concept of dual relationship extends to teacher-student relationships. That is, it is regarded as unethical by the American Psychological Association for teachers, supervisors, and other individuals in places of responsibility to become sexually or romantically involved with students. While perhaps not as stringent as with patients, boundaries regarding business and social relationships must be maintained between professor/supervisor and student.

Finally, in routine clinical functions the concept of dual relationship is currently understood to extend to differentiating the functions provided. For example, the individual therapist or professional who performs an examination for a court hearing or some other proceeding should not be the individual who is currently treating the client. Likewise, an individual who performs a forensic examination should not assume treatment of that patient unless there is a high degree of certainty and assurance that he or she will not be required to return to court for additional testimony. The point is that examinations that are used for decision making must be performed in a totally objective manner, and one's psychotherapy should not be jeopardized or undermined by the possibility of requirements to make evaluative statements or draw conclusions in a court proceeding.

Misrepresentation

The ethical principle of misrepresentation is very important for beginning therapists to understand. It is unethical for a professional to misrepresent his or her level of training or current status as a provider of care. There was a time when physicians, for example, were referred to as "doctor" from the first day they began medical school classes. The idea was to inculcate in them a sense of being professional physicians. However, recent legal decisions have made it clear that it is inappropriate to refer to a medical student as a doctor. This title implies to the patient a level of training, experience, and licensure that is not accurate for that individual. The same is certainly true for psychology trainees. Trainees must clearly communicate to the client their status as a student or trainee in a program leading to a particular degree and the fact that they are supervised in their work. Likewise, a therapist should not make exorbitant claims about the wealth of experience he or she has had and promise unrealistic outcomes from the treatment.

Further, as professional mental health providers we must be realistic about the limitations of our methods. This means that when we conduct psychological testing and assessment, instruments must be chosen that are appropriate for the client and the interpretation of the data must be in keeping with research and normative information regarding the instruments employed. Interpretations that cannot be supported by appropriate data are not acceptable. The purpose of administering tests should be carefully explained to the client as should the results. Any questions that the client has about the results should be answered. The treatment methods employed should be described and questions answered in order for the patient to determine whether he or she wishes to be involved or not. Extravagant claims for success or dire predictions for refusal of treatment should not be made unless thay can be substantiated explicitly by data.

It is extremely important that the therapist be aware of cultural and ethnic differences among people and take these into account in performing assessment and treatment. Pertinent information can be obtained from your supervisor, from the literature, and from other individuals of the same ethnic and cultural background. It is inappropriate to assume that white middle-class standards apply to all groups. In particular, the therapist must be very cautious about giving specific advice to clients about major life decisions. For example, it is appropriate for a therapist to discuss marital problems the client has. It is inappropriate for the therapist to advise the patient to get a divorce. It is appropriate for a therapist to help an individual think through a career choice or a job change, but it is inappropriate for a therapist insist that the client begin a certain career path or quit a particular job. Such considerations become particularly important when the client's religious beliefs are involved in the decision making. For example, one's desire to use contraception or get an abortion may well be in conflict with religious beliefs. In such situations the therapist as a health professional is ethically bound to provide appropriate information but as a mental health professional is also prohibited from giving specific advice—particularly advice that may be in conflict with the religious beliefs of the client (or, in the case of a young person, with those of the parents and guardians). Situations of this sort are often highly complex and it is not possible to give simple guidelines for all of them. Needless to say, such circumstances should be carefully discussed with your supervisor.

PROFESSIONAL BURNOUT

When students complete classroom instruction and begin the task of providing care to actual patients, they enter an arena that is at once highly exciting, stimulating, and rewarding, but also intense, strenuous, and emotionally draining. Physical and emotional burnout are real dangers.

Certain basic principles are involved in preventing burnout. For one, the therapist should take care to have sufficient recreational, relaxation, and other meaningful activities and relationships beyond professional work that provide perspective and stability for one's life. Likewise, the professional should have a network of colleagues who provide perspective, support, information, feedback, consultation, relief, and so forth as needed in order to continue to function optimally. Obviously, one should be careful not to assume cases or attempt to perform duties in clinical situations which one is not prepared to handle confidently. Burnout comes very quickly if one attempts to function beyond one's realm of competence.

Managing one's time and case load is very important. Different individuals have different energy levels and some can handle more cases than others. However, one should be careful not to assume responsibility for more cases than he or she can reasonably handle. Therapists should be sensitive to biological rhythms and schedule patients when they are likely to be effective, avoiding times of the day when they cannot be productive. Likewise, the therapist should schedule the day and patients in such a way as to maximize effectiveness. Knowing when to refer cases is an important part of avoiding burnout. If one has several very difficult cases and another case of that sort is referred, it is best to decline that referral and suggest that this patient be treated by another individual.

Obviously, effective professionals will update their skills and organize their professional life so that they are able to capitalize on abilities and perform duties that are rewarding so that they can continue to be effective and avoid burnout. More extensive discussions of the problem of burnout can be found in several books available on the topic (Cherniss, 1980; Farber, 1983; Malach, 1982; Pines, Aronson, & Kafrey, 1981).

As a beginning mental health professional you are starting on a significant and rewarding career. The chapters to follow will provide you with much additional information and guidance. A word to the wise: Use your supervisor often and take his or her direction readily.

REFERENCES

American Psychological Association. (1992). Ethical principles of psycholgists and code of conduct. *American Psychologist, 47*(12), 1597–1611.

Cherniss, C. (1980). *Staff burnout: Job stress in the human services.* Beverly Hills, CA: Sage.

Farber, B. A. (1983). *Stress and burnout in the human services profession.* New York: Pergamon Press.

Malach, C. (1982). Burnout is the cost of caring. Englewood Cliffs, NJ: Prentice-Hall.

Pines, A. M., Aronson, E., & Kafrey, D. (1981). *Burnout: From tedium to personal growth.* New York: Free Press.

Schofield, W. (1964). *Psychotherapy: The purchase of friendship.* Englewood Cliffs, NJ: Prentice-Hall.

▶ 2

Finding a Training Placement and Making the Transition from Student to Trainee

THERESA WOZENCRAFT

OBTAINING A TRAINING PLACEMENT

The success students experience in obtaining a placement at a training site and making the transition into the practice realm depends to a large extent on the knowledge they have about the training site and their roles as trainees. For example, students should be aware of the site's professional and business practices, site personnel, and the expectations faculty and site personnel have of trainees. In addition to demonstrating competence in the field of study, students must demonstrate specific professional behaviors. This chapter will provide information students need not only to obtain a placement, but also to function effectively during the training experience.

University Protocol

How students begin the process of placement at a training site will depend on the academic department's protocol. Before students begin the training experience, the faculty member who serves as the campus training coordinator will inform them about who takes responsibility for each step of the placement process (Boylan, Malley, & Scott, 1988). One of several options may apply: (1) students may be responsible for finding their own placements, (2) the training coordinator may be responsible for assigning students to placements, (3) students may be given a list of placements they can pursue, (4) placement site personnel may come to the university and interview all potential applicants during an internship/practicum placement day, or (5) some other arrangement may be utilized by the institution. In many cases the training coordinator will assign students to their sites, with students having minimal responsibility for the actual placement. If this is the case, then students need only make certain they complete the application process on time and follow the directions of the training coordinator. If students are not assigned, then they should clarify whether they are free to explore placements, schedule interviews, and make final choices. They should also ascertain from the training coordinator whether some sites select applicants earlier than others and what time frames should be considered for the exploration and application process.

DETERMINING TRAINING NEEDS

For many students the primary consideration in choosing a site will be the match between their training needs and the training opportunities offered by the site. How do students determine training needs? The preparation of the *vita* (an extensive résumé) allows students to review experiences and strengths, as well as to note categories of experience they have not had or which are not sufficiently developed. The vita can be read by the training coordinator, who can help assess training needs.

EXPLORATION OF TRAINING SITES

When to Start Exploring

Students who are required to obtain their own placements (usually master's and doctoral students) need to begin their exploration of potential sites well in advance of when they are planning to begin the training experience. Master's students should plan to begin exploring sites 2 to 6 months ahead of time. Applying to two to four sites is recommended, so students will want to thoroughly explore five or six sites. Doctoral students seeking placement in a pre-doctoral internship are advised to begin exploration a full year in advance of the desired beginning date. Application to six to eight internship sites is desirable, so exploration of at least ten sites is advisable.

How to Explore Training Sites

Students should next consider where and how to get the information that should be obtained during exploration of sites. For simplicity, information sources can be categorized as internal and external—internal being from the site and external being from outside the site. Both kinds of sources can be useful in finding and successfully negotiating the training situation.

Internal information sources include literature from the site and information from site staff. The training coordinator will tell students whether it is appropriate to write or to call for information. Never pay an unexpected and uninvited visit to a site, even just to get information. Before writing or calling a site, obtain the name of the on-site supervisor (Belar & Orgel, 1980). Most agencies have multiple practica and thus several practicum supervisors, making an envelope addressed to "Practicum Supervisor" a piece of undeliverable mail. When calling, it is common to speak with the secretary rather than the supervisor to request information about the site. When writing or calling, ask for information on the site, an application, and the due date for application material.

Carefully review the information received and write down any follow-up questions you have. It would be useful to see whether the training coordinator or a senior student can answer any of these questions. By doing this, students avoid having unnecessary or inappropriate questions for the site supervisor or staff. Students can then call the site supervisor to obtain answers to the remaining questions. The site supervisor may elect to refer students to a trainee currently completing the training experience at that site. Because of the importance of the impression created during the initial contact, do not seem to interrogate the site staff. The appropriate tone to convey is that one is interested in learning more about the site and in determining if there is a good match.

There are other options for obtaining information to answer one's questions; specifically, the student may use external information sources, such as university faculty, students who have completed or are completing a placement at that site, practitioners in the community, and published directories of internships. These sources provide objective, albeit more impression-based, information on a site. External sources can also be approached more informally, and questions about sites can be asked with more candor. All questions should be positively framed, however, as these same external sources for the student may also be sources of information about prospective trainees for the site. An informal directory of local practicum sites may be available from the training coordinator. The training coordinator and perhaps other faculty members should be able to describe the sites and comment on the nature and quality of the site experience. Students (past or present) will be able to give a detailed and useful description of the supervision they received, the training experiences available, and the client populations typically served. Professionals in the community can comment more generally on site characteristics.

Matching Training Needs to Site Characteristics

Once information on the site has been gathered, it is time to compare training needs with training experiences available. Students may wish to consider the following areas (Boylan, Malley, & Scott, 1988) when exploring the suitability of the site to their training needs:

* Types of experiences available to students (crisis intervention, short-term and long-term therapy, case management, individual and group)
* Site personnel (disciplines and theoretical orientations represented, credentials)
* Professional associations of the site (accrediting bodies, affiliations with other agencies)
* Professional practices of the site (recordkeeping, in-services, staffings)
* Site stability (staff turnover)
* Client population characteristics (SES level[s], gender, ethnicities, ages)
* Administrative support (library, computer facilities, secretarial/clerical services, phone, office space and desk)
* Opportunities to participate in ongoing research or grant writing
* Quality and quantity of supervision (individual, group, and co-therapy)

SECURING A TRAINING SITE

The Application Process

After reviewing sites, students are ready to begin the application process. Check for limits on how many students from one program may apply to each site and communicate with classmates and the training coordinator throughout the exploration and application process. When completing the applications, compose a checklist of the materials required by each site. Two commonly requested types of materials for those applying to predoctoral internships are letters of recommendation and transcripts. Letters of recommendation and transcripts should be requested 3 to 4 weeks in advance of the earliest application deadline. A vita and a cover letter should also be prepared and accompany the application.

Vita Preparation

Content.   The first section of the vita should include all basic personal information, the name of the university, and degree program. The vita should also include all professional experience, supervised practice courses, volunteer work, and any other practica. Research experience and publications or presentations should be included, as well as involvement in extracurricular activities such as a psychology club or a service organization. Scholarships, honor society memberships, and awards may be highlighted briefly. The last page of the vita should include references who may be contacted. Students should always ask potential references whether they feel comfortable serving in that capacity. Generally, references are individuals who are familiar with your professional and academic performance over the period of at least 1 year. A sample vita is provided in Chapter 12.

Style.   Clarity, conciseness, organization, and consistency are the keys to a professional vita. The vita sections should be clearly demarcated. Use technical elements such as headings, underlining, bold lettering, spacing, and indentation to make a neat and organized document that is internally consistent. Internal consistency of the vita is achieved by using comparable technical elements to demarcate the subsections of each section. Avoid long, unbroken blocks of text, which tend to be less appealing to the eye. An additional technical concern is whether to use an ascending or descending chronological sequence. A descending sequence (from most recent experiences to those that occurred longest ago) is commonly used and serves to highlight the experience most pertinent to the site staff.

Course Summary Addendum.   Students may or may not be expected to prepare a course summary sheet to accompany the vita. A course summary sheet gives brief descriptions (one or two sentences in length) of all courses taken to date. A twist on the course summary sheet would be to add a sentence describing how the course contributed to one's ability to participate in the training experience.

Cover Letter

A cover letter should accompany each typed (never handwritten) application and its attachments (i.e., vita and other requested materials). The cover letter should present three important considerations. The first of these is how one's interests and skills match the experience the practicum has to offer. The second is how one's strengths could be useful in that practicum (Brill, Wolkin, & McKeel, 1985). A third consideration included in a cover letter is how one might expect to grow if accepted at the site. Alternatively, this information can be presented in a statement of interests or goals, if that is requested. In that case the cover letter would serve to briefly introduce oneself, to report which materials are enclosed and which are coming directly to the site (e.g., transcripts, letters of recommendation), and to thank the site for considering the application. If no statement of interest is requested, then the cover letter should include all of these considerations within one to one and a half pages.

Students may wish to include additional, unrequired materials with their application packets. Some sites ask for voluntary contributions of work samples, while others do not solicit this material. In the latter case, asking the site supervisor whether they would like any additional information would be appropriate. A well-written research paper, publication, or poster presentation would be appropriate to submit.

HOW TO INTERVIEW

Regardless of whether one is seeking a training experience at the undergraduate or the graduate level, an interview is likely to be part of the experience. Interviews may be held by telephone or they may be in person and on site. Sometimes, if distance is involved, preliminary interviews are held by telephone and then students who make the cut to the final group being considered are interviewed in person. Ask the training coordinator how interviews are granted—by invitation or request. Although being assertive and demonstrating interest in the site are important, it is equally important to honor each site's selection process. If it is up to students to request an interview, include an interview request in the cover letter.

There are several ways to prepare oneself for the interview. First, practice the interview with fellow students and get feedback on nonverbal and verbal presentation. Videotaping mock interviews allows one to evaluate mannerisms and vocal behaviors. Obtain advice from the training coordinator on how to change mannerisms that detract from an effective presentation (Belar & Orgel, 1980).

Other pre-interview preparations are to (1) know what the site personnel do in terms of practice and research, (2) review letters of recommendation (if possible), and (3) memorize one's vita. Knowing one's own professional strengths and weaknesses is important. Think about how to word weaknesses so that they are presented as areas needing further growth and development rather than unchanging deficiencies (Hersh & Poey, 1984).

At the interview itself, students have two tasks. Students must demonstrate that they are competent and knowledgeable, as well as interested in and knowledgeable of that particular site. Generally, the questions students answer will demonstrate the former and the questions students ask will demonstrate the latter. Hersh and Poey (1984) offer this advice about the underlying message that should be apparent in the questions students ask: "The best questions are those that reflect motivation to learn and take part in many work activities" (p. 3). The advice given by Hersh and Poey (1984) suggests that it is best to avoid questions that make it seem that students are trying to limit their experience to only what they see as interesting. Hersh and Poey (1984) recommend that some questions, among others, not be asked:

How long does a trainee work each week?

Will I be able to take time off to work on my thesis/dissertation?

Will I be able to work around my work schedule?

Would it be possible for me to focus completely on assessment (therapy, substance abusers, etc.)?

NEGOTIATING PLACEMENT OFFERS

Post-Interview Letter to Site

Appropriate follow-up behavior can contribute to the likelihood of being offered a position. It is desirable to send a follow-up letter to the site supervisor indicating appreciation for the interview opportunity and briefly mentioning one or two aspects of the site that were of particular interest. If the interview was conducted by a committee, the letter should be sent to the committee in care of the site supervisor. The letter should be no longer than three-fourths of a page and should state appreciation succinctly and sincerely.

How to Accept or Reject Placement Offers

Accepting, rejecting, and holding offers for predoctoral internships is regulated by the Association of Psychology Internship Centers (APIC). Current regulations should be provided to doctoral students by their directors of training. For master's level or undergraduate training experiences, the training coordinator will advise students about protocol. Typical professional courtesy in the acceptance/rejection process is outlined here for those with no official guidelines. If offered placement at a site that is not first on one's list, it is appropriate to defer accepting for a day or so, if the first choice site is about to make its offers. Being honest about the reason for asking to defer an answer is important. Sounding too disinterested in an offer that is not a first choice might be a mistake as many students are not placed at their first-choice sites. Remember, the agency may be unwilling to accept a deferral, or may ask for a briefer deferral interval. It is appropriate at this point, when "holding an offer," to contact the first choice site and make them aware of the situation. Once you have made a choice, you should notify all sites of the final placement decision. Send an acceptance letter to the placement site, indicating acceptance of its offer and anticipation of beginning the training experience.

TRANSITIONS

Beginning the training experience can be both thrilling and terrifying at the same time. Beginning trainees will likely find themselves looking forward to engaging in the helping process. They will also be likely to find themselves questioning how much they know and if they can apply it to real-life situations. Students will be less anxiety-ridden if they keep in mind that the training experience is a continuation of the learning experience—an opportunity to translate knowledge into action. This section will address how to lower the stress associated with this transition and also how to adapt to the site as quickly as possible. Students can prepare in advance for many of the changes that the training experience will bring. There are three changes in particular for which students may want to prepare: (1) changes in learning mode, (2) changes in role and social environment, and (3) changes in culture.

Changes in Learning Mode

The learning process in the classroom is one that encourages conceptual growth. Students are taught to understand and mentally manipulate concepts. They are asked to apply knowledge in certain activities and on tests; however, they are primarily responsible for understanding the concepts. In a training experience, on the other hand, beginning trainees are expected to apply the concepts at a nearly continuous pace. This interface between understanding concepts and applying them is a challenging one, and many beginning trainees find themselves mentally exhausted in the early weeks of the training experience.

Another surprise to many beginning trainees is the self-instruction that is expected during the training experience. Trainees participate in their own training by reading documentation and literature, observing service provision, and providing services. Most beginning trainees, in the author's experience, report that they had to perform tasks for which they did not believe they were adequately prepared. This is different from classroom exercises, for which students are able to practice before being graded. Keep in mind that *doing* is a learning experience and that perfection is not expected on the first few attempts at a new skill. Preparing as much as possible through reading and role-play practice is a major responsibility of the trainee. Beginning trainees should remember that the supervisor will not allow a trainee to do something that causes irreparable harm to another person. In light of the energy that it takes to learn in a new mode and at an accelerated pace, it is wise for beginning trainees not to put too many other mental demands on themselves in the first weeks of the training experience.

Changes in Role and Social Environment

The role and social environment changes that beginning trainees experience are related to each other and thus are discussed together here. Trainees will be partially assuming the role of a mental health professional. During the training experience they will have the opportunities and responsibilities of a trainee rather than a full-fledged professional. Clients will be made aware of the trainee's status as a supervised student. Students will also be assuming the role of supervisee, learning to receive close supervision and constructive criticism.

For beginning trainees the social environment will become that of the professional mental health work environment. That social environment will consist of a new set of folkways and mores. The professional social environment will often involve being treated more like a staff member than a student observer—a gratifying experience with challenging implications. Functioning effectively in the professional social environment will call for students to learn, among other things: (1) the ethics of the discipline, (2) the chain of command, (3) how to work as part of a multidisciplinary team, and (4) how to follow the policies and procedures of the site. Specific recommendations on how to function effectively within the new role and social environment will be discussed in the following sections.

Learning about Role and Social Environment Changes

Preparing for the changes in role and social environment eases the transition period of the first few weeks and enhances the quality of the entire training experience. Part of the preparation is being aware of the kinds of changes outlined above. A second part of the preparation is learning about the new role and the site's social environment through students who are just completing or have recently completed (in the past year or two) a training experience at that site. Determining who's who and what's what before arriving can help to minimize the information overload that normally occurs in the first week. Some of the information obtained from other students will be heard again in orientation and during the first few weeks. Hearing it from senior students in a relaxed atmosphere should assist beginning trainees in remembering more of what is heard in the first few weeks and allow them to deal more effectively with the novel information that is presented. This priming can help trainees start the training experience with more confidence. Students will need an hour or so of the senior student's time, so offering to take him or her to lunch might be a good way to obtain the information needed in a way that respects that student's schedule. Table 3.1 provides a list of areas of inquiry (Boylen, Malley & Scott, 1988).

Adequate preparation will ease the transition into the training experience. As students begin and continue in the training experience, they will find challenges that cannot be or were not anticipated. Some of these issues will be addressed in the following section.

TABLE 2-1   Questions about Role and the Site's Social Environment

1. What is the chain of command at the agency? Who will supervise? Who is the supervisor's boss? What are the names of some of the other people in administrative positions with which one should be familiar?

2. Who are the professionals with whom one will come into contact most frequently? What are their professional disciplines?

3. Who are the support staff with whom one will be working? Will they do for a trainee any of the clerical tasks that they do for permanent staff? With which clerical tasks may one ask for their assistance?

4. What is the layout of the building in which one will be working? Will there be several buildings? Which areas are off-limits?

5. What types of paperwork will one be expected to do? What is the time frame for each type of paperwork?

6. What types of equipment will one be expected to be familiar with and able to use?

7. What are the procedures for storing confidential data on paper and on computer floppy or hard disk? How are phone calls handled in relation to requests for information about clients?

ESTABLISHING ONESELF SUCCESSFULLY IN THE TRAINING EXPERIENCE

Learning New Roles

Being successful in the training experience is based on success in integrating new roles. Student, professional, and practitioner roles must all be integrated into the beginning trainee's cognitions and behaviors. As previously discussed, the student role changes because there is a greater focus on active learning. The professional and practitioner roles must be observed and modeled from site staff, as well as constructed from one's own knowledge base and previous experiences.

Student Role

Students will be engaged in a new set of learning activities during the training experience. The types of activities will not be the only change in the learning experience. How students learn as trainees will be as different as what they learn.

How Training Activities Are Determined

As part of the learning experience, trainees participate in a wide variety of activities at the training site. These activities vary from site to site, so it would be futile to attempt to list all of them here. What is relevant is understanding how the activities of a trainee are determined. The supervisor, the training coordinator, the agency, the ethics of the profession (American Psychological Association, 1992), and the trainee's experience will play a role in the determination of specific activities. The agency administration and the supervisor will make most of the decisions regarding activities. Legal, ethical, and practical considerations will govern much of their decision making. For example, the agency must consider its funding guidelines and the credentials required of those who may provide certain services. Apart from agency dictates, the supervisor must consider what trainees can do independently in a short amount of training time. Also, the skill and proficiency with which students handle initial, sometimes mundane tasks will give the site supervisor a message about the feasibility of training them to perform increasingly complex tasks.

The training coordinator will have input about previous academic performance, training needs, and the amount of challenge that can be handled. Trainee input varies; at a minimum, trainees should be able to indicate which of the opportunities available interest them the most.

Ethical Limitations on Activities

The ethics of the profession govern what trainees can do independently and what they must do under supervision. The types of experiences students are allowed to engage in will, to a great extent, vary with the amount of education and training, as well as experience, with which students enter the training experience. For example, undergraduate students will not be allowed to independently provide therapy or many types of assessment. Ethics governing client rights may also limit participation in activities. The supervisor must also consider what trainees can observe or do without interfering with the therapeutic process or the client's rights. For example, the supervisor must have the client's permission before a trainee may observe a session. Not to obtain permission would be to breach confidentiality. If the client decides not to give permission for a session to be observed, the supervisor must respect the client's decision. Depending on the setting, clients may or may not have the opportunity to decide whether they work with a trainee or a staff member. In some settings a condition of receiving services is being willing to be seen by a trainee.

Typical Activities Engaged in by Trainees

Undergraduate students will often be allowed to do some assessment procedures on their own, such as administering and scoring self-report instruments. Undergraduate students may be allowed to engage in more activities independently if they complete their training experiences in social services agencies such as the state-based Child Protective Services or Juvenile Probation Office, or private agencies such as the Mental Health Association or Court Appointed Special Advocates. Social service agencies frequently employ people at the bachelor's level and encourage hands-on experience and independent work for their trainees. This sort of training experience may be preferred by undergraduate students who will be entering the job market right away, as it will provide a network for future employment opportunities. Social service agencies are more likely to give undergraduate students the opportunity to: (1) provide case management, (2) make referrals to community resources, (3) provide education and training to clients or volunteers, and (4) provide supportive client counseling. An example of one such agency might be a state mental health/mental retardation center, which may allow undergraduate trainees to play a large role in case management activities.

Graduate students will likely be allowed, under supervision, to administer, score, and interpret assessments on which they have already trained. Additionally, graduate students can expect to learn to administer, score, and interpret assessments with which they are not familiar. The same circumstances hold true for therapy training experiences. Students at all levels may also be allowed to independently provide client education and orientation services.

Modalities for Learning New Skills and Knowledge
The modalities for learning at the training site are largely different from those utilized in the classroom. Three modalities commonly used at training sites are self-instruction (reading), vicarious learning (observation, role play practice, co-provision of services), and independent provision of services. Observation of a staff member (conducting assessment or therapy, for example) is commonly used by supervisors as a training tool, particularly early in the training experience. After observation, the next most commonly utilized learning tool is generally co-provision of services. Students are encouraged to share in service provision by making comments or performing certain tasks. Generally, students would begin by making a few comments and receiving feedback or coaching on these after the session. As trainees become more comfortable and learn how to work with the staff member (usually but not always their supervisor), they are invited to play a larger role in service provision. For example, they may model the supervisor's actions and undertake explaining the purpose of and how to complete self-report instruments. Eventually, when the supervisor believes the trainee is ready, independent work will be allowed.

Professional Role

In addition to learning about the practice of psychology, students will also be learning about the professional behavior of psychologists. Some of what students will be learning applies to professionals in any discipline, whereas some applies only to psychologists. The professional behavior that is psychologist-specific will be discussed throughout the chapters of this book. This section will deal primarily with generic professional behavior, with some attention to professional behavior of psychologists. In conjunction with the latter, a few key behaviors expected of beginning trainees will be reviewed.

Working within the System

In general, all professionals work under a code of expected behavior, which allows them to function more effectively in service delivery. To this end, working within the system is one of the rules by which a successful professional lives. Working within the system means using the structures that are already in place and utilizing the strengths of the staff. Working within the system accrues benefits for both trainees and their clients. It benefits trainees because they are seen as resourceful team players, and it benefits clients because they need to learn to utilize the system in order to assist themselves in the future.

How do trainees use the structures and utilize staff strengths to work within the system? The answer to that question lies partially in the information they gathered before and at the beginning of the training experience. Just knowing what services are provided by the agency and who provides them allows trainees to work within the system more effectively. Trainees can learn more about this by asking various staff members about their roles and the services of their departments and writing this information down for later reference.

Working within the system also means getting things done the way the system dictates, no matter how much trainees disagree with that system. Although many systems are cumbersome, policies and procedures must be followed by all in order to ensure some predictability in that system. A part of professional growth is learning how to use bureaucracy to the client's advantage, a skill that most staff have attained and are willing to teach to trainees.

A conflict is another opportunity for personal growth. When a trainee has a conflict with the system or a staff member, it is recommended that the conflict be used as a growth experience, rather than trying to change the system or those who work in it (Boylan, Malley, & Scott, 1988; Dimick & Krause, 1980). Often, conflicts between staff and trainees are based on the trainee's unrealistic expectations or lack of knowledge. Defensiveness is a substantial impediment to professional growth. Being open to new ways of viewing relationships or policies can help trainees enhance the training experience and increase their adaptability. Those who do not have the ability to adapt and learn about themselves may wish to consider another profession.

Specific Behaviors Expected of Psychology Trainees

As mentioned previously, there are certain behaviors expected of psychology trainees. One set of behaviors revolves around being a guest at the site. A second set of behaviors revolves around being a student in training. It is important to remember that trainees are seen as temporary members of the staff. Just as a guest in the household asks the host before eating something from the refrigerator, trainees need to know whom to ask for clearance before beginning an activity. Supervisors will generally cue trainees on this, but sometimes trainees will need to make this judgment on their own. If a trainee is working in a multi-unit facility, it is always a good idea to touch base with someone in the department or unit before beginning work there, even after a supervisor has approved the activity. This shows respect for the staff and gives them a chance to provide up-to-date information that may help the trainee work more effectively. At the initial check-in, the trainee should ask if there is anyone else with whom to meet, thus allowing identification of the point persons with whom contact should be made. In addition to meeting the ethical mandate of cooperating and communicating with other professionals working on a client's treatment, another dividend of checking in is that trainees learn more about who does what, when, and where, thus making it possible to utilize the system more effectively.

The American Psychological Association (1992) ethical standards mandate the practice of a trainee identifying herself or himself as such to other professionals and to all service recipients. An introduction of oneself to a staff member might be similar to the following:

> Hello, my name is _____ _____. I am a student in the _____ program at _____University and I am doing my practicum in psychology here at _____ for the next_____ months. My supervisor is _____ and she/he has asked me to introduce myself to the staff with whom I'll be working. I understand that I will be working with you and your staff throughout my time here, and I would like to visit with you at your convenience to talk about how I can best be of service.

An introduction of oneself to a client is similar, but with more explanation of one's supervised status:

> Hello, my name is _____ _____. I am a student in the _____ program at _____ University and I am doing my practicum in psychology here at _____ for the next _____ months. Since I am a student in training, I must be supervised. My supervisor is _____ , and she/he will be supervising my work with clients. I will share with her/him what we have discussed and she/he will make some suggestions to me

about how to approach our work together. Do you have any questions about my supervision or training?

In sum, being a professional includes having good interpersonal skills, being able to work efficiently, recognizing one's limits, being willing to learn from others and grow, and having a respect for others and their needs.

Practitioner Role

Becoming a practitioner brings its own set of issues and challenges. Solway (1985) discusses the potential crisis that can occur as a student's identity shifts from academic to practitioner—from thinker to doer. The potential for crisis arises when students have achieved competency in the student role and desire to attain the same level of competency as a practitioner.

Solway (1985) points out that the need to be autonomous and the needs to be supervised and accept student status are in conflict throughout most of the training experience. In a sense, the training experience is the adolescence of professional and practitioner development (Kaslow & Rice, 1985). Kaslow and Rice (1985) believe that the development of students during training parallels Mahler's separation-individuation process. Students tend to need more personal and professional support at the beginning of the training experience; later in the experience they become more independent and want consultation as opposed to the supervision previously sought. Personal, professional, and institutional stresses that students are likely to experience can lead to lowered functioning. More specifically, students may find themselves unable, at the beginning of the training experience, to perform previously mastered tasks as well as usual (Kaslow & Rice, 1985). Completing the preparation outlined in the preceding sections should facilitate a higher level of performance and a better quality of training experience.

SOCIAL ENVIRONMENT

In addition to changes in role, the trainee must also adapt to changes in the social environment. Rather than being among familiar students and professors, the trainee is surrounded by an unfamiliar multidisciplinary team of professionals. Additionally, the trainee should anticipate working with people (both staff and clients) from cultured groups different from his or her own.

The Multidisciplinary Team

In order to work effectively in the new social environment, the trainee must have an appreciation of the functions of the members of a multidisciplinary team. The new environment will include members of other professions who have different types of training and ethical codes. This variety of perspectives should be an experience that enhances clinical training. Social workers, psychiatric nurses, counselors, psychiatrists, and psychologists (typical members of a multidisciplinary team) each bring something different to the treatment team. To enhance one's understanding of the multidisciplinary team, one might ask representatives of the various disciplines how they view a patient/client case and what types of contributions they make to that client's treatment. The keys to success in interacting with members of other professions are to treat everyone with respect, regardless of their level of education, and to respect differences in perspectives.

Social workers, psychiatric nurses, case managers, psychotherapists, counselors, substance abuse counselors, psychiatrists, educational diagnosticians, speech therapists, occupational therapists, physical therapists, recreational therapists, art therapists, music therapists, and, of course, psychologists are the professionals with whom students are most likely to interact. The educational backgrounds and typical duties of each of the types of professionals with whom students may work are discussed in the remainder of this section.

Social workers may work in positions at the bachelor's level (B.S.W.), the master's level (M.S.W.), or the doctoral level (D.S.W. or Ph.D.) . Master's- or doctoral-level social workers may receive licensure from a state licensing agency. In many states, bachelor's level social workers are also eligible for licensure. Social workers are employed in a wide variety of positions and settings. Bachelor's-level and master's-level social workers are often employed by government and private agencies to do case management, resource and referral (community services broker), and protective services. Doctoral-level social workers typically are found in academic or administrative positions. Due to changes in training and broadening of the social work field over many decades, social workers are as likely to do therapy as they are to do human welfare or protective services work. At the master's or doctoral level, social workers conduct therapy in private practice as well as other settings. Social workers with whom students might come into contact will do different types of work, depending upon the setting and the social worker's level of education (Morales & Sheafor, 1995). For example, at private and public psychiatric hospitals, students are likely to find social workers doing individual and group therapy, as well as social histories. At medical hospitals, social workers frequently are employed to help patients access community resources. At mental health centers, social workers usually have the primary duties of therapy and case management.

Psychiatric nurses are trained in nursing and address the medical and psychosocial needs of psychiatric patients. Psychiatric nurses may have a bachelor's degree or master's degree in nursing; some have a master's degree in psychiatric nursing. The nurses generally are in charge of carrying out the psychiatrist's orders for medication and for charting the physical health of the patient. At psychiatric hospitals, psychiatric nurses often manage the wards on which they work.

Licensed professional counselors (L.P.C.s), who may also call themselves counselors, therapists or psychotherapists, have a master's or doctoral degree in counseling or in counseling or clinical psychology. (Note: The terms *therapist* and *psychotherapist* are not protected titles under the law in most states and may be used by a person with a degree or with no degree or training.) The L.P.C. is a post-degree license that, in the states in which it is offered, allows these individuals to do private practice. They work in mental health centers, psychiatric hospitals, hospitals, government social service agencies, nursing homes—basically the same places where master's-level social workers are employed. Licensed professional counselors do individual and group counseling and therapy, as well as some types of assessment. The specific activities allowed vary by each state's laws governing mental health occupations.

Substance abuse counselors have education and training in substance abuse treatment. They may not necessarily have a bachelor's degree, but they may take workshops and/or college classes to fulfill the educational requirements for a state credential. Substance abuse counselors work in both inpatient and outpatient settings, assisting clients with learning how to abstain from the substance being abused, how to prevent and recover from relapse, and how to utilize self-help and other new support systems. Other mental health professionals may seek certification in substance abuse counseling in order to meet specific job requirements.

Psychiatrists are physicians who specialize in psychiatry after they complete medical school. The specialization period, residency, typically lasts 4 to 5 years. Psychiatrists are trained to deal with the medical aspects of human behavior and mental illness. They work primarily with patients who have disorders requiring medication, although they may also do therapy. At mental health centers, psychiatrists typically perform assessments, prescribe medication, and monitor medication effectiveness. Psychiatrists in inpatient settings are generally the heads of multidisciplinary treatment teams and perform basically the same functions there as they do in outpatient mental health centers. Many psychiatrists engage in some private practice in which they provide therapy. In most government mental health agencies, psychiatrists are hired primarily to manage medication regimens and direct treatment teams, while master's-level service providers practice therapy.

Psychologists are doctoral-level mental health service providers. Clinical, counseling, and school psychologists are those with whom students would be most likely to come into contact. Psychologists must be licensed by a state board in order to provide services. In some states, persons with a master's degree may be referred to as psychologists if they work in a state-exempt agency such as a state hospital or were grandparented when licensure was initially developed. (Grandparenting generally involves allowing a person to become licensed based on years of experience rather than obtaining a certain degree.) Psychologists provide assessment and therapy services at institutions such as medical and psychiatric hospitals, outpatient clinics, probation and parole agencies, and school systems. Psychologists also work in administrative positions such as chief of psychology service at a hospital or executive in a managed care agency. Psychologists may also write grants, conduct research, and develop programs.

There are a number of other professionals who are sometimes part of a multidisciplinary team but with whom students are likely to make infrequent contact. These professionals will be discussed more briefly. If students work within a school system or rehabilitation hospital, they may work with an *educational diagnostician*. This individual generally has a master's degree in education and provides assessment of educational aptitude, skills, and achievement. *Speech therapists* are also employed by school systems and rehabilitation programs, among other agencies. They provide diagnostic and therapeutic services for those who have learning disabilities, physical problems, or injuries interfering with the production of speech.

Occupational therapists, physical therapists, recreation therapists, art therapists, and music therapists are primarily employed by medical hospitals, psychiatric hospitals, rehabilitation hospitals, or public or private clinics. All of these therapists generally have at least a bachelor's degree. *Occupational therapists* teach people who have physical limitations to be able to perform daily living tasks (e.g., cooking, cleaning, hygiene, and dressing). *Physical therapists* assist people with physical limitations resulting from injury, disease, or physical malformation. They help these persons to improve strength, coordination, balance, and motor skills. *Recreation therapists* assist people in finding ways to relax and express themselves; as well as develop hobbies. Recreation therapists may or may not incorporate art and music into the repertoire of avocational activities they teach. *Art and music therapists* teach people to express themselves and to develop new skills and hobbies by using a variety of artistic media.

All of the professionals just described contribute to mental health service provision. Each professional group does its own assessment and intervention. Each group also has its own ethical and professional standards. Most groups share ethical standards similar to, but not identical to, those promulgated by the American Psychological Association (1992).

DIVERSITY ISSUES AND THE TRAINING EXPERIENCE

Working effectively with groups of persons different from one's own group is an important part of professional and practitioner development. Each staff member and client will be unique in terms of gender, culture, race, ethnicity, lifestyle, sexual orientation, and age. Each of these domains contributes to how individuals view and act upon professional and practitioner issues. These domains will also contribute to assessment and intervention issues encountered in working with clients. These domains have at times been collectively referred to as *diversity;* a term that will be used in this chapter. Any of these domains might contribute to what people say and do in given situations, based on values and beliefs that differ from group to group. For example, attitudes, values, and beliefs underlying behaviors illustrate cultural and ethnic differences. People from various cultures and ethnicities may behave and think differently because of differences in such areas as (1) the importance/lack of importance of time, (2) present versus future orientation, (3) competition versus cooperation orientation, (4) loci of control and responsibility, and (5) structure and function of social relationships (Dana, 1993).

Each of the diversity domains may affect students in a number of different professional relationships. An additional challenge is understanding both "within-person" and "between-persons" interaction of domains. For example, a client may be a lesbian Hispanic professional, while the trainee may be an African American man and the supervisor may be a gay Caucasian man. Not only must the trainee understand how this Hispanic woman views her sexual orientation, ethnicity, and professional lifestyle choice (within-person interaction), but he must also consider how each person's uniqueness, including the trainee's own, affects the perspective taken on issues, behaviors, and values being addressed (between-persons interaction). For example, a question to ask oneself is "How does the client view me as an individual?" Another question is "How do the ways in which the client and/or the supervisor differ from me affect my thoughts about and behaviors toward them?"

Being aware of myths, stereotypes, and facts associated with each group can help students manage interpersonal interactions more effectively. This awareness is accomplished through reading, having experiences with others from groups different from one's own, and asking questions of persons from different groups (for the purposes of clarification and knowledge expansion). Most persons prefer to be asked questions rather than having unwarranted assumptions made about them.

It is important to remember that there is as much within-group variation as there is between-group variation. Degree of acculturation to the majority culture and degree of identification with cultural heritage will determine the degree of expressed identification with the reference group. Behavior and physical presentation (dress, jewelry, etc.) may provide clues to identity in relation to cultural heritage; however, listening to what a person says will tell trainees even more. Identifying a person's culture based solely on physical appearance (e.g., skin color, facial features) can be a serious error. Assumptions and stereotypes are often tied to physical traits, ignoring the contributions of acculturation and identification with the reference group.

Keeping an open mind will help trainees not only recognize stereotypes they may hold, but also to add more in-depth, experience-based information to their understanding of individual differences among those of the same group.

Each diversity domain will be addressed individually at this point, even though, as trainees have seen, more than one domain applies to any one person at any one time. This chapter will address diversity as it relates to the trainee maximizing his or her learning experience and success while in training; other chapters will address diversity issues in supervision and clientele. Due to the broader nature of this chapter, it is not possible to include specific information on each domain of diversity. Rather, the purpose of this section of the chapter is to orient trainees toward the issues and ways to address them.

Gender

Gender issues play a role in both the client–therapist relationship and the supervisee-supervisor relationship (Hartman & Brieger, 1992; Powell, 1993; Stoltenberg & Delworth, 1987; Taylor, 1994). It is important for the trainees to use the training experience as an opportunity to learn more about how gender roles influence human behavior and attitudes, both within and across gender. Trainees can learn more about these issues by asking their supervisor about the influence of gender roles, observing basic behavioral/attitudinal differences in male and female clients, and reading about gender differences. Research data suggest that supervisors' stereotypes of men's and women's roles and behaviors may contribute to different expectations of their male and female supervisees (Pleck, 1976). If a trainee believes that he or she is being treated by a supervisor in a stereotyped or sexually harassing way, it would be appropriate to discuss this with the training coordinator. Training also affords trainees the opportunity to become aware of their own gender stereotypes and to work to eradicate them.

Race and Ethnicity

Jackson (1992) stated that it is important to recognize ". . . racial and ethnic diversity in language, culture, values, motivations, perceptions, and other psychological variables. . . ." (p. 84). First, the hurdles that ethnic and racial minority persons face will be discussed here. Second, Jackson's strategies for dealing with the hurdles will be presented.

One hurdle may be the lack of persons of similar ethnic background present at the training placement, thus limiting the number of role models. Jackson (1992) relates that many non-Caucasian employees were lost during Reagan's presidential years because of "last hired–first fired" layoffs in the social services. These persons typically had joined social service agencies later than their Caucasian counterparts; thus, they were laid off in disproportionate numbers. A second hurdle may be the timing of non-Caucasian persons joining a primarily Caucasian staff. According to Jackson, when one non-Caucasian person joins a staff, there is acceptance and integration of that individual into the team. When more than one such person joins a staff within a short time, Jackson believes there is less acceptance by, and sometimes even negative reactions from, the Caucasian group. In the latter situation, there is more likely to be segregation but no problems with courtesy and professional functioning. What is missed is the opportunity for those of different backgrounds to learn more about each other, which affects long-term professional and practitioner functioning.

A third hurdle can be described as the "devaluing experience." Jackson (1992) reports that non-Caucasians have experienced more devaluing when sharing information than have their Caucasian counterparts. This devaluing may come through being ignored, not receiving credit for a contribution, being interrupted, or having a contribution to a conversation suddenly terminated. Due to this devaluation of their contributions, these individuals may exhibit the following behaviors when they are in an interaction with one or more Caucasian persons:

> . . . (a) simply refusing to participate verbally, (b) racing in a hasty but disorganized manner to make a complete statement before being cut off, (c) speaking only to support a point already expressed by a majority group member, and (d) giving thought to the message that this is the majority group's organization and only they make decisions for it, which angers and interferes with one's thinking. (p. 84).

This vicious cycle prevents meaningful dialogue between the two groups and reinforces stereotypes, prejudice, and noncooperative stances between races and ethnicities. Pope-Davis, Menefee, and Ottavi (1993) provide a resource for Caucasians desiring an increased awareness of Caucasian racial identity attitudes and how to use that awareness to grow in acceptance and understanding of different races, ethnicities, and cultures.

What can non-Caucasian trainees do to maximize the positive quality of their training? Jackson (1992) suggests that trainees find a mentor who can help with issues such as insecurities, defensive behavior that is self-defeating, and withdrawal or self-segregation. A second suggestion is to look for programs that have non-Caucasians on professional staff. Third, trainees can look for programs that demonstrate through their organizational behavior that racial differences are valued. If differences are valued, it should be apparent during the interview that segregation is not occurring among the staff.

A fourth suggestion is for trainees to consider seeking professional or personal counseling to deal with training-related issues (concerns or conflicts) that might impair professional functioning. Jackson's suggestions maximize the chances of the non-Caucasian experiencing success in a Caucasian-majority setting. Flexibility and openness to change can help both trainees and staff to succeed in dealing with ethnic and racial differences.

Lifestyle

As mentioned previously, within-group differences are often as pronounced as between-groups differences. Within races and ethnicities, individuals can vary considerably in terms of lifestyle choices. Lifestyle choices may go with or against the grain of the practices of the gender, race or ethnicity, of the individual. Lifestyle choices include such decisions as whether or not to marry, when to marry, whether or not to have children, when to have children, whether and which religious affiliation to take, and how and where to live. Lifestyle variables are an important part of diversity because of the expectations of others in the reference group. For example, a Mexican American woman may be expected by her reference group to be affiliated with the Catholic faith, marry before age 25, and to have children in her 20s. If that woman makes different lifestyle choices, it may affect the way she views herself and the way the reference and external groups view her. Lifestyle issues can impact the worldviews of trainees, supervisors, and clients. For example, first-generation (attending college) trainees are likely to make lifestyle choices that differ from those of the previous generation and even perhaps the current generation. Students may find support in each other and from new professionals who have recently undergone the experience of making and following through on lifestyle choices different from those of their reference group.

Sexual Orientation

Homosexuality is perhaps the most misunderstood and unaccepted domain of diversity. Many of those from various races, ethnicities, and cultures do not accept homosexuality. Homosexual persons in American culture have made strides toward gay and lesbian rights, but they remain a stereotyped and feared minority. Many gay and lesbian trainees may find it difficult to share their sexual orientation, when it is appropriate to do so, because of these societal sanctions. It is important for gay or lesbian trainees to be comfortable with their orientation, as well as to feel accepted by colleagues. No trainee should be discriminated against on the basis of sexual orientation, nor should the training experience be altered because of one's sexual orientation. If trainees believe they are experiencing discrimination on the basis of sexual orientation, they should feel free to approach the training coordinator to discuss these concerns. Heterosexual trainees must deal effectively with their own stereotypes and fears of gay and lesbian persons and not allow these to interfere with their working relationships. Respectful expression of one's concerns to a trusted staff member or the training coordinator may assist the trainee in working more effectively with persons from this population.

Age

Age is an often overlooked domain because it is a part of every person's life. The role of age is partially defined by domains such as race, ethnicity, and gender. Age is an important consideration because it may affect, among other issues, the way people view themselves, the goals they have, their civic and familial roles, and the values they hold. Trainees may learn more about life issues affected by age by reading developmental psychology texts, consulting with supervisors, and recognizing that those with exactly the same racial, ethnic, and cultural background can differ in their worldviews because of age-related issues.

Diversity in all its domains affects the trainees. All those working in the field of psychology are charged with the ethical responsibility to accept diversity and to understand it before work is undertaken with those who are different from themselves. Learning about diversity can be accomplished through reading about and having personal contact with persons from different groups. Trainees must challenge themselves to examine their ideas about those different from themselves and to revise stereotypical, overgeneralized ideas.

MAXIMIZING THE TRAINING EXPERIENCE

In the interest of maximizing the benefits of the training experience, it is useful to consider the findings of a study investigating perceived worth of internship activities (Steinhelber & Gaynor, 1981). The population for this survey was a group of former pre-doctoral interns in clinical psychology. In reflecting upon their internships, psychologists believed that their most valuable experience was outpatient adult work of all types (individual and group, testing, and intakes). This study also found that psychologists valued their exposure to, and training in, a variety of theoretical approaches to psychotherapy. This study may suggest a way to maximize the long-term benefits of training by being sure to obtain adult outpatient work experience. Students who are interested in pediatric psychology should not be discouraged by this advice. Gaining some proficiency with adults is important because it is necessary to work with the adult caretakers of the children who are the primary clients. Another recommendation that can be deduced from this survey is that obtaining experience in many different realms was considered useful. Narrowly focused interests do not appear to serve even the doctoral student's best interest in the future.

EMERGING AREAS OF CONCERN

Two areas will continue, in the near future, to demand the attention of the mental health establishment. Diversity will continue to be an issue of concern and optimally also an area in which much will be learned (Hills & Strozier, 1992). Trainees of the future should emerge from their programs better prepared to work effectively with diverse groups as a result of more systematic training and education on domains of diversity. It is imperative that diversity issues be taken into consideration for effective therapeutic work and accurate assessment (Dana, 1993).

Managed health care and health care reform have changed and promise to continue to change the nature of mental health services (Winegar, 1992). With the emphasis on cost-effective provision of quality services, it is foreseeable that trainees may be utilized more consistently to provide basic services to clients. This could yield a training experience in which students have many more opportunities, resulting in a broader base of experience. This trend toward cost-effectiveness in health care may also engender a market demand for individuals trained at the bachelor's and master's level in psychology. Managed mental health care emphasizes the utilization of community resources, making the growth area in the job market likely to include private or public agencies offering low-cost services. Brief interventions are also considered a necessity; thus, behavioral treatment techniques will likely be one of the interventions of choice (Armenti, 1993). Other brief therapies, such as solution-oriented therapy and brief dynamic therapy, will also be likely to be used more often. Education and training in the brief therapy area seem to be necessities for any student hoping to apply psychology to the mental health needs of others.

Experience with clients from diverse backgrounds and training in the behavioral approach to treatment will be even more important to the success of future practitioners than they are to those currently practicing. Informed and proactive students will be certain to include these two areas in their education and training.

INFORMATION SOURCES

If more information on the process of obtaining an internship is desired, an excellent reference is *Internship Training in Professional Psychology* (Dana &

May, 1987). Two excellent references on the pragmatics of the training experience are *Practicum and Internship Textbook for Counseling and Psychotherapy* (Boylan, Malley, & Scott, 1988) and *Practicum Manual for Counseling and Psychotherapy* (Dimick & Krause, 1980). Both books include forms for tracking the trainee's experiences, as well as self-exploration exercises that promote professional development.

A thorough source for information on issues related to diversity and professional training in psychology is the book *Toward Ethnic Diversification in Psychology Education and Training* (Stricker et al., 1990). Although this book contains chapters that are directed toward faculty members in training programs, it is useful in pointing out issues with which all those trained in psychology will deal. The Jackson (1992) and Hills and Strozier (1992) articles referenced in this chapter provide much information on diversity in a limited number of pages. Further, the reference sections of these articles provide access to some of the seminal research in the area of diversity.

A number of books for the novice are available on managed health care. Giles (1993) and Winegar (1992) have prepared books that introduce the practitioner to this area. Armenti (1991, 1993) has written articles that assist the practitioner in negotiating the new terms that direct the provision of mental health services.

REFERENCES

American Psychological Association. (1992). Ethical principles of psychologists. *American Psychologist, 47*(12), 1597–1611.

Armenti, N. P. (1991, May). The provider network in managed care. *the Behavior Therapist, 14*(15), pp. 123–128.

Armenti, N. P. (1993, January). Managed health care and the behaviorally trained professional. *the Behavior Therapist, 16*(1), pp. 13–15.

Belar, C. D., & Orgel, S. A. (1980). Survival guide for intern applicants. *Professional Psychology, 11*(4), 672–675.

Boylan, J. C., Malley, P. B., & Scott, J. (1988). *Practicum and internship textbook for counseling and psychotherapy.* Muncie, IN: Accelerated Development.

Brill, R., Wolkin, J, & McKeel, N. (1985). Strategies for selecting and securing the predoctoral clinical internship of choice. *Professional Psychology: Research and Practice, 16,* 3–6.

Dana, R. H. (1993). *Multicultural assessment perspectives for professional psychology.* Needham Heights, MA: Allyn & Bacon.

Dana, R. H., & May, W. T. (1987). *Internship training in professional psychology.* Washington: Hemisphere.

Dimick, K. M. & Krause, F. H. (1980). *Practicum manual for counseling and psychotherapy* (4th ed.). Muncie, IN: Accelerated Development.

Giles, T. R. (1993). *Managed health care: A guide for practitioners, employers, and hospital administrators.* Needham Heights, MA: Allyn & Bacon.

Hartman, C., & Brieger, K. (1992). Cross-gender supervision and sexuality. *Clinical Supervisor, 10*(1), 71–81.

Hersh, J. B., & Poey, K. (1984). A proposed interviewing guide for intern applicants. *Professional Psychology: Research and Practice, 15*, 3–5.

Hills, H. I., & Strozier, A. L. (1992). Multicultural training in APA-approved counseling psychology programs: A survey. *Professional Psychology: Research and Practice, 23*(1), 43–51.

Jackson, J. H. (1992). Trials, tribulations, and triumphs of minorities in psychology: Reflections at century's end. *Professional Psychology: Research and Practice, 23*(2), 80-86.

Kaslow, N. J., & Rice, D. G. (1985). Developmental stresses of psychology internship training: What training staff can do to help. *Professional Psychology: Research and Practice, 16*(2), 253-261.

Morales, A. T., & Sheafor, B. W. (1995). *Social work: A profession of many faces.* Needham Heights, MA: Allyn & Bacon.

Pleck, J. H. (1976). Sex role issues in clinical training. *Psychotherapy: Theory, Research and Practice, 13*(1), 17–19.

Pope-Davis, D. B., Menefee, L. A., & Ottavi, T. M. (1993). The comparison of white racial identity attitudes among faculty and students: Implications for professional psychologists. *Professional Psychology: Research and Practice, 24*(4), 443–449.

Powell, D. J. (1993). "She said . . . he said": Gender differences in supervision. *Alcoholism Treatment Quarterly, 10*(1–2), 187–201.

Solway, K. S. (1985). Transition from graduate school to internship: A potential crisis. *Professional Psychology: Research and Practice, 16*(1), 50–54.

Steinhelber, J., & Gaynor, J. (1981). Attitudes, satisfaction, and training recommendations of former clinical psychology interns: 1968 and 1977. *Professional Psychology, 12*(2), 253–260.

Stricker, G., Davis-Russell, E., Bourg, E., Duran, E., Hammond, W. R., McHolland, J., Polite, K., & Vaughn, B. E. (1990). *Toward ethnic diversification in psychology education and training.* Washington, DC: American Psychological Association.

Stoltenberg, U., & Delworth, C. D. (1987). *Supervising counselors and therapists.* San Francisco: Jossey-Bass.

Taylor, M. (1994). Gender and power in counselling and supervision. *British Journal of Guidance & Counselling, 22*(3), 319–326.

Winegar, N. (1992). *The clinician's guide to managed mental health care.* New York: Haworth Press.

▶ 3

Working with Supervisors

SANDRA D. NETHERTON   LARRY L. MULLINS

Professional training in clinical and counseling psychology, as well as in many other professions, requires at least two basic processes. First, students must be educated in the scientific body of knowledge of the profession. Second, students must be trained in the acquisition of skills and experiences in the clinical application of that knowledge. Neither component alone is sufficient to the development of a well-trained professional in clinical psychology.

Through the typical educational processes most students have considerable experience in the acquisition of psychological knowledge and learning new information. They also have had numerous opportunities on oral and written examinations for demonstrating that the knowledge has been acquired and retained. On the other hand, students are less frequently required to demonstrate competence in the application of that knowledge in "the real world." This is one reason students may perceive working with clients and supervision as anxiety-provoking. However, learning the processes involved in applying psychological principles to work with clients can be one of the most satisfying and rewarding experiences of professional development.

Feeling apprehensive about being "supervised" and monitored in clinical activities is certainly reasonable. It is essential, however, that the student make a concerted effort not to allow fear to become a barrier to the supervisory process. The supervisory relationship can be developed and used to optimize learning, productive interactions, and professional growth and development. In fact, supervision has been described by recent graduates as one of the most valuable aspects of training in contributing to their perceived competence as psychotherapists (Bradley & Olson, 1980). This chapter will outline the basic processes involved in the supervision of clinical psychology trainees, define the roles and functions of the supervisor and supervisee, explore some of the barriers that frequently interfere with the supervisory process, and, finally, make suggestions for maximizing the opportunities afforded by this aspect of professional training. Because the supervisee may be functioning within one of several stages of professional development, the terms *supervisee, trainee, student,* and *therapist* will be used interchangeably in this chapter.

NATURE AND PURPOSE OF SUPERVISION

Students in clinical psychology are typically educated in several aspects of personality theory, human development, psychopathology, clinical assessment, diagnostic processes, and therapeutic skills and techniques. Working with clients is sufficiently complex, however, that additional measures must be taken to ensure that professionals in clinical psychology are trained and supervised in the application of this knowledge to clinical work. In essence, it is a giant step from understanding psychological principles and theories to utilizing that knowledge to effect therapeutic change in the lives of clients.

The role of the supervisor is generally undertaken by an advanced member of the profession who thereby promotes the professional development of a less experienced supervisee. The student is provided with opportunities to provide services and gain experience under the guidance and support of the supervisor, who assists the trainee with clinical activities. However, the level of training required to be considered "more advanced" and to qualify as a supervisor is not always clear.

Although clinical psychology has clearly recognized the importance of supervision and has taken steps to monitor this process, relatively few guidelines have been provided for the training of supervisors. For example, few graduates have had a course or seminar on supervision (McColley & Baker, 1982). Occasionally trainees may be given the opportunity to "supervise" less experienced students. These opportunities, however, are often restricted because of the trainees' professional status and the constant monitoring of the supervision by a more experienced supervisor. For this reason, students may find that novice supervisors may have a limited understanding of the supervisory process and some misconceptions about the requisite skills for being an effective supervisor.

Supervision of clinical work is sufficiently paramount to the training processes that governing bodies have established clear guidelines for supervision and the level, type, and quality of supervision required for licensure, certification, and accreditation (e.g., American Psychological Association, 1986). These standards detail the number of hours of direct supervision provided to supervisees, as well as the number of hours that supervisees must be engaged in clinical activities. In all cases, however, supervision is *not* optional.

As a profession, clinical psychology has largely adopted an "apprentice" model as a means of training students in the standards and guidelines of clinical practice. The apprentice model establishes a unique relationship between the supervisor and student. Through this relationship students are trained in the provision of clinical services, the training process is monitored to ensure client welfare, and supervisors function as "gatekeepers" to those individuals entering the profession (Bernard & Goodyear, 1992). In order to meet these lofty goals, the individuals involved in this complex relationship should have a clear understanding and appreciation of the roles and functions of the individuals involved.

SUPERVISORS' ROLES AND FUNCTIONS

Defining the Supervisory Relationship

One of the most important aspects of supervision is the nature of the supervisory relationship. The initial meeting with the supervisor can serve several valuable functions, including the development of a specific set of goals for supervision and a plan for achieving those goals. Similarly to the relationship established in psychotherapy, the development of a working alliance between supervisor and trainee can be an important tool in achieving the goals of supervision. Trainees are encouraged to discuss with the supervisor their theoretical orientation, the anticipated structure of supervision, the medium that will be used for supervision, the evaluation process, and how specific goals are expected to be achieved.

It is important for developing clinicians to remember the multitude of functions assumed by a supervisor in clinical practice. Supervisors are typically available during scheduled and informal times to assist students in conceptualizing clients' problems, examining the advantages and disadvantages of treatment options, evaluating the effectiveness of interventions, and monitoring clients' progress. Supervisors are also available to assist with emerging crises and facilitate progress when therapy has stagnated. Supervisors are charged with numerous duties that entail several significant challenges and potential risks. Ultimately, the supervisor is professionally, ethically, and morally responsible for the clinical services provided by their students. It is imperative that students appreciate the enormous responsibility assumed by the supervisor in this relationship.

Ensuring Client Welfare

Some authorities in the field believe that the primary function of supervisors is to ensure quality client care (i.e., Loganbill, Hardy, & Delworth, 1982). Supervisors must, at all times, take the necessary precautions to see that clients' welfare and safety are ensured. In fact, the principle of vicarious liability establishes that supervisors can be held legally and ethically responsible for any harm done by a supervisee in clinical practice under their supervision.

Supervisors and students are obligated to inform clients of the nature of the training and the supervisory relationship. Clients must always be aware of the professional status of the trainee and the trainee's role in providing clinical services and monitoring the clients' diagnosis and treatment. It is also important that clients read and execute forms that detail informed consent to treatment via this process.

As a means of ensuring client welfare, supervisors must *always* be aware of the status of each client's diagnosis, treatment course, and current level of psychological functioning. In almost all cases, supervisors will appreciate being kept informed of a client's current status. Supervisors may differ, however, as how much information they need to feel comfortable supervising a case. It is also likely that this level of information may differ with respect to the type of client being treated and the nature of the proposed treatment plan.

Promoting Professional Ethics

One of the most challenging aspects of clinical practice may prove to be the acquisition of the ethical standards and associated behaviors of the profession. Providing a thorough appreciation of the complexity of ethical considerations is typically accomplished during the initial stages of supervision. Supervisors may attempt to accomplish this function by encouraging trainees' empathy for clients, providing experiences that will augment trainees appreciation of ethical principals, requiring trainee's to reflect on the motivation behind the ethical decisions made, and providing opportunities for following through on ethical decisions (Rest, 1984).

Professional standards also require that supervisors ensure that trainees are clinically functioning within areas in which they are competent. Competency implies that students have particular skills, knowledge, and appreciation for working with specific problems and populations, including ethnic and culturally diverse groups. Competency is generally attained through formal instruction and supervised experience in particular areas of clinical practice. Competency should, of course, be maintained and enhanced over time through additional reading, consultation, and training.

In some cases, supervisors may find that trainees' personal issues or biases have a significant effect on their abilities to work with clients. One of the most important supervisoral responsibilities is to assist trainees to become aware of this influence and minimize its effect on the therapeutic process. However, it is important to remember that supervision is not psychotherapy. It is true that many aspects of the supervisory relationship parallel those found in psychotherapy, but it is not appropriate for supervisors to do "counseling" with supervisees for personal problems. Supervisors and students should be aware of the limits of supervision and, if appropriate, students should be encouraged to seek counseling with another professional.

Evaluation of Supervisees

In almost all situations, supervisors will be required to evaluate supervisees' performance. The aspects of student functioning that might be examined and evaluated include (1) effectiveness in establishing relationship with clients, (2) diagnostic abilities, (3) accuracy of case conceptualizations, (4) ability to develop appropriate and comprehensive treatment plans, and (5) effectiveness in implementing proposed interventions. Trainees may be evaluated with regard to their knowledge of ethical and legal standards for professional activities, their documentation of professional duties, their utilization of supervision, and their abilities to interact with other professionals. Students may also be evaluated on their ability to understand and monitor personal responses to clients and effectively work with clients while minimizing interference caused by any personal issues.

It is essential that supervisors provide students with clear information about the evaluation process. Supervisees should understand the expected activities, anticipated levels of competency, and consequences for failure to achieve training goals. Supervisors should provide trainees with ongoing positive and negative feedback regarding their performance. It is also helpful to delineate the mechanism by which this feedback will be provided, how frequently the feedback will be forthcoming, and who will have access to the feedback. Keith-Spiegel and Koocher (1985) noted that failure of supervisors to provide trainees with timely and accurate feedback is one of the most frequently occurring ethical complaints emanating from the supervisor-supervisee relationship.

Promoting Professional Development

Finally, the most important task and guiding goal of supervisors throughout the supervisory process is to promote the professional development of their trainees. An essential aspect of this process is to assist supervisees in the development of a sense of professional identity and appreciation for theoretical frameworks.

The roles and functions previously described may vary considerably depending on the supervisor. A supervisor's training in supervision, perspectives on the importance of supervision, theoretical orientation, and previous experience as a supervisor will certainly influence the supervisor's approach. Similar factors will also influence the nature of a supervisee's contribution to the supervisory process.

SUPERVISEES' ROLES AND FUNCTIONS

Supervisees in clinical practice assume enormous responsibility. Trainees should be encouraged to reflect on this position of responsibility and the level of commitment required by virtue of engaging in clinical practice. It is understandable, and perhaps not unexpected, to be somewhat intimidated and humbled by this responsibility. Trainees should discuss any concerns or reservations they may have about assuming this role with their supervisor. Optimally, supervisors will be in a position to process these concerns with students and accomplish this so as to relieve students of some of the misperceptions that might be present—as well as facilitating their view of being competent to assume this responsibility and effectively function as mental health professionals.

Providing Clinical Services

In many cases, supervisees will be required to assume a direct role in providing professional services to clients. It is assumed that the students will be learning and gaining new experience through this endeavor. Trainees may be working with a new client population or learning new therapeutic techniques and interventions. Under these circumstances it is understood that the supervisees are in the process of acquiring a new set of skills and need mentorship. Clearly, it would be unrealistic to expect trainees to function effectively without encountering certain therapeutic obstacles. It is important, however, that students communicate with their supervisor about problems that have occurred, anticipated problems, and proposed changes in diagnostic or treatment plans.

A supervisee's job is to learn, and learning often requires taking calculated risks and making mistakes. These mistakes, failures, and even successes will never occur, however, if a supervisee resists these opportunities. It is important, therefore, that the student enter this experience with a willingness to learn, to try new techniques, and to be open to new experiences and ideas. This is no small task because it can be very anxiety-provoking to risk failure and expose oneself as "incompetent" to supervisors and peers. One of the most essential tasks of trainees is to use this opportunity to grow and develop as professionals, and, as some have said, there is little true growth without risk or failure.

It should be equally emphasized that under absolutely no circumstances should trainees attempt to provide services that are beyond the scope of their professional competence. Trainees must recognize their level of skill and expertise and consistently function within those limitations (American Psychological Association, 1990). Of course, trainees (and supervisors) may learn and utilize new skills with adequate training and supervision. If students feel uncomfortable or uncertain about their level of training and supervision in a particular area of clinical work, these responses should be discussed with the supervisor, a colleague, or other professional in order to clarify the nature of the hesitancy and the appropriateness of engaging in these activities under the given circumstances.

Trainees must also understand that the quality of the supervisory experience will largely depend on their own investment in the process. Students who fail to devote time and energy to their clinical work and preparation for supervision may derive minimal benefit from the supervisory experience. On the other hand, trainees who seek out additional readings, spend time processing therapeutic issues, struggle with diagnostic formulations as well as case conceptualization, and devise treatment strategies and plans *before* supervision will find the process significantly more valuable, instructive, and educational. Preparation for and investment in supervision are valuable strategies trainees can use to maximize the supervisory experience.

Personal Awareness

Every supervisee and professional will have personal issues that affect clinical work. When clinical services are provided by a professional, there are innumerable ways that the professional's personal issues and biases may affect the therapeutic process. It is impossible to avoid this situation, but it is imperative that steps be taken to minimize the potentially negative effects of these personal issues on the clinical services provided to clients. Supervision is one of the mechanisms established by the profession to address this problem.

Supervisees may find this process challenging, interesting, uncomfortable, or even frightening. It is essential, however, that students be willing to examine how *relevant* personal thoughts, feelings, or behaviors might be influencing clinical activities. Some supervisors, for whatever reason, may exceed the limits on this process. It is not necessary, however, to reveal information that is not pertinent to trainees' professional development and affecting trainees' clinical activities (Schaeffer, 1981).

Upholding Professional Standards

Supervisees should abide by professional standards in clinical activities and must have the self-confidence, assertiveness, and professional support to follow through with legal and ethical behavior. From an ethical perspective, there may be occasions in which students may feel uncomfortable with the structure or functioning of the supervisory relationship. In these situations, students should initially discuss the issues directly with their supervisor to clarify the nature of the problem and gain additional insight into the process involved. Under these circumstances considerable effort should be expended to resolve the conflict within the supervisory relationship. If this approach fails, supervisees might request a meeting with their supervisor and the supervisor's supervisor. A thoughtful discussion and professional examination of the issues involved will generally result in successful resolution of any difficulties. Only when these options have been thoroughly explored and a reasonable resolution is not found should other alternatives be considered. For example, trainees might consult with their university practicum supervisor. Ultimately, if these measures fail, it may be necessary for a student to terminate the practicum experience.

THE LOGISTICS OF SUPERVISION

The actual mechanisms by which the supervisory process is accomplished will depend on numerous factors. Training opportunities are often available in a variety of settings, with diverse clinical populations, and with various supervisors.

Supervision Vehicles

Although it has been repeatedly emphasized that supervisors will monitor the clinical activities of students, it should be noted that this monitoring can occur via a variety of methods. Each of these methods is associated with particular advantages and disadvantages that supervisors and trainees should be aware of so that thoughtful, considered selection of the optimal method occurs to maximize the benefits of supervision (Bernard & Goodyear, 1992).

Self-Report Method
The self-report method of supervision is probably the most basic, the most commonly used, and the oldest form of supervision. In some respects, the self-report method may also be the most difficult means of supervision. In this approach, trainees report to their supervisor the information relevant to clinical activities. This method of supervision relies very heavily on

supervisees' ability to report accurate, perceptive information regarding the interactions that have occurred over the course of treatment. Thus, students are in a position of assuming considerable responsibility for perceiving, understanding, conceptualizing, and reporting on therapeutic processes. The self-report methods may be perceived by trainees as one of the least threatening forms of supervision. When the self-report method is used, there is generally no direct observation of students' skills, limited alternative perceptions of the therapeutic processes, and limited auditory and visual information from sessions available to the supervisor.

Process Notes

Some supervisors rely almost solely on the process notes prepared by their trainees for supervision. The use of process notes encourages students to reflect on the content of the session, the student–client relationship, and the interventions implemented. Because direct access to sessions is not possible, this approach has many of the same disadvantages as using the self-report method.

Taping

Advances in technology have included considerable growth in the use of audiotape and videotape in supervision. Each of these taping methods allows supervisors more direct access to the content of the clinical activities of trainees. Supervisees may initially find it somewhat uncomfortable to be audiotaped or videotaped, but this discomfort generally fades over time. If a student has very strong reservations, it is important to discuss concerns with the supervisor and possibly negotiate alternative means of supervision until taping becomes more acceptable.

Trainees must ensure that clients are informed about any form of taping that will occur. Clients should be given a complete explanation of the purposes for the taping, who will be allowed access to tapes, and what precautions will be taken to ensure client confidentiality. In addition, supervisees' assume responsibility for storing tapes in a secure location and erasing tapes when they have served their purpose. In general, most clients express little resistance to taping when they are informed about the limits of confidentiality and how tapes will be used in supervision.

Audiotaping can be accomplished in almost any clinical setting and by almost every supervisee. This methods provides considerable advantages for supervisors because the tape can be reviewed at any time, material can be reviewed numerous times, and specific segments of a tape can be preselected for discussion during supervision.

Audiotapes and videotapes have the advantage of flexibility. These tapes might be reviewed separately by the student and the supervisor before supervision. Particular aspects of a session might be selected for discussion—

for example, points at which progress seemed to stagnate or especially productive aspects of the session. The selection of both positive and negative
aspects of a session for discussion is encouraged to ensure that supervisors
have opportunities to confront problems, as well as acknowledge successes.

A major advantage of videotaping is that it gives supervisors clear visual information about sessions. Supervisors have the opportunity to observe clients, interpret body language, and note changes in nonverbal behavior. These are incredibly valuable aspects of the therapeutic process that
give supervisors opportunities to instruct supervisees on the importance of
these factors and the utility of this information in clinical work. Videotape
also allows trainees to gain an additional perspective on their role within the
session. Supervisees can assume a more detached perspective and evaluate
their own functioning more objectively. Unfortunately, using videotape requires considerably more physical space and some level of comfort with electronic devices. In some cases it may also be financially unfeasible to use videotaping equipment.

In Vivo Observation

Supervision can also be accomplished through the live observations of a session by the supervisor. Advantages associated with this type of supervision
include the wealth of information available to the supervisor and the opportunity the supervisor has to provide immediate feedback about the observations. The feedback provided may range from post-session discussion with
the supervisee to having the supervisor enter the room and provide input to
the supervisee and the client. In some cases, the supervisor may choose to
interrupt the session via telephone, a "bug in the ear" (a hearing aid device
through which the supervisor can talk to the trainee), or even knocking at
the door to provide immediate suggestions for intervention. The use of live
supervision may not always be feasible, however, due to limitations on coordinating the schedules of the supervisor, trainee, and client.

Supervisory Styles

Supervisors, like most individuals, will evidence considerable variability in
their perceptions of supervision, their expectations for the student, and their
approach to supervision. Many approaches to supervision have been discussed, and it is likely that there are as many approaches to supervision as
there are supervisors. There are, however, several basic approaches that generally account for the basic styles that supervisors may use. As might be
expected, many of the basic approaches used by supervisors in clinical psychology parallel theories of psychotherapy (Leddick & Bernard, 1980).

Supervisors may rely solely upon their approach to psychotherapy or
counseling to structure the supervisory process. For example, a supervisor

who utilizes a psychodynamic approach might be expected to focus on the trainee's resistance to supervision, encourage the examination of dynamics that might reflect intrapsychic conflict, and assist in the resolution of these conflicts to promote more effective psychotherapeutic work with clients.

Client-centered supervisors would tend to focus more on the personal growth and understanding of the trainee fostered through the supervisory relationship. Supervisors who use this type of approach may frequently use reflective statements to encourage students to explore and understand interpersonal and intrapersonal needs and behaviors. The ultimate goal of this process is to enhance trainees' work with clients.

Some approaches to supervision may be much more directive than the psychodynamic or client-centered styles. Supervisors who adhere to a behavioral approach will primarily use reinforcement and shaping to teach appropriate skills. In this respect, it is more likely that a supervisor and trainee will discuss specific behaviors to be learned and modified, develop specific strategies for the modification of the behaviors, and periodically review the progress made in attaining these goals. The focus of supervision will be primarily on the acquisition of specific skills and knowledge relevant to the therapeutic process. Supervisors who use a cognitive-behavioral approach, will put more emphasis on the thoughts supervisees may have about their abilities to work with patients and the modification of faulty ideas that might interfere with the acquisition of appropriate skills.

Supervisory Models

An alternative means of conceptualizing the supervisory process relies on the developmental perspective (i.e., Loganhill, Hardy, & Delworth, 1982; Stoltenberg, 1981). This approach emphasizes the systematic growth of supervisees through a series of stages and the application of appropriate interventions by supervisors to promote and enhance the growth of the students. The developmental view also maintains that the supervisors grow and develop similarly to the trainees. Developmental theories of supervision often focus on the recommended interventions to be provided to students at each level of development. For example, early in a trainee's clinical experience it is often important to provide more structure, guidance, and support than during subsequent levels. As the supervisee gains experience and confidence, less direction and support are necessary, and it becomes increasingly important to provide the trainee with increased autonomy and independence.

The developmental process of supervision may be influenced by a variety of individual factors associated with the supervisors and the students. In addition, the nature of the clinical setting, the client population, and the specifics of a particular case may affect the developmental nature of the supervisory process. For example, more advanced trainees may require additional supervision and guidance when confronted with a client in crisis or an especially challenging patient population.

Clinical Setting

Occasionally supervisors and their students may be functioning in different geographic settings. Although many standards recommend—or in some cases require—that supervisees and trainees function within the same primary setting, this type of arrangement is sometimes impossible. When supervisors and students are functioning in different contextual settings, additional measures may need to be taken to ensure that an adequate level of supervision is maintained. Supervisors might need to coordinate supervision with another supervisor who is physically located at the site of service. Coordinating these services may necessitate that information is shared with multiple supervisors on a given case; thus, facilitating communication between supervisors, clarifying primary responsibilities for supervision and evaluation, and specifying the requirements for the off-site supervisor (e.g., participation in meetings to discuss student performance) are vital.

PROBLEMS ENCOUNTERED IN SUPERVISION

Whose Clients Are They?

A major potential problem in clinical supervision is that of identifying who has the primary clinical, ethical, and legal responsibility for clients. In the traditional supervisor-supervisee relationship a client is assigned to a practicum student or trainee. Typically, the student assumes the role of primary therapist for that client, meeting directly with the individual and delivering some type of psychotherapeutic service. The supervisor, however, assumes responsibility for the *direction* and *course* of psychotherapy, especially with a novice student. Thus, the student and supervisor are both responsible for the client. Additionally, the therapeutic relationship is a shared one. The supervisor assumes ultimate responsibility for the clinical services provided to the client; the trainee acts as an agent of the supervisor, who determines the nature and the course of the services provided.

Such a complex relationship translates into the need for flexible collaboration with the supervisor. The trainee will be on the "front line," directly offering services to the client. The supervisor provides ongoing expertise, guidance, and support. Because of this unique relationship, one of the major challenges in supervision is for the trainee to maintain responsibility for the client while remaining comfortable with the available help and support of the supervisor. The student must also be sensitive to the fact that the supervisor rarely has direct contact with the client; even with the use of audiotape or videotape, the supervisor typically does not or cannot review every moment of the therapy hour, nor do these media always capture the richness of the therapeutic encounter. This lack of firsthand experience makes it critically important that there is clear, direct, and frequent communication between the trainee and the clinical supervisor.

Fear of Evaluation

Perhaps the most common problem encountered in supervision is the students' fear of negative evaluation by their clinical supervisors. Virtually all supervisees desire to present themselves as competent in dealing with therapeutic issues. The trainees are, of course, critically aware of their supervisors and the evaluative nature of the relationship. With rare exceptions, this places additional pressure on students. In addition, there is the desire to present themselves as "psychologically healthy" (e.g., confident, self-assured) to their supervisor. Many students harbor secret fears that their personal shortcomings will become apparent during the intense process of supervision.

Such fears of evaluation can potentially lead to specific problems. First, students may be predisposed to omit or hide information from the supervisor lest they be judged incompetent—they may not disclose information that took place in a session because they might appear "inept." As a result, their supervisors are left with incomplete information and a distorted view of the therapeutic process. These kinds of omissions or distortions may seriously compromise the supervisory process.

A second common fear of supervisees is of therapeutic failure with a client. As a rule, most trainees are strongly committed to seeing their clients progress toward treatment goals. Should that not occur (or not occur quickly), trainees may be vulnerable to self-criticism and self-denigration. In addition, there may be an intense fear that a client will terminate early, with the subsequent internal attribution that the termination was the direct by-product of "inadequate or poor treatment." Students may also fear that a client will criticize them for their relative lack of experience and expertise. On some occasions, clients will indeed confront the student clinician. Care must be taken by the supervisor and trainee to address the student's fears of therapeutic failure in order to establish appropriate expectations for therapeutic response. The student also needs to be prepared to therapeutically respond to various subtle or not so subtle communications about competence or experience by a client.

Stylistic and Orientation Conflict

Obviously, supervisors present with very different supervisory styles, expectations, and goals for their students. They vary tremendously on dimensions of directiveness, didactic style, method of supervision (e.g., audiotape versus written transcription), and degree of control over the direction of treatment. Worthington (1987) has noted such conflict revolves around whether supervision should be *proactive* versus *reactive*. A supervisee may share a very consistent style and set of expectations and goals concerning such issues. Conversely, one may be at extreme odds with the supervisor on some of these dimensions. For example, students may desire a supervisor who is somewhat nondirective and allows for considerable therapist control of the direction of treatment, yet find themselves in a supervisory relationship in which the supervisor is autocratic and directive.

An important question here is whether students should learn and adopt the supervisors' orientations, or whether the supervisors should adapt to the students (Worthington, 1987). Importantly, supervisors and trainees may have quite different professed orientations to treatment. For example, a supervisee may have adopted a strong cognitive-behavioral framework to treatment, while the supervisor bases his or her approach on a traditional psychoanalytic perspective, which may give rise to considerable theoretical conflict over the course of work with a given client. Although most training programs encourage students to learn therapeutic processes of various theoretical orientations, diverse therapeutic stances may lead to dissent over the course of treatment. This problem may be exacerbated if students harbor strong beliefs about the suitability of a given orientation for a particular client or client problem. Some of this difficulty may wane as students gain experience, as supervisors may be more likely to give the students greater freedom with experience (Stoltenberg, 1981).

Ethical and Moral Conflicts

Situations may also arise in the supervisory context when ethical conflicts emerge with clients. For example, a given client may suddenly present to the supervisee with suicidal ideation. The client may be quite distraught, have exhibited poor judgment in the past, yet be noncommittal to the extent of explicit intention to attempt suicide. Or a new client may present information that there has been sexual misconduct on the part of a former therapist. The client may indicate feeling quite confused and victimized. The client may question the trainee as to how to best resolve this painful issue. In each of these complex dilemmas the student is faced with serious and potentially onerous therapeutic tasks.

In each of these scenarios, consultation with a supervisor is obviously needed. However, what happens when in the course of supervision, it is apparent that the student and supervisor have quite different ideas about how to resolve the ethical problem? For example, what if the supervisor believes that the suicidal ideation of the client is not particularly serious, and that an attempt is not imminent, while the student believes that the client is *quite* serious about taking his or her life and may well do so if not hospitalized? Or what would occur in the case of the sexually victimized client if the supervisor told the trainee to ignore the allegations, as the supervisor believed they were "false memories" and part of the client's personality disorder, while the supervisee believes the client and wants to proceed with further discussions of the incident?

Such dilemmas, while perhaps occurring rarely, exemplify how extremely sensitive and anxiety-provoking ethical dilemmas can be. A number of guidelines may help, taking into account that both students and supervisors have particular liabilities and responsibilities. First, students must realize that the ultimate ethical, moral, legal, and professional responsibility for the client remains with the supervisor. Therefore, in almost all cases the supervisors' decisions should be followed and respected. If a particular therapeutic action seems warranted, the student must be able to present the case *directly* to the supervisor, stating the advantages and disadvantages of particular therapeutic actions. If the conflict does not become resolved this way, the trainee may need to follow the "chain of command" and arrange a joint consultation with the clinic director or director of clinical training. Consultation with the supervisor's supervisor should always be done with the supervisor's knowledge and permission. In this manner, additional expertise can be brought to bear on the clinical dilemma. Ultimately, the student may choose to resign from the case and/or the practicum placement if the conflict cannot be satisfactorily resolved.

The possibility also exists that, on occasion, moral conflicts may arise with either clients or with the supervisor. For example, a pregnant client may wish to pursue an abortion, while the trainee personally believes such behavior is morally inappropriate. Although a complete discussion of these issues is beyond the scope of this chapter, it should be noted that such moral conflicts can indeed occur in the therapeutic context and need resolution. Most therapeutic schools in psychology argue for the need to remove personal morality from the therapeutic context. That is not to say that the student does not have a right to have such beliefs; he or she merely does not have a right to share or act upon personal values or beliefs in the therapeutic context. Similarly, the supervisor does not have the right to act upon his or her morality in the supervisory context. The trainee should, however, have the opportunity to process personal reactions or responses to clients' morality within the supervisory relationship. Discussing these issues with the supervisor should assist the trainee in formulating plans to address the conflict while maintaining the client's best interests. One reasonable alternative under these conditions might be to refer the client to another professional.

Finally, a note is in order on sexual harassment on the part of the supervisor. Because of the inherent power inequity in the supervisor–supervisee relationship, opportunities are abundant for abuse. A number of researchers have commented on the high incidence of sexual harassment and misconduct on the part of academicians and other supervisors with students (Fitzgerald et al., 1988). In keeping with the American Psychological Association (1990) guidelines, such behavior is prohibited and considered to carry inherent personal risks. In fact, professionals are prohibited from engaging in dual relationships whereby the roles and responsibilities of those involved in the relationship become unclear or change so that the nature of the relationship is altered. Such behaviors should be promptly reported to the appropriate person or committee for action. (See also Chapter 1 for a more detailed discussion of ethical considerations.)

Involvement with Multiple Supervisors

With certain clients a supervisee may provide therapeutic contact over the course of a number of semesters. In most educational contexts, supervisors will rotate by semester. Thus, with long-term clients a supervisee may well end up with two, three, or even more supervisors.

A trainee working with the same client and the same presenting problem may have different supervisors with different orientations, styles, and advice. Such rotation of supervisors obviously adds to diversity of experience for the student. In some cases, however, this may prove to be problematic, especially if supervisory styles are quite diverse. The student has the responsibility to monitor the therapeutic process and to ensure that differences in supervisory input do not result in fragmented delivery of treatment. The student may potentially alleviate part of this difficulty by carefully describing the theoretical stance used with a given client at the initiation of a new supervisory experience.

ENHANCING THE SUPERVISORY PROCESS

At this point it should be clear that the nature of the supervisory experience will be primarily determined by individual characteristics of the supervisor and the trainee. Because trainees are the intended audience for this chapter, the following section will focus on suggestions students might use to improve this aspect of professional training. Trainees should realize that the overall quality of supervision received will depend, in large part, on the trainee.

Establishing Expectations for Supervision

To enhance the supervisory process, it is helpful for the trainee to engage in a number of activities before supervision begins. First, it is often wise to gather information about a particular supervisor. This might include talking to other students who have had a given supervisor and soliciting their perspectives on his or her orientation, style, and attitude about supervision. Such perspectives may inform the student about possible stylistic similarities and/or differences.

Second, if at all possible, arrange a meeting with the supervisor to discuss his or her perspective on supervision. It is helpful to have generated a list of questions, such as "What methods of supervision do you engage in?" "What is your theoretical approach to supervision?" "What modes of feedback do you prefer?" "How much contact with the student do you expect?"

Finally, it is helpful to define clearly for yourself your personal expectations for supervision with a given supervisor. What new knowledge base is sought with a particular supervisor? What types of new client problems would facilitate the therapist's professional development? Taking the time to articulate personal expectations will diminish the likelihood of conflicts in the supervisory process.

Choosing a Supervisor

Unfortunately, students often do not have the option of selecting a given supervisor or may find that they made an error in judgment when they selected the supervisor. If supervisors are assigned or there are a limited number of supervisors available, this problem may be unavoidable. If students have a choice of supervisors, it is important, as already mentioned, to identify personal expectations and clarify their professional needs. Trainees will need to assess further what educational experiences are going to be most helpful and, based on that assessment, what supervisor will maximize the possibility of fulfilling those needs. Trainees may need to take certain risks in this regard. Although it may be "safer" to choose a supervisor who is known to be "lax," having supervisors who will challenge existing skills and contribute to further knowledge is the primary goal of the experience.

Communication

Honest communication may be the most critical aspect of supervision. For supervision to be beneficial (rewarding to the trainee and to the client), clear, direct communication must take place. It is helpful for trainees to inform supervisors about positive aspects of supervision, for example, information that was particularly valuable, a helpful level of supervisor availability, or a supervisor's beneficial insights and understanding. Giving positive feedback to supervisors is a excellent means of letting them know what has been helpful, what you have valued about supervision, and what you might like to have more frequently.

Some communication, especially about negative aspects of supervision, may not be particularly comfortable or pleasant. Examination of goals, expectations, problems, and conflicts in the context of an uneven power relationship is difficult and may elicit very uncomfortable feelings. However, unless such discussion takes place, the likelihood of future problems in supervision is greatly enhanced.

Conflict Resolution

Despite all efforts to maintain and facilitate communication, problems may occur within the supervisory relationship. When a conflict arises, it is helpful for a trainee to first clearly define the nature and boundaries of the problem. In other words, it is imperative that the student separate his or her feelings from a given problem and objectively and operationally define the stated problem. Second, it is often helpful for the student to utilize a "cost-benefit analysis" approach in looking at the particular conflict. What are the relative advantages and disadvantages of tackling a conflict directly with a particular supervisor? Conducting such an analysis may help the supervisee determine whether the issues are or are not worth raising at a particular point in time. On the other hand, such an analysis may lead the trainee to feel even more strongly that there is a need to discuss particular problems, and that the potential benefit is quite high.

Finally, it is essential that a student be able to consult with other supervisors. Consultation with others should always be done with the knowledge and consent of the primary supervisor. Surreptitious consultation is highly likely to eventually be discerned and perceived as malicious. Consultation should take place with other supervisors who are known to be fair and experienced. Ideally, such consultations should take place in the physical presence of the primary supervisor.

FUTURE DIRECTIONS IN SUPERVISION

Considerable advancement in our understanding of the supervisory process has occurred in recent years. As has been pointed out, clinical supervision is a complex, multifaceted phenomenon; much remains to be found out about the intricacies of supervision and training of students. It is probably safe to say that the basic question is not whether supervision is beneficial, but rather what type of supervision is best for what type of student with what type of client problem with what particular therapeutic modality (Stoltenberg, McNeill, & Crethar, 1994). Carefully designed empirical studies are in order to address these issues.

Importantly, little is yet known about the training of supervisors themselves. The current literature would suggest that formal training in supervision rarely takes place, with only about one-third of psychology interns receiving any type of supervisory didactics (Hess & Hess, 1983). Thus, most supervisors are probably self-taught, learning through the modeling of previous supervisors. Theoretical models of supervisor development have begun to emerge (e.g., Alonso, 1983; Hess, 1983) that may spur further research in this area. Worthington (1987) comments that such models are largely descriptive, and much more information is needed about such issues as how supervisors behave at different theoretical levels, how they learn their craft, and whether critical incidents can positively or negatively influence their development.

Notably, two other contemporary trends in clinical practices may potentially influence the nature of supervision: managed mental health care and prescriptive treatments. Managed health care will undoubtedly dictate *length* of treatment, and the advent of a federal health care authority sanctioning treatment protocols may dictate the *type* of treatment offered. Students will be expected to offer short-term treatment while adhering to a particular theoretical bent. Hypothetically, supervision may increasingly become much more didactic, structured, and proactive to meet the demands of the health care/ counseling marketplace.

Technological advances may also continue to significantly impact on the process of supervision. Use of videotapes, live supervision "bugs," and computer simulations are increasingly utilized by supervisors as teaching tools. Fiberoptic systems on many college campuses and laser disc technologies may continue to enhance the quality of supervision by allowing more direct observation and recording of actual client–therapist interactions. These strategies may also potentially hasten the development of the novice therapist, who will have direct access to such forms of technology.

Finally, culturally sensitive approaches to counseling are increasingly being experienced in the context of our ethnically diverse population. All supervisors must have an appreciation for such therapeutic issues for the sake of the client and supervisee. As well, the increasing numbers of ethnically diverse counselors increases the need for cultural sensitivity in the supervisory process itself.

REFERENCES

Alonso, A. (1983) A developmental theory of psychodynamic supervision. *The Clinical Supervisor, 1,* 23–36.

American Psychological Association (1986). *Accreditation handbook*. Washington, DC: Author.

American Psychological Association (1990). Ethical principles of psychologists. *American Psychologist, 45*, 390–395.

Bernard, J. M., & Goodyear, R. K. (1992). *Fundamentals of clinical supervision*. Boston: Allyn & Bacon.

Bradley, J. R., & Olson, J. K. (1980). Training factors influencing felt psychotherapeutic competence of psychology trainees. *Professional Psychology, 11*, 930–934.

Fitzgerald, L. F., Shullman, S. L., Bailey, N., Richards, M., Swecker, J., Gold, A., Ormerod, A. J., & Weitzman, L. (1988). The incidence and dimensions of sexual harassment in academia and the workplace. *Journal of Vocational Behavior, 32*, 152–175.

Hess, A. K. (1983). Growth in supervision—stages of supervisee and supervisor development. *The Clinical Supervisor, 4*, 51–67.

Hess, A. K., & Hess, K. A. (1983). Psychotherapy supervision: A survey of internship training practices. *Professional Psychology: Research and Practice, 14*, 504–513.

Keith-Spiegel, P., & Koocher, G. P. (1985). *Ethics in psychology: Professional standards and cases*. New York: Random House.

Leddick, G. R., & Bernard, J. M. (1980). The history of supervision: A critical review. *Counselor Education and Supervision, 19*, 186–196.

Loganbill, C., Hardy, E., & Delworth, U. (1982). Supervision: A conceptual model. *The Counseling Psychologist, 10*, 3–42.

McColley, S. H., & Baker, E. L. (1982). Training activities and styles of beginning supervisors: A survey. *Professional Psychology, 13*, 283–292.

Patterson, C. H. (1983). A client-centered approach to supervision. *The Counseling Psychologist, 11*, 21–25.

Rest, J. R. (1984). Research on moral development: Implications for training counseling psychologists. *The Counseling Psychologist, 12*, 19–29.

Schaefer, A. B. (1981). Clinical supervision. In C. E. Walker (Ed.), *Clinical practice of psychology: A guide for mental health professionals*. New York: Pergamon Press.

Stoltenberg, C. D. (1981). Approaching supervision from a developmental perspective: The counselor complexity model. *Journal of Counseling Psychology, 28*, 59–65.

Stoltenberg, C. D., McNeill, B. W., & Crethar, H. C. (1994). Changes in supervision as counselors and therapists gain experience: A review. *Professional Psychology: Research and Practice, 25*, 416–449.

Worthington, E. L. (1987). Changes in supervision as counselors and supervisors gain experience: A review. *Professional Psychology: Research and Practice, 18*, 189–208.

4

Establishing Rapport and Developing Interviewing Skills

PETER J. GIORDANO

The skills involved in rapport building and interviewing will be some of the most fundamental clinical abilities you will develop in your training and throughout your professional career. These skills pervade all of your clinical work. They are the foundation on which other, higher level skills are based. These skills take time and effort to develop. It is a myth to assume that you either have these abilities or you do not. The "natural ease" your supervisor or other more experienced clinicians display in their clinical work is in part a result of years of experience resulting in a certain level of comfort in a variety of clinical situations.

Before we think about interactions in an interview with a client, let's first consider ordinary interpersonal interactions. Whenever you meet a person for the first time, one of the initial interpersonal tasks is to establish a sense of rapport, that feeling of relationship or connectedness, with the other individual. Actually, it is not your responsibility alone to make this happen; it is a dyadic responsibility. This rapport building is even more critical if you hope to have an ongoing alliance, with the aim of achieving some mutually agreed upon goal. This process starts immediately and will affect the future character of the relationship. Some relationships may get off to an almost effortless start, and others take more time to evolve.

Similar dynamics are part of any relationship you seek to establish in your clinical work, although, because of the unique nature of your chosen profession, the challenge of rapport building often falls largely on your shoulders. Whether you view yourself as the "expert" or the "collaborator," you are still seen by your client as an expert in interpersonal relationships (Sullivan, 1954), and you are expected to behave accordingly.

In addition to issues of rapport, this chapter will discuss topics related to developing interviewing skills. Establishing rapport is discussed first because without it little of worth may occur in your interviewing activities. If your client feels psychologically uncomfortable, other inteviewing techniques may have limited impact.

Thus, these topics are important because many of your clinical activities grow out of how you relate to your client and to other important members of the client's context (e.g., family members). For example, if you are testing a child for possible mental retardation, you will ultimately need to share the results and your recommendations with the child's parents. Depending on the assessment results, it may take extreme sensitivity and skill to convey results accurately. Let's now consider issues of rapport building in greater depth.

ESTABLISHING RAPPORT

Rapport is the sense of mutual trust and harmony that characterizes a good relationship. It is a relationship quality that must be carefully nurtured, because it is critical to the success of your clinical work. There will certainly be clinical relationships you encounter in which the development of rapport seems effortless. More typically, however, rapport takes time to develop and you must carefully work to help it evolve.

There are many things you can do to contribute to the sense of rapport, some of which are behavioral and others attitudinal. Rogers' (1957) classic work highlights the importance of a particular clinical attitude by arguing that the effective clinician will be empathic, genuine, and show unconditional positive regard. While we may debate if these attitudes are sufficient to be effective, there is little doubt that they are necessary and that they contribute to a trusting and harmonious relationship. Thus, even in the initial contact with your client it is important to be empathic and caring.

It may sound simple to exhibit these qualities, but a moment's reflection indicates that this is not the case. You will undoubtedly encounter clients who bore, anger, repulse, arouse, or frustrate you. Depending on your theoretical orientation, you may label these feelings as countertransference or as something else. Regardless of the label, however, the feelings are real and they are common to all who do clinical work. Do not feel guilty or alone if you experience them. In fact, it is inevitable that you will experience them.

Be careful not to deny these feelings. Acknowledging them is the first step to removing their power to damage the quality of the developing relationship. Discuss these feelings with your supervisor so that you can learn to manage them. The important point at this juncture is to be aware that such feelings can inhibit the development and maintenance of rapport in the initial interview situation.

Brenner (1982) also argues that regardless of training, theoretical orientation, or typical treatment methods, there are certain characteristics of the clinician that contribute to effectiveness. I believe that these personal characteristics largely contibute to the development and maintenance of rapport. According to Brenner, helpers should be empathic, demonstrate composure, be ready to discuss everything, be willing to encourage, and remain purposeful in their actions. All of these characteristics are obviously important in a longer term clinical relationship, but they are also relevant to your initial contacts with a client.

If your task is to complete an initial interview, for instance, and then to refer the client to someone else, you will still need to establish a good working relationship with the individual. In fact, clients may be indirectly evaluating the entire clinical facility and all the professionals who work there through their initial contact with you. If they experience a lack of understanding or a reticence on your part to discuss important issues, they may generalize this experience to others in the setting and never return, even if they know they would not be seeing you.

One caveat is important here. What I have written in this chapter reflects my biases and my clinical style. The way I work as a clinician is a direct outgrowth of my personality, my experience, and my clinical training. As Corey (1991) notes: "... you ... are your very best technique. There is no substitute for developing techniques that are an expression of your personality and that fit for you" (p. 437). Do not uncritically accept what I write. Through your training and experience, find what works best for you. Discuss your clinical style and behavior with your supervisor. He or she may offer alternatives to my suggestions and give specific feedback based on his or her observations of your clinical style. Above all, be yourself, and then continually strive throughout your career to improve your technique.

DEVELOPING INTERVIEWING SKILLS

The Setting and Some Procedural Issues

The responsibilites in your practicum work depend to a significant degree on the nature of your field placement. In some settings you may only do assessments of one sort or another. In other settings you may engage exclusively in therapy. And in others you may be responsible for both of these activities. Common to all placements, however, is the need to do some type of interviewing.

There are a variety of interview types, including diagnostic interviews, intake interviews, case-history interviews, mental status interviews, pretherapy interviews, and crisis interviews (Nietzel, Bernstein, & Milich, 1994; Phares, 1992; Weins & Matarazzo, 1983). Further, interviews can be structured or unstructured. Structured interviews, as the name implies, are designed to standardize the interview, with the aim of increasing the reliability of the information obtained . The Schedule for Affective Disorders and Schizophrenia (Endicott & Spitzer, 1978) is one example of a structured interview. Mental status interviews are also generally done in a structured format. These interviews are designed to assess intellectual, emotional, and neuropsychological functioning and cover such areas as thought content and process, memory, sensorium, affect, mood, insight, judgement, appearance, orientation, psychomotor activity, state of consciousness, and intellectual resources (Cohen, Swerdlik, & Smith, 1992). The Mini-Mental State Exam (Folstein, Folstein, & McHugh, 1975) is an example of a structured mental status interview. Chapter 6 of this book contains a more thorough discussion of mental status interviews and other structured screening procedures.

In contrast, unstructured interviews give greater latitude regarding the type and the sequence of questions. For example, a clinician may assess relevant areas of mental status in a more informal and flexible format than with a structured mental status exam. Regardless of interview type and format, however, all interviews share the characteristic that information is to be gathered during the process.

This chapter will use as its model the intake interview in a relatively unstructured format, since this is the type you will most likely be doing. The intake interview is often the first type of interview a client experiences, and on the basis of the intake a variety of recommendations may be made, including psychological testing, psychotherapy, a medication consultation, or further diagnostic interviewing.

Regardless of your clinical responsibilities at your placement, keep in mind that each clinical setting will have its own procedures for doing things. As a trainee in any setting it is important to learn the procedural rules and follow them carefully. Your careful attention to procedural guidelines will ease your transition into the setting and will help the staff appreciate the contributions you have to offer. For example, for intake interviews, settings typically ask you to turn in your written report in a specified amount of time.

Settings may also vary in how the initial contact is made with clients. In some settings you may be the person to have the clinical contact with a client, from the time the appointment is made until your contact is terminated.

Thus, you may make the initial phone contact to schedule the appointment, see the client for the intake interview, follow the client for testing and/or psychotherapy, and terminate at the end. In other settings you may first see the client only after someone else has done the intake and referred the client to you, and in others you may be given some brief clinical information obtained over the phone by someone else prior to your initial appointment. The specific procedures of your setting will be explained to you by your supervisor or by administrative staff. If you are unsure of how to proceed, ask someone. However, always keep in mind that clinical and administrative staff are often extremely busy and you do not want to overburden them with unnecessary questions, especially those that can be answered by consulting a policies and procedures manual.

The Initial Interview—General Considerations

Given that you are acquainted with procedures at your clinical setting, the time will come when you meet your first client. All clinical settings have a reception area where clients are seated while waiting for their appointment. Some of these areas are quiet and private; others are more like major thoroughfares. Also, depending on the setting and time of day, the waiting area may be full of people or your client may be the only one there. Once you have identified your client, your first task is to introduce yourself. Simply identify yourself by name and invite the individual back to your office. It is tempting to engage in small talk while walking back to your office, but I recommend against this practice. With small talk you may inadvertently set the wrong tone for your interview. Further, you may begin to elicit information that is best suited to the privacy of your office.

A story may illustrate this latter point and highlight the intricacies of this initial contact. Not long ago I walked into the reception area of the outpatient clinic where I was working and introduced myself to the young African American man who was waiting to see me. I knew very little about this person, as the practice of the clinic was to obtain only basic information over the phone prior to the intake interview. When I walked into the waiting area, I extended my hand, introduced myself as Dr. Giordano, and asked, "How are you today?" This phrase is a common social convention, although it really is not appropriate when first meeting a client in a mental health facility, because it is a question that elicits answers that are best discussed in the privacy of an office, not a public waiting area. However, at that moment I forgot this fact. In response to my question, Mr. Jones (a pseudonym) stood up, avoided my handshake, looked me squarely in the eye, and said, "I'm a black man living in America. How good could it be?" It was a brutally honest and passionate remark in response to my question. Unfortunately, I never should have posed the question when and where I did.

To make a long story short, the remainder of the interview was a disaster. Some might argue that his behavior was inappropriate; I think it was a congruent response to my ill-timed question. In my office I learned that Mr. Jones was extremely angry about the racism he was experiencing particularly at work, and he felt little rapport with me as a white psychologist. We candidly discussed the obvious fact that he was black and I was white. He intimated that he would prefer a black therapist. We discussed this important issue, and he agreed to a referral to another clinic (the clinic where I was working had no African American clinicians). Was the "failure" of this intake session completely a result of my inappropriate "How are you?" I don't think so. However, I did not help the situation by making what seemed at the moment to be a minor faux pax.

The Initial Interview—Specific Skills

There are a variety of strategies for developing interviewing skills. Some skill-building approaches are structured; others are not. Hackney and Cormier (1988), for instance, provide a number of structured practical exercises for the development of skill in this area. Others advocate more of a learn-by-experience approach. What follows here are some practical suggestions for beginning to develop basic skills for effective interviewing. The guiding principle in all these suggestions is, as noted before, to be yourself, and to work diligently to improve your interviewing skills.

Beginning the Interview

Even in relatively unstructured interviews, clients look to you for some direction, and rapport is facilitated by helping them feel at ease. Keep in mind the perspective of your clients when they first come to see you. They are walking into a strange place, will sit down with a person they have never met before, and will be asked detailed questions about their most private experiences. Thus, they are likely to be nervous and uncertain about the whole situation. Given the inherent stress of this situation for clients, it is no wonder that about half of the clients who come for an intake interview never return for follow-up appointments (Baekeland & Lundwall, 1975). How you handle the interaction in the initial moments may do much to put your clients at ease and therefore facilitate the entire interview process, as well as the likelihood that they will return for further help.

An effective question for getting the interview started is simply to ask, "What brings you to the mental health center/hospital/clinic today?" This question usually draws forth information pertaining to the presenting problem, which is typically a good place to begin. As details are fleshed out from there, you can then delve into relevant topics. One of the challenges of the intake interview is the breadth of information to be covered. Major themes of the intake usually include the presenting problem; current household composition; educational, family, social and psychiatric history; substance use and legal history; history of mental illness in the family; and general physical status (e.g., any serious medical conditions?). Often much of this information will emerge as you talk with clients about their present difficulties and life circumstances. However, at times you may need to be deliberate or structured in your questions. If an adult client alludes to a "wild adolescence," for instance, you may need to follow up with a question like, "A moment ago you mentioned a wild adolescence. When you say wild, what do you mean? Did you use drugs, have frequent sexual partners?" If your clients indicate they used drugs, it would be wise to inquire about the types and frequency of drugs used and if they are currently using. Sometimes clients volunteer such information and sometimes you need to ask directly. In either case you are learning something about the interpersonal style of your client.

Given the range of information that can be revealed, sometimes it is essential to take notes to remember what clients are telling you. For example, if you are taking a family history, it can be extremely difficult to remember siblings, genders, and ages. When taking notes, however, continue to pay careful attention to the needs of your clients. When I first start to jot down some notes, I usually say something like, "If you don't mind, I'm going to write down some of what you say so that I'll be able to remember it better." I have never had a client object.

Verbal Behavior

We take for granted the meaning of what we say to people. We have all had the experience, however, in which what we thought we said to someone is not what they heard. Such experiences point to the complexities of verbal communication. Since interviewing is to a large degree a verbal activity, we need to pay careful attention to what we say and what our clients say. When talking with your clients, be sure to talk in language they can understand. (More will be said about this issue later.) Also, as you speak with them, you will be implicitly making a global estimate of their level of intelligence, and it is important to offer your questions and comments at a level appropriate for their understanding.

Asking questions is an important part of an interview. Early in the interview it may be useful to keep questions relatively unstructured or open. For example, when asking a married female client about her marital relationship, you might ask, "How would you describe your relationship with your husband?" This question is sufficiently open to give your client latitude in responding to it. Later in the interview, however, or as an immediate follow-up to her answer, it may be necessary to gather more specific data about the relationship. For example, if your client says something like, "Well, I guess I would say our relationship is pretty good, but we do fight sometimes," you could follow up in a more structured way by asking, "Earlier (or a moment ago) you mentioned that your relationship with your husband is pretty good, but sometimes you fight. How often would you say that you fight?" And, "What issues do you fight over?" and so on. Your particular use of questions will depend on how you like to structure things. Some clinicians like to keep things relatively structured throughout much of the interview and others are more comfortable with a relatively unstructured format. Both styles can elicit a great deal of information in a comfortable interpersonal atmosphere. Experiment with different styles and do what works well for you.

Nonverbal Behavior

It is no mystery that our communication depends only in part on what is said. Important information is embedded in our nonverbal behavior as well. The skilled clinician pays careful attention to these important cues. How and where you sit, your level of eye contact, the tone and rate of your speech, your facial expressions, how you dress or wear your hair, and your gestures all convey information about you to your client. For example, as you talk with a client who is crying, the tone of your voice may convey much more information than what you say. A soothing, quiet, slow-paced tone of voice may do much to help the client feel safe in the presence of strong affect. Because nonverbal behavior is so important, some training programs now videotape their trainees when interviewing. The information gathered from these tapes can be enlightening and can lead to increased self understanding. If your training program does not require this practice, I highly recommend it. Of course, written permission from clients to videotape is required, as is careful attention to confidentiality issues.

In a similar vein, the nonverbal behavior of your clients can yield important information about them as persons. Their posture, body movements, eye contact, style of dress, physical appearance, and rate and quality of speech all convey aspects of their personalities, their cultural background, the effect of their behavior on others, and the nature of their symptoms. For example, a person who is verbally reporting depression may confirm this report through congruent nonverbal behavior. Or, conversely, a client may report feeling fine about the death of a loved one, while displaying nonverbal behavior that conveys anxiety.

Assessing Strengths

Often the purpose of interviewing is to understand what is going wrong in the lives of your clients. However, it is easy to become completely focused on the pathology of clients and to lose sight of their strengths. All clients, even ones who are significantly disturbed, have personal assets. At some point in the inteview it is important to spend at least a little time thinking about this issue. If nothing else, your attention to this topic conveys to your clients that you are interested in them as whole persons, not just as diagnostic categories.

Dealing with Silence

Moments of silence are very difficult to deal with when first learning to interview. In your nervousness you may feel compelled to fill up every interview moment with dialog. Keep in mind, however, that silence during the interview may mean different things, some of which are important for your clients to experience.

On one end of the spectrum, moments of silence can indicate that your client is resistant to exploring some issue. In the initial interview you may not wish to press the issue of what your client seems to be avoiding, while noting to yourself that your client is reticent to discuss the issue. Later, assuming you continue to follow the client, it may be useful to confront more directly. On the other end of the spectrum, silence may occur when your client is deep in reflective thought, letting some memory, awareness, or affect "sink in." Obviously, the silence is serving a different function in each case. In the former it may be impeding the progress of the interview, and in the latter it may be facilitating it.

The important issue for you as a beginning interviewer is to become aware of your own comfort level with silences, so that you can be better equipped to handle them when they inevitably occur.

Closing the Interview

At some point it will come time to close the interview. Sometimes the interview flows so that when time is up, there is a sense of completion, a natural stopping point. At other times, when the interview is over, you still may have a good deal of material to cover. For example, in a traditional intake interview it may be difficult to cover the range of topics needed to write an adequate intake assessment report.

One of the most difficult situations is when the interview time is over but your client is in emotional turmoil. Perhaps an emotionally charged issue surfaced near the end of the hour. In this situation it is best not to end abruptly and send the client out of your office still in tears or otherwise upset. Yet the reality is you may have another appointment scheduled immediately after this one.

Assuming that your client is not suicidal and in need of crisis intervention, there are some useful strategies for handling this type of situation. One strategy is to be proactive in the interview. In other words, having an awareness of time may help you avoid getting in the situation in the first place. For instance, if a client starts to bring up an emotionally charged, complex issue with 3 minutes remaining, you can politely say something like, "You know, this sounds like a very important issue that we need to discuss. However, I'm aware that our time is about up and it might be best if we waited to discuss this next week, when we have more time to give it the attention that it deserves." In this way you acknowledge that the issue is important and also that it would be more fruitful to discuss it later.

If your client is already emotionally in pieces when the interview time is over, it is useful to give the client a few moments to collect himself or herself before leaving.

RAPPORT AND INTERVIEWING PITFALLS

The general suggestions here should help you get started with your interviewing. As you will discover, interviewing is always interesting and filled with new situations. This section of the chapter describes potential problems or pitfalls that are common to the beginning interviewer. Many of the pitfalls described are problems that undermine rapport and therefore contribute to a breakdown in trust and harmony.

In the best of all possible worlds you will feel comfortable with every client you meet. However, we do not live in the best of all possible worlds, and you will encounter many clinical situations in which you feel a lack of connection with the person you are interviewing. If you think about the work you are doing, this phenomenon makes perfect sense. The persons who come to see you are there because they are encountering difficulties in daily living. They may be depressed, anxious, psychotic, or personality disordered, to name a few possibilities. Any of these conditions makes it difficult for the person to deal effectively with others. Further, by the time most individuals make the decision to seek professional help, they are at the point of feeling overwhelmed. They are lacking a sense of self-efficacy to deal effectively with their problems. Thus, in addition to your own self-consciousness as a novice clinician, you must deal with the self-consciousness, anxiety, and uncertainty of your client. Keeping in mind that your primary task is to attend to the needs of your client, your work is cut out for you.

Here are some suggestions for dealing with the potential awkwardness of this first session. First, be willing to acknowledge your anxieties to yourself and to your supervisor. Your supervisor will remember what it was like in those initial sessions, and your willingness to be frank about your nervousness is a mark of maturity. Second, give yourself permission to be not perfect. A corollary to this suggestion is to have a sense of humor about yourself. In your first interviews you will likely behave in ways that feel alien. Remember not to take yourself too seriously. You inevitably will see improvement in your interviewing skills.

You do not learn to cook by reading recipe books; you learn by making the recipe, and then ultimately by experimenting to discover your unique preferences. The same principle obviously applies to clinical skills. As helpful as this book may be to your development as a clinician, there is no substitute for actual practice. It is helpful, however, to keep in mind some common pitfalls with which all trainees, and even experienced clinicians, struggle.

The Authenticity Pitfall

In an excellent review of the literature pertaining to the clinical relationship, McConnaughy (1987) argues, as have others, that the most important instrument to effect change in a helping relationship is the person of the clinician. McConnaughy confesses,

> For me, it was important to acknowledge that I could not be my supervisors, I could not be the authors whose techniques I read about, I could not be the master clinicians I observed on videotape or on stage. I could only be myself; I could only do what felt comfortable and solidly connected to who I am. (p. 303)

What McConnaughy refers to is the problem of authenticity, of being yourself. McConnaghy applies this issue to psychotherapeutic work, but the same concerns are relevant to the beginning interviewer.

It is common to feel a sense of dis-ease, of inauthenticity, of social awkwardness as you learn to develop interviewing skills. After all, you are working hard to find your interviewing persona. I agree with McConnaughy that you cannot be your supervisor or anyone else for that matter; you can only be yourself, and, as obvious as that seems, it is a common pitfall not to be yourself. Or, to put it another way, it is common to feel that you are not yourself.

There is probably good reason for this common experience. You are worried about a host of factors in your initial interviews, all of which make it difficult to relax and be the person that you spontaneously are otherwise. You are concerned with obtaining a good deal of information from your client. You may be thinking about how you are sitting or your facial expressions. Are you conveying enough empathy, too much empathy? Will your client return for his or her next visit, and if he or she doesn't, is it your fault? Your mind may be filled with thoughts, questions, and insecurities that interfere with the usual process of simply being you. When you feel this way, acknowledge it as part of the learning process and then try to reorient your attention away from yourself and to the needs of your client. As noted before, with time you will become better at being yourself and at giving undivided attention to your clients.

The Jargon Pitfall

A related problem is that in your search for your clinical identity you may find yourself using unnecessary jargon when talking with your client. Such jargon may be tolerable when conversing with student colleagues, professors, or supervisors, but generally it is not appropriate for talking with your client. Remember that your initial task is to build rapport. The use of big words may sound impressive to you but may communcicate nothing to your client—worse, it may alienate your client. For example, when interviewing a depressed person, you could possibly ask, "Are you anhedonic?" Such a question is likely to be meaningless even to a client of above average intelligence. A far less pretentious and more effective way to obtain the same information would be to ask, "Do you ever feel like you don't enjoy things the way you used to? Perhaps you have a hobby that was once a lot of fun, but now you really don't feel like doing it?"

Of course, there is a balance here as well. You don't want to talk down or be condescending to your clients. Try to speak their language, but don't fake it either (the authenticity pitfall). If you were born, raised, and college educated in New England and then attend graduate school and undertake training in the South, where you interact with a client population of largely rural Southerners, don't try to act Southern. Even though your clients may be psychologically distressed, they are still very perceptive and will surely pick up on your lack of authenticity. Be yourself and allow your clients to respond to you as you are, not to some facsimile of who you are. If differences between yourself and your client seem to be impeding progress, it is useful to discuss these with your client in a nondefensive manner. I also recommend discussing such issues with your supervisor, as they are very important.

The Ignoring Reality Pitfall

It is an interesting phenomenon that in your desire to appear professional, you may do things that you would not ordinarily do. I remember my first diagnostic interview with an adolescent. The interview took place in a residential school for violent teenagers, and, since it was my first interview, my supervisor was observing. The room where the interview took place was large, and my supervisor was seated about 10 feet from where the client and I were. The physical set-up was not ideal, but it was the best room available for training purposes.

About midway into the interview the phone next to me began to ring. The office was not mine and therefore I decided not to answer it. In my eagerness to be the ever "composed" clinician, I simply acted as if the phone was not ringing. It seemed like a benign decision. I sat there and continued to try to interview this young man, without showing the slightest indication that I heard the phone. Had the phone rung only four or five times, my decision to ignore it may have been fine. However, the phone continued to ring for what must have seemed like an eternity to the client, and I steadfastly ignored it, persistent in my vain attempt to appear "professional." My supervisor did not answer it because he was seated a good distance away and because it was "my interview." However, he pointed out later that it would have been much better had I simply said "excuse me" and taken the call, stopping the incessant ringing. A simple acknowledgment of reality would have allowed the interview to flow far more smoothly.

You may encounter similar situations in your early clinical work. Agencies, clinics, and inpatient units are busy places. There can be large numbers of staff and clients trying to function in small quarters. You may work in a different office each week or each day, and confusion may ensue regarding who is working where. Or you may be in the office that has the only copy of the agency's TAT (Thematic Apperception Test), and someone else needs it and comes in for it. You may be in the middle of an important part of an interview and the phone may ring or someone may knock on the door or walk into the room, not realizing that it is in use. These situations are not optimal, but they happen. The TAT incident happened to me not long ago. A colleague recently shared with me similar situations at the hospital where he practices. He has been in the middle of interviews and therapy sessions when a member of the custodial crew walks in and tries to empty the wastebasket or mop the floor.

When faced with such bizarre circumstances, it is important to maintain your composure and candidly acknowledge reality. In actuality, such situations are a great opportunity to model effective coping and interpersonal skills in the midst of what could otherwise be an extremely frustrating situation. Dealing tactfully with the intruder while maintaining a sense of professionalism with your client models a mature response.

The Slave to the Intake Form Pitfall

The function of your first interview with a client will determine to some degree your behavior. As we already noted, there are a variety of initial interview types, each with its own set of challenges. One particular problem for an initial intake interview is the breadth of information you feel compelled to collect. It is a daunting task to cover relevant areas while also paying attention to rapport and relationship building issues. You may need to assess the client's presenting complaint, including a detailed description of intensity, duration, and situational specificity of symptoms; social, psychiatric, occupational, and educational history; family constellation; mental status and general level of intellectual functioning; history of drug abuse; and legal history. To cover all these areas adequately in a limited amount of time takes great skill.

One possible coping strategy is to become a slave to the intake form, committing yourself to cover it all, no matter what. After all, you may suspect that your supervisor will be impressed to know that you were able to obtain all that information in a mere hour to an hour and a half. At what possible cost, however? Yes, you may have obtained a good deal of information, but at the same time you sacrificed rapport with your client. We have all sat in interviews or had conversations that were hurried. Typically, we feel a lack of rapport and that our thoughts are not valued. This situation is not one that you want to create with your client.

In the preceding scenario you have become caught up in completing the task without due consideration to the process. An alternative strategy is to go to the opposite extreme by paying exquisite attention to the process of establishing rapport, to the neglect of obtaining relevant information. In this case your clients may feel listened to; however, they may have little sense of why they talked with you. This extreme nondirective strategy may also allow clients to avoid talking about important and troubling aspects of their experience.

Also, during supervision your supervisor may ask about information you did not obtain in the interview. We have already seen that the amount of data to be gathered in an initial interview is considerable. If your supervisor begins to ask you about questions you failed to ask, do not become defensive. Candidly acknowledge that you failed to ask the question. Supervisors want trainees who are open and teachable, not individuals who are defensive and unwilling to admit oversights. For instance, if you fail to ask a client about substance use history and your supervisor questions you on these issues, you can straightforwardly say something like, "You know, we never really got into those sorts of issues and I completely forgot to ask about it. I'll make a note to follow up on that the next time we meet." Or you could say, "Wow, I never thought to bring it up. She seemed just so young and naive that I never would have considered she might use drugs. But you're right. It's worth checking on and I'll do that next time." Obviously, the particular circumstances surrounding the interview will determine the essence of what you say to your supervisor. The guiding principle is to be straightforward and nondefensive in responding to your supervisor.

A final strategy is to find a balance between these two alternatives, by paying careful attention to the nuances of the relationship without losing sight of the ultimate goal of the interview. Above all, do not become a slave to the intake form. If need be, you can always schedule a follow-up appointment for further evaluation. On the other hand, avoid small talk and be efficient with time.

The Diagnostic Label Pitfall

You are probably aware of the benefits and liabilities of diagnosis. Diagnosis is important in that it can help organize clinical information, enhance communication among professionals, aid in the conduct of research, or suggest treatment strategies (Turner & Hersen, 1984). On the negative side, diagnosis can create the illusion of explanation (it is merely description), contribute to a self-fulfilling prophesy, or obscure the individuality of the client.

This latter point may seem abstract, but it is a real problem and one to keep close in mind. Rosenhan's (1973) classic and controversial "pseudopatients" study serves to remind us of the potential problems with diagnosis and labeling. You may recall that Rosenhan and seven of his cohorts all reported to different hospitals complaining of hearing voices saying the words "hollow," "empty," and "thud." Beyond this false report and the falsification of their names and vocations, all eight pseudopatients truthfully responded to interview questions and all were admitted as inpatients to the hospital. The length of hospitalization ranged from 7 to 52 days, with an average of 19 days, and on discharge all were diagnosed with schizophrenia in remission. This diagnosis was made despite the fact that all the pseudopatients behaved normally while on the unit. After all, like real psychiatric patients, the pseudopatients did not know when they would be discharged and therefore they tried to act as sanely as possible. Yet, despite their normal behavior, these patients could not overcome the diagnostic label, and their normal behavior tended to be interpreted in terms of their diagnosis. For example, on one occasion a pseudopatient walked the halls out of boredom and a staff member asked if he was anxious. One obvious implication of this study is that diagnostic labels can potentially alter our perceptions of our clients.

A personal story may also illustrate the potential impact of a diagnostic label. In my first practicum with an adult population, one of the first clients I interviewed was a 55-year-old woman. The information I received prior to the interview was contained in a short form that had been completed by the office staff with information obtained over the telephone. The form indicated the client's age and that she was depressed. My supervisor was sitting in on this interview, which, from the bit of information I had in front of me, seemed to me to be a fairly straightforward one. After all, I thought I knew a fair amount about depression. After several minutes into the intake interview, I began to wonder, however, if I really knew anything about depression. I was becoming increasingly frustrated with my inability to obtain relevant information from the client. I was having extreme difficulty following her responses. I thought I was asking her all the "right" questions. "Were you having any difficulty sleeping? Noticing any change in your appetite? Feeling sad or blue? Having any crying spells?" But I was getting nowhere and feeling more and more inadequate. Luckily, I had a wonderful supervisor: kind, patient, and able to recognize a trainee in trouble. After about 20 minutes of observing my interview, he asked if I would mind if he asked Mrs. Smith a question or two. With relief, I gladly consented. "Mrs. Smith," he asked, "have you noticed lately that you've had some problems with your memory? Do you ever seem to get confused at the grocery store or while you are out driving your car?" At this point it was becoming clear to me that Mrs. Smith's primary problem was not depression at all. She was showing signs of significant cognitive impairment, more consistent with a diagnosis of presenile dementia than with major depression alone. I had been completely duped by the diagnostic impression given on the form. In my mind, Mrs. Smith walked into my office as a diagnostic category, not as an individual.

I assume that today, with more clinical experience under my belt, I would not be as easily fooled by the label, but the Rosenhan study makes me wonder. Further, certain labels may carry more weight than others when it comes to stereotyping someone. How would it affect your impression of a client when conducting an intake interview if you were informed that the client had a previous diagnosis of borderline personality disorder, or multiple personality, or that he or she had a WAIS-R IQ of 84 or of 135? This information would likely affect your perception of the client. All of us are affected in this way. It is helpful to acknowledge this tendency, so as to minimize its potential impact.

For the reasons given here, my bias in working with adults is to avoid obtaining client information prior to the initial interview. I prefer to formulate an impression based on what I learn in the interview and later compare this impression with other data when or if they become available. But not all clinicians operate this way. Others prefer to have relevant clinical information before the initial contact. Agencies and hospitals also may vary in how much client information is obtained prior to the initial contact. In some cases only a referral question is available, while in others a fair amount of history is available at the time of the intake interview.

Moreover, in some instances it is very desirable, if not imperative, that the interviewer has relevant information ahead of time. When working with children or adolescents, for instance, there are many cases in which you simply do not establish sufficient rapport and get enough information to adequately evaluate the problem. Prior information from parents, teachers, or others who have observed or interacted with the child for a period of time can be essential. Further, a delay of a week or two until additional interviews are completed may be harmful to the welfare of the child or adolescent client.

Am I more objective because I choose to limit prior information in my work with adults? Of course not. It is a matter of personal preference. I have tried it both ways, and I prefer not to know. And, of course, there are certain circumstances when I do have prior information. I encourage you to discuss this matter with your supervisor, to obtain his or her perspective. It is possible to have prior information and not be blinded by it. The important point is to remain aware of the potential effects of prior information.

The Reassurance Pitfall

The initial interview is difficult for a variety of reasons. We have already discussed the complexity of your behavior and the potential impact it may have on the client. The initial interview can also be difficult because you may speak for an hour or more about all that is going wrong in the life of the client. You are assessing the client's symptoms, family and social situation, history of psychiatric problems, and so on. The enormity of the problems may seem overwhelming.

With experience, you are able to detach somewhat from the suffering of your client, and be more objective, while still remaining empathic and compassionate. If a physician became emotionally wrought over every suffering patient, his or her effectiveness as a physical healer would be greatly reduced. The same applies to the "psychological healer." Accurate empathy communicated clearly to your clients is essential; however, don't mistake pity and extreme emotional involvement for empathy. Being empathic means seeing the world through the eyes of your clients—experiencing their subjective world as if you were them, without losing the "as if" quality. It is this quality that helps you remain objective about your clients, and this objectivity facilitates your ability to help them. As soon as you become lost in the intensity of their feelings, you become far less effective. When conducting an effective interview, you want to understand and feel with your clients, but not feel sorry for them. Understanding will facilitate rapport; pity will not.

At the end of the initial interview it is sometimes tempting to offer reassuring remarks to the client. If a female client, for instance, has been in an abusive relationship and has come to your clinic because she has recently separated, is caring for two young children while trying to keep a full-time job, is fearful that her husband may try to hurt her, and is significantly depressed, you may feel compelled to tell her that you admire her strength in coming to the office and that you are sure everything will work out. The first part of your remark is fine. Clients can benefit from an appropriate amount of encouragement or reinforcement for their efforts. However, the latter part may convey that perhaps you did not listen carefully enough to understand the depth of her problems, otherwise you would not offer such a glib remark. When the temptation comes to offer reassurance at this early stage, it may reflect more of a need to comfort yourself than to comfort your client.

At the same time, it is appropriate and perhaps beneficial to reassure your clients that you intend to work with them and stick with them in an effort to resolve their problems. You are not saying that you are sure that their problems will go away (you do not know that). You are conveying that you will be a constant in their lives as they try to work through troubling issues. This type of reassurance is appropriate because your clients have likely been let down by others in the past, and knowing that you are committed to helping them is good for them to understand. Of course, if you will not be following the client after the initial interview, you would need to qualify your remarks.

The Apology Pitfall

When confronted with real problems in real lives, things suddenly become very complex, far more complex than your textbooks are able to communicate. In addition to learning first hand about the complexities of persons and their problems, you are trying to understand how your placement site operates, how supervision works, how the health care system functions, and how to keep records and write reports.

In the midst of all this new learning some clients may ask about the level of your training or may comment that you seem "awfully young to be doing this type of work." If you are interviewing a married couple and you happen to be single, the couple may try to discount your ability because you are not married. If you have no children of your own but are talking with a client or couple about parenting issues, you may be called on this. You may be asked by a client, "So how much experience do you have working with folks with PTSD?" or "Have you ever seen combat?" If your answer to the first queston is "None" and to the second "Never," then the dilemma is obvious.

There are several possible avenues to deal with these or similar situations. One option is to apologize for your marital, parental, or experiential status. Along these lines, you may take some comfort in the research suggesting that length of clinical experience makes little difference in clinical effectiveness (Christensen & Jacobson, 1994; Smith & Glass, 1977). However, I do not recommend discussing this research with your client. Such a discussion would evade the real issue. Another option is to try to defend your status by arguing that, well, you are in an excellent training program or you have excellent supervision, or some other "excuse." I do not recommend taking this course of action either.

The best strategy is to discuss the issue openly with your clients. If they have raised the issue (actually, many never will), it may be a legitimate concern to them, in which case you need to address it head on for their sake. Or it may be an attempt by a client to evade other, more important clinical issues. In either case an open, nondefensive posture is most useful. Simply be honest and straightforward. For example, regarding the parenting question, you might say,

> You are right. I don't have children of my own, although I did help with my younger brothers and sisters as I grew up and I have worked with kids in other settings. However, because you are a parent and I am not, you may need to help me understand how a parent feels in

certain circumstances. With your input and my understanding of principles that psychologists have learned from research and practice over many years, I am in a better position to be of help to you.

A similar response can be given for the PTSD question or any other client inquiry about your competence.

The guiding principle is to take the question seriously and to answer it honestly and nondefensively, while also conveying that you have confidence in your ability to be helpful. Your client will likely appreciate your candor, which may actually enhance your trustworthiness in his or her eyes.

ETHICAL ISSUES

Understanding ethical principles and issues is one of your most important responsibilities as a psychologist in training. It is also incumbent upon you continually to refine your understanding of ethical issues throughout your professional career. One of the most interesting aspects of ethical decision making is that in most cases the issues are not clear cut. You must bring your knowledge of ethical principles, your understanding of legal statutes, and your clinical experience to bear on understanding complex situations to make sound decisions. If you ever are in doubt regarding an ethical dilemma, consult with a supervisor or professional peers about the decision-making process. To be sure, some individuals engage in ethical violations because they are acting with conscious intent to do so; many, however, act inappropriately because of lack of knowledge about ethical principles (Keith-Spiegel & Koocher, 1985). There is no place in the practice of psychology for the former category, and we should make every effort to avoid finding ourselves in the latter.

The Ethical Principles of the American Psychological Association (APA, 1992) provide the foundation for an understanding of ethical behavior. This document reflects the complexity of contemporary clinical practice, and it has changed over the years to reflect the evolution of our practice. In other chapters of this book you will find ethics discussed as they pertain to the specific topic of the chapter.

With regard to your initial contact with a client in the first interview, the ethical issue of confidentiality is probably the most important. This issue is so important and complex that it is of serious concern to many practitioners, according to a national survey (Haas, Malouf, & Mayerson, 1986). Therefore, it is worth considering in some detail.

What follows here is a brief description of the nature of confidentiality and its limitations. Read and understand what is written here. However, before you see your first client, have a good discussion with your supervisor to be sure that you clearly grasp the principle of confidentiality and its limitations. In addition, the administrative staff of many agencies and hospitals will give you formal training on how to keep proper records that maintain confidentiality as well as on when and how you are obliged to break it. This training is important because agencies may differ in their policies regarding these issues. Furthermore, legislation regarding confidentiality and its limitations may differ from state to state, and it is important that you understand the law in the state where you are training.

Now let us turn to your initial interview. At the outset of the interview it is common practice to describe to your client the principle of confidentiality. Assuming that your clients are adults, you may tell them something to the effect that whatever they tell you will be held in strict confidence. You will discuss this material with no one, except your supervisor who will need to hear case material to be of help to you in your training. Depending on the practices of your placement site, you may also be sharing details of this case with a treatment team or some other type of case conference. However, this sharing of information stays within the agency and is a part of your training and of sound clinical practice. Experienced clinicians do the same thing, although perhaps not as routinely as you do while in training.

You will also make it clear to your clients that if you need to release any information to anyone else, you will obtain their written consent. For instance, if a client has been referred for evaluation by a probation officer, you must obtain the client's written permission to release information back to the probation officer.

Confidentiality, however, has its limitations, and it is also important to explain these to your clients. There are at least four limitations to confidentiality. First, if in your judgment your client is in danger of harming himself or herself, you are obligated to break confidentiality to ensure client safety. Thus, you may need to initiate hospitalization, which will involve the release of relevant information to a hospital. The agency where you are training will likely have a procedure for this carefully worked out, and you should follow it to the letter, with the aid of your supervisor.

Second, if you suspect child or elder abuse by your client, then you must break confidentiality to report your suspicion to the appropriate authorities. Keep in mind that it is not your responsibility to investigate or to substantiate the abuse. If you have reason to suspect that abuse is occurring, you should break confidentiality to report it.

Third, your records may be subpoened by a court. In some cases it is important to inform your client at the outset of this limit on confidentiality. For example, if you are interviewing a parent who is currently in a child custody battle, your records may be subpoened later as part of the court proceedings.

Finally, as a result of the *Tarasoff v. Board of Regents of the University of*

California legal case, you are now ethically, and in some states legally, bound to break confidentiality if your client threatens to harm someone else. In this situation, breaking confidentiality includes informing the person who has been threatened. The Tarasoff case set a landmark legal precedent for what is now known as the "duty to warn" or "duty to protect" limit on confidentiality.

In 1969 a counselor at Cal Berkeley's student counseling center was seeing a male client who threatened to kill his girlfriend, Tatiana Tarasoff. The therapist informed the campus police of the threat and they took the client into custody for questioning. He was released a short time later because he appeared "rational." The potential victim was never warned of the threat, and 2 months later she was murdered by the client. The family of Ms. Tarasoff brought suit against the university for not warning their daughter, and the California Supreme Court ruled in their favor in 1976. This ruling has generated a great deal of controversy in the clinical community and it will likely continue to do so (Fulero, 1988; Knapp & Vandecreek, 1982; Knapp, Vandecreek, & Shapiro, 1990). The legal and ethical implications of the "duty to warn" mandate are complex and should be discussed with your supervisor.

There are two other important considerations at this juncture. First, it is not necessary to explain these limits to your clients in detail. Usually, it is sufficient to briefly describe confidentiality and its limits in language that your clients can understand. Second, if you are interviewing children or adolescents under legal age, other considerations apply. For example, you will still want to explain the idea of confidentiality to the child or adolescent; however, you will need to do so in age-appropriate language. In addition, children and adolescents technically do not have confidentiality. Their parent or guardian has a right to demand information. Most clinicians are able to work out a contract with the parent that allows them a significant degree of discretion in what they report. However, the parents can, at any time, demand more. If you are seeing children or adolescents, be sure to discuss these issues with your supervisor.

DIVERSITY ISSUES

Most models of interviewing, psychopathology, and psychotherapy are built on a white, middle-class client population and value system. The very real issue for mental health professionals, however, is that we live in a society of great racial, ethnic, and cultural diversity. When you conduct a clinical interview, the interaction of your own race, gender, ethnicity, socioeconomic status, or sexual orientation with that of your client is a dimension that may dramatically influence establishing rapport and other dynamics of the interview situation. The need is great to become sensitive to and skilled in dealing with issues of diversity. However, many training programs still do not offer systematic training with regard to these dimensions of clinical practice (Allison et al., 1994).

In their excellent book on working with culturally different clients, Sue and Sue (1990) detail the cultural barriers to effective interviewing and therapeutic communication. These barriers develop out of differences regarding culture-bound, class-bound, and language values. Because of cultural differences, for instance, you and your client may differ with regard to verbal, emotional, and behavioral expressiveness; the value placed on psychological insight; the importance of self-disclosure; and typical patterns of interpersonal communication. Similarly, since inteviewing is largely a verbal activity, cultural differences in language usage can be barriers to effective interviewing.

All interviewers should become skilled in communicating with clients from different cultures. In particular, if you are working in a clinical setting where the culture, race, or ethnicity of the client population is typically different from your own, you should familiarize yourself with the culture of your clients. For example, if you are white and are working in an agency with a large Hispanic population, then it is incumbent upon you to educate yourself about the cultural values of your Hispanic clients. The implications of this activity for rapport building and effective interviewing are obvious. While a detailed discussion of issues of diversity is beyond the scope of this chapter, the reader is encouraged to consult the Sue and Sue (1990) book for further elaboration, and to refer back to Chapter 2 of this text.

CONCLUSIONS

Clinical interviewing is exciting and rewarding work. It is also hard work, and it takes time to perfect your skills. This chapter has outlined some pertinent issues to consider as you begin to develop rapport-building and interviewing skills. The time and effort you put into the development of these skills will pay big dividends, as they are fundamental to many other clinical activities.

Two themes should have emerged as you read this chapter. First, regardless of your theoretical orientation or the techniques you like to use, your most important asset is yourself. You can be no one else, and all of what you do flows out of who you are. Second, commit yourself to a lifetime of professional development and education. Refining your understanding of the nuances of rapport building, interviewing, ethical issues, and issues of diversity is a lifelong process.

REFERENCES

Allison, K. W., Crawford, I., Echemendia, R., Robinson, L., & Knapp, D. (1994). Human diversity and professional competence: Training in clinical and counseling psychology revisited. *American Psychologist, 49,* 792–796.

American Psychological Association (1992). Ethical principles of psychologists and code of conduct. *American Psychologist, 47,* 1597–1611.

Baekeland, F., & Lundwall, L. (1975). Dropping out of treatment: A critical review. *Psychological Bulletin, 82,* 738–783.

Brenner, D. (1982). *The effective psychotherapist: Conclusions from practice and research.* New York: Pergamon Press.

Christensen, A., & Jacobson, N. S. (1994). Who (or what) can do psychotherapy: The status and challenge of nonprofessional therapies. *Psychological Science, 5,* 8–14.

Cohen, R. J., Swerdlik, M. E. , & Smith, D. K. (1992). *Psychological testing and assessment* (2d ed.). Mountain View, CA: Mayfield.

Corey, G. (1991). *Theory and practice of counseling and psychotherapy.* Pacific Grove, CA: Brooks/Cole.

Endicott, J., & Spitzer, R. L. (1978). A diagnostic interview: The schedule for affective disorders and schizophrenia. *Archives of General Psychiatry, 35,* 837–844.

Folstein, M. F., Folstein, S. E., & McHugh, P. R. (1975). "Mini-Mental State": A practical method for grading the cognitive state of patients for the clincian. *Journal of Psychiatric Research, 12,* 189–198.

Fulero, S. M. (1988). Tarasoff: 10 years later. *Professional Psychology: Research and Practice, 19,* 184–190.

Haas, L. J., Malouf, J. L., & Mayerson, N. H. (1986). Ethical dilemmas in psychological practice: Results of a national survey. *Professional Psychology: Research and Practice, 20,* 48–50.

Hackney, H., & Cormier, L. S. (1988). *Counseling strategies and interventions* (3d ed.). Englewood Cliffs, NJ: Prentice-Hall.

Keith-Spiegel, P., & Koocher, G. (1985). *Ethics in psychology: Professional standards and cases.* New York: Random House.

Knapp, S., & Vandecreek, L. (1982). Tarasoff: Five years later. *Professional Psychology: Research and Practice, 13,* 511–516.

Knapp, S., Vandecreek, L., & Shapiro, D. (1990). Statutory remedies to the duty to protect: A reconsideration. *Psychotherapy, 27,* 291–296.

McConnaughy, E. A. (1987). The person of the therapist in psychotherapeutic practice. *Psychotherapy, 24,* 303–314.

Nietzel, M. T., Bernstein, D. A., & Milich, R. (1994). *Introduction to clinical psychology* (4th ed.). Englewood Cliffs, NJ: Prentice Hall.

Phares, E. J. (1992). *Clinical psychology: Concepts, methods, and profession* (4th ed.). Pacific Grove, CA: Brooks/Cole.

Rogers, C. R. (1957). The necessary and sufficient conditions of therapeutic personality change. *Journal of Consulting Psychology, 21,* 95–103.

Rosenhan, D. (1973). On being sane in insane places. *Science, 179,* 250–258.

Smith, M. L., & Glass, G. V. (1977). Meta-analysis of psychotherapy outcome studies. *American Psychologist, 32,* 752–760.

Sue, D. W., & Sue, D. (1990). *Counseling the culturally different* (2d ed.). New York: Wiley.

Sullivan, H. S. (1954). *The psychiatric interview.* New York: Norton.

Turner, S. M., & Hersen, M. (Eds.) (1984). *Adult psychopathology and diagnosis.* New York: Wiley.

Wiens, A. N., & Matarazzo, J. D. (1983). Diagnostic interviewing. In M. Hersen, A. E. Kazdin, & A. S. Bellack (Eds.), *The clinical psychology handbook* (pp. 309–328). New York: Pergamon Press.

▶ 5

Psychotherapy

JULIA SHIANG   BOB LANDRY

BRUCE BONGAR

The process of learning to become a competent, skilled psychotherapist takes knowledge, time, dedication, and self-awareness. This process is by no means an easy one. In our experience, the requirements to become a competent and efficient therapist include: (1) mastering a body of knowledge that includes theories of human development, models of disease, and interventions for change; (2) integrating this knowledge with practice of actual skills that promote change; (3) having the discipline to develop new interpersonal skills that foster effective relationships as well as staying flexible and open to new ideas/hypotheses about clients; and (4) cultivating an awareness of oneself as an effective change agent. This process takes both practice and the integration of self with intellectual knowledge.

The purpose of this chapter is to review a number of characteristics of the psychotherapeutic relationship that have been found, through clinical practice and research findings, to promote adaptive change in the client. Another purpose is to assist the beginning therapist in the task of translating psychological theory into practice. Basic guidelines for decision making in the beginning phases of psychotherapy will be provided. Our focus will be on interpersonal forms of therapy—whose express purpose is to improve the client's relationships with other people. Two case examples of clients who suffered major losses and come from different cultural backgrounds, a Caucasian and an Asian woman, will help illustrate our main points. Where possible, we will include research findings that may help orient the therapist toward considering those factors that appear to be most salient for decision making in the therapeutic process. Other chapters in this volume address specific considerations that relate to psychotherapy, such as assessment, the development of rapport and interviewing skills, screening exams, and other topics.

DEFINING PSYCHOTHERAPY AND THE THERAPEUTIC STANCE

Since modern psychotherapy began, its precise definition has proven somewhat elusive. One type of definition focuses on the interaction between two people. Whitaker and Malone (1953) suggest that whenever one individual is engaged in an interpersonal relationship with another and functions in such a way as to increase the integrative adaptive capacity of the latter, then psychotherapy has taken place. This interaction can occur regardless of the intent of those in the relationship. A more formal definition is provided by Wolberg (1954), who suggests that psychotherapy is a form of treatment for problems of an emotional nature in which a trained person deliberately establishes a professional relationship with a client with the object of removing, modifying, or retarding existing symptoms; of mediating disturbed patterns of behavior, and of promoting positive personality growth and development. The relationship is seen as the core of the therapeutic process, and this relationship is to be deliberately planned, nurtured, and guided by the therapist. In both these definitions, reciprocal human interaction between the client and the therapist is emphasized.

The therapeutic process is an interpersonal approach that requires, above all else, the development of a relationship that is therapeutic to the client. This does not mean that therapists are all giving, always available, and accept whatever occurs. It does mean, however, that therapists are responsible for establishing the "therapeutic" environment of the relationship; they must work within their own personal understanding of self to form an alliance with their client, who brings to the setting particular, often maladaptive ways of functioning. We might think of this process as the attempt to match pieces of a rather fluid puzzle. Each part has its own shape, and the task is to fit them together largely for the benefit of one part of the puzzle. This then requires therapists to mold and shape themselves into stances that on one hand do not reenact dysfunctional patterns and on the other hand provide new ways of being more functional in the interpersonal realm. For example, if a client is angry or hostile, the therapist must take a neutral, curious stance rather than a "typical" reaction to anger; "getting back" at the client through undermining, distancing, and the like, will most likely reenact the client's usual nonadaptive patterns. The ability of therapists to take a functional stance and to genuinely feel neutral will depend, to a great degree, on their own personal growth, especially in the area of reflecting on their own projections. With such a stance, therapists are more available to resonate to the particular affective experiences of the client and the ways in which the affect is triggered and maintained, as well as how it is specifically being used in the therapy.

These interactions take place within the confines of a specific setting, and the therapist brings to the work a specific "orientation." Therapies are actually based on assumptions of implicit definitions of human "goodness" (and corresponding "badness") and how people change. Many of the Western-based psychotherapy models presently in use, and the assumptions upon which they are based, are built on views of humanness that are distinctly North American–Eurocentric and individualistic. The goals of therapy in this model are individuation, separation, and achievement. In recent years there has been a recognition that other models of human behavior exist. For example, most Southern European, Asian, and African definitions of humanness assume that individuals define themselves with reference to others (Markus & Kitayama, 1992). In fact, there is an increasing body of evidence that indicates that women in the United States define themselves in terms of others (Gilligan, 1982). Therapies based on relational models place greater emphasis on group dynamics, family interactions, and self-in-context. Prescriptions for change will differ depending upon whether the therapeutic orientation is based on an individualistic approach or a self-in-relationship approach.

LEARNING TO BE A THERAPIST

Learning to be a therapist can be compared to learning to drive a car to an unknown place. It's not clear when to put on the brakes and when to accelerate, whether to take this street or this boulevard—sometimes we're not even sure there is a destination. The beginning therapist is generally unsure how to handle the many layers of information and how to test hypotheses. Developmental and pathological theories provide the therapist with a general orientation to the presentation of the problem, but they do not provide the ability to make here-and-now decisions. Unfortunately, suggestions from supervisors made at the beginning of the process of learning to provide psychotherapy feel much like directions received in a post-war military review. They provide optimum solutions for the last client, but often do not fit the chaos of the present client's situation.

The beginning therapist has to define the parameters of the new role and learn how to balance different aspects of this new responsibility. Some of these issues include how to maintain a professional stance while allowing the client to share very intimate details of his or her life, how to stay focused on the client's process while paying attention to one's own emotional reactions, and how to keep the larger goals in mind while keeping straight the many details that surface. It can be uncomfortable to sit with someone in emotional pain, and it can be uncomfortable to not respond to a client's desire for an immediate solution. The beginning therapist often responds to the pressure to "do something" and assume responsibility for fixing the client. This is an overwhelming self imposed burden. The desire to fix things is a deeply ingrained part of our culture, and it creeps into the therapist's thinking in subtle ways. However, this need to "fix" the situation can, in certain situations, perpetuate the client's problems. Therapeutic change is generally based on the development of an intense interpersonal relationship. The process of therapy will at times create strong emotions, memories, and fantasies in the therapist. The beginning therapist must learn to understand these in himself or herself and use them in a way that is constructive for the client. Personal therapy for the therapist can be very important in developing the necessary self-understanding.

Managing their own anxiety is one of the most important skills that therapists can master. A feeling of incompetence is normal for a beginning therapist. Much of it is generated by self imposed expectations—the expectation that the client will be "cured," the expectation that the therapist will rescue the client from his or her problems. These types of expectations can distract the therapist from attending to what is actually happening with the client in the session. The experience of learning psychotherapy can feel like an emotional roller coaster. Stimulus is coming from everywhere—from the client, the supervisor, the institution, and oneself. Suddenly perceptions are confused: The client's progress is seen as a reflection of one's own abilities, one's own emotions based on positive and negative input from supervisors find their way into the session, and the therapist is tempted to quit the whole endeavor.

Self-imposed expectations are often simply unrealistic and unreasonable, as the beginning therapist who perseveres will learn. As we have stated earlier in the chapter, the process of learning takes knowledge, self-awareness, dedication, and practice.

Structuring the Session

Every therapeutic relationship is unique. In a typical session three or four themes will be discussed and elaborated. The therapist must find a balance between working with what the client brings into the room and bringing the client back to the focus of therapy. Over the course of therapy the balance of this process will change. In the early sessions the therapist must take responsibility for building the relationship. In the middle sessions more confrontation is sometimes called for if the client is avoiding key issues.

It is the therapist's responsibility to keep track of the flow and passage of time in the session. A client who is expressing an unusual amount of affect during the session will need help getting to a place of calmness so that he or she can leave the office ready to move onto the next task of the day. While the beginning therapist sometimes wonders how he or she is going to fill the hour, the reality is that it is much more difficult to stop on time. Often, to the chagrin of the therapist, many important issues come to the surface toward the end of the session. Clients will sometimes drop a "bombshell" just as they are leaving the session. This is usually an expression of their ambivalence about discussing the topic, although it is sometimes used as a way to extend the session. If the new topic does not constitute an emergency situation, it is best to tell the client, "This sounds important. We should discuss it first thing next week."

ADDRESSING THE NEEDS OF CLIENTS

Duration of Therapy

When clients enter psychological treatment, they generally do not anticipate that their therapy will be prolonged, but instead believe that their problems will require a few sessions at most (Garfield, 1978). Indeed, clients typically come for psychological treatment seeking specific and focal problem resolution, rather than general personality "overhauls," as was assumed in providing the forms of long-term therapy of the past (Koss & Shiang, 1994).[1] The duration of therapeutic contact, regardless of the therapeutic orientation of the therapist, is a median number of six to eight sessions (Garfield, 1986). Research has found that 75% of those clients who benefit from brief therapy do so in the first 6 months of contact (Lambert, Shapiro, & Bergin, 1986). This finding suggests that in most cases a short-term or brief therapy will provide the types of interventions that help the client become more functional. While there are clearly situations in which long-term therapy is merited, most therapies are likely to be provided on an intermittent basis over the course of a lifetime (Cummings & Vandenbos, 1979). Another pattern of care that is increasingly seen, especially in health maintenance organizations (HMOs), is that of intermittent care in which clients engage in therapy for short periods of time, terminate as problems are resolved, and then reenter treatment when problems recur (Cummings & Vandenbos, 1979; Siddall, Haffey, & Feinman, 1988). Recent financial pressures to limit the payments for psychotherapy to a predetermined number of sessions have resulted in a practice climate in

---

[1] Sections of this chapter were adapted from Koss and Shiang (1994).

which many insurance companies advocate therapy modalities that are, in fact, brief or crisis treatment approaches.

Principles of Brief Therapy

The set of principles that guide most forms of brief therapy (Koss & Shiang, 1994) are:

1. Therapeutic goals are based on the view that clients are capable of making change throughout their lifespan.
2. The time required to achieve these goals is limited.
3. The development of a working alliance between therapist and client is required to achieve the goals in a stated period of time.

The technical aspects that support these principles include:

1. The careful selection and exclusion of clients
2. Rapid and early assessment of the client
3. Therapist actions that promote the underlying principles, such as the maintenance of focus, high therapist activity, therapist flexibility, promptness of intervention, and addressing the termination

It is not possible to do justice to describing the complexities in various aspects of the process of learning the knowledge, "art," skills, and self-understanding that are required to develop into a competent psychotherapist given our limitations on space. However, a number of excellent books have been published; we suggest the reader consider: *Doing Psychotherapy* (Basch, 1980), *Learning Psychotherapy* (Bruch, 1974), *The Art of Psychotherapy* (Storr, 1980), as well as some works that, despite being "old," still contain much wisdom: *The Teaching and Learning of Psychotherapy* (Ekstein & Wallerstein, 1972), *Psychotherapy* (Dewald, 1964), and *How Psychotherapy Heals* (Chessick,1969). We also suggest the reader consider several writings about clients and therapists: *The Taboo Scarf and Other Tales* (Weinberg, 1990), *The 50-minute Hour* (Lindner, 1982), and *I Never Promised You a Rose Garden* (Green, 1964).

MAKING INITIAL TREATMENT DECISIONS

Having established rapport and obtained information about how the clients present themselves and their particular constellation of problems (see earlier chapter), therapists next face many decisions:

1. What overall systemic principles should guide the treatment of their client?
2. Which format (family, individual, group, child, etc.) should be used?
3. Which theoretical orientation will provide the client with the most efficacious course of therapy?
4. Which client variables must therapists consider first?
5. How should the therapist act in order to establish a therapeutic alliance?
6. Are there special considerations that need to be addressed at the end of therapy?

We would like first to present two case examples to illustrate these considerations.

▶ CASE EXAMPLE

Sandra

Sandra is a 26-year-old Caucasian woman who has just ended a relationship with her boyfriend of 2 years. She comes into the clinic stating that she'll never be able to have a satisfying relationship, that she often "sabotages" her intimate relationships. She says that she breaks into tears "for no reason," doesn't want to sleep, that she's lost 10 pounds in the last 3 weeks, has no appetite, and just can't seem to get rid of the idea that she will never be able to have a long-lasting relationship. At the same time she says she wants to be independent and will continue living alone even though her sister has offered a room in her home for a while. She's missed several days of work in the last week. The precipitating factors that bring her into treatment are the recent break-up with her boyfriend and the death of her father 2 months ago. She also reports that she occasionally has thoughts of suicide.

▶ CASE EXAMPLE

Clare

Clare is a 28-year-old Chinese American woman who is deciding whether to break off her engagement with her fiancée. She has been experiencing intermittent stomach pain, has been feeling sad, and has missed several days of work in the past 2 weeks. She has just been offered the possibility of moving across the country to a new job position. She realizes that it is a good job opportunity but also that it would be an "easy" way out of her problems

(Cont.)

▶ CASE EXAMPLE   *(Continued)*

with her fiancée. She states that her parents will be extremely unhappy when she lets them know she is going to end her engagement. She says she is worried that her parents will be disappointed in her.

Clinical Considerations of Case Examples

In Sandra's situation we must first assess her level of suicidal ideation. If she has an active plan, she will need to be hospitalized. If she does not, we would immediately consider a diagnosis of some form of depression (American Psychiatric Association, 1994). The data that lead us to this way of thinking are based on her self-report that she has suffered several recent losses and that she has had recent appetite changes, loss of weight, sleeplessness, emotional instabliity, and days missed from work. This diagnosis provides us with a working hypothesis on which to map further information as well as a language that can be useful for communicating with other mental health workers. Her presentation of the wish to be independent helps the clinician consider what types (individual, group, family) of therapy would be amenable to her. The way she talks about her problems helps us consider what forms of therapy (e.g., interpersonal, cognitive-behavioral) might be useful in the long run. We do not yet have critical information about the quality of "problems" in her interpersonal interactions. This information must be gleaned from the clinician's interactions with the client, her reporting of patterns with others in the past, and corroborating information from other sources.

In Clare's situation we are not sure whether her problems stem from physical concerns or psychological concerns. We know that the beliefs and values of traditional Chinese culture emphasize the continuum of the mind and body so that psychological problems are often normally expressed in the physical realm. So, while she might reasonably be treated psychologically, it is first necessary to send her to a physician in order to rule out any physical disorder. If she has no physical complications, we can gather more information in the following areas: (1) physical symptoms, (2) problems with her fiancée, (3) concerns with her parents when she lets them know that she is thinking about breaking off her engagement, and (4) anticipation of loss (her fiancée, parents' concerns, and present position at work). Clare's feelings of sadness and loss may be related to concerns in these areas. The need for additional information in the areas of relationships and family expectations is based on knowing that, in general, Clare's concerns related to self-in-relation to others may be more salient for her self-definition than for Sandra's.

We will consider culture-specific diagnoses such as neurasthenia (Kleinman & Kleinman, 1985) and the *DSM-IV* diagnosis of "depression" while realizing that physical concerns may be part of the "normal" expression of sadness for more traditional Chinese Americans. Our knowledge base in working with people of different cultures in the United States is not yet highly developed and consultation with other clinicians may be required.

We will use these two prototypical case examples throughout the remainder of the chapter to illustrate our points.

General Systems Issues: A Model for Considering Client, Treatment, Interaction, and Intervention

The practice of psychotherapy takes many different formats (individual, group, family, case management, crisis management, referral, etc.) in many different settings (hospitals, community clinics, mental health centers, private practices, etc.), each with its own set of specific institutional rules. At the outset of psychotherapy all these factors come into play and influence the course of therapy. Unfortunately, many decision-making processes that may be standard procedure at the institution in which the therapist is working may not necessarily be geared to provide the most efficient and effective course of therapy for a specific client. The therapist must make a number of decisions within a short time frame that will influence the development of his or her relationship with the client.

A model that considers four therapeutic variables: has been proposed by Beutler and Clarkin (1990). Called *systematic eclectic psychotherapy*, it recognizes that "effective treatment is a consequence of increasingly fine-grained decisions. No effective treatment can be developed from information that is available at one point in time nor from decisions made on the basis of a static set of client characteristics" (Beutler & Clarkin, 1990, p. 20). The four classes of variables that should be considered in the treatment decision process are: (1) client predisposing variables, (2) treatment contexts, (3) relationship variables, and (4) strategies and procedures of psychotherapy (Beutler, Consoli, & Williams, 1995). These classes of variables have the following characteristics: (1) Each is part of an overall system and is therefore temporally and sequentially related to the others, (2) the variables are "activating" characteristics that describe both weaknesses and strengths (e.g., client expectations and coping style can help determine to what degree a client will engage in the therapeutic process), (3) the outcome of the interaction between the client's presentation and prior helping agencies must be considered at every decision point for further interventions, and (4) both individual characteristics as well as the situational context of client and therapist must be considered.

The specific strategies and procedures suggested in the systematic eclectic model relate to the outcomes of the assessment of client factors, treatment context, and client–therapist relationship. Determinations are made on such variables as (1) the client's optimum arousal levels, (2) a more or less directive stance of the therapist in providing interventions, (3) types of overall goals for therapy (symptomatic or thematic), and (4) the tasks of therapy as largely behaviorally based or insight-based. Some of these decisions are made at the outset of therapy, while others change from session to session.

In this method specific aspects of the client's presentation (variables such as optimum arousal, problem complexity, resistance potential, diagnosis, coping style) are evaluated. A client may present with a high level of anxiety or arousal. This client will need to be helped to lower his or her level of arousal in order to work effectively with the therapist. If it is also determined that the client's problems are circumscribed and maintained by inadequate knowledge, then symptomatic relief is set as a goal for therapy. If, on the other hand, it is determined that the behaviors are long-standing and repetitious across unrelated situations and based on unresolved past conflicts, then a treatment that focuses on recurrent patterns, life themes, and the social systems in which the problems occur may be more useful for the client. Next, the therapist, within the confines of his or her institution, decides whether or not treatment, is necessary. If so: What format (individual, group, or family)? For how long and how often? Where (are other institutional supports necessary, such as hospitalization)? What modality (medical, psychoeducational, psychosocial, and so forth)? The third set of variables that influence the outcome of therapy relate to the client–therapist relationship. See Table 5-1 for a list of the sequence of decisions and the possible strategies.)

TABLE 5-1   Selection of Strategies

Problem Complexity	
Behaviors are situation-specific	Behaviors are thematic, occur across unrelated situations
Chronic habits and transient responses	Symptoms have a symbolic relationship to initiating events
Symptoms are relatively isolated	Repetitive behaviors result in suffering rather than gratification
Behavior repetition is maintained by inadequate knowledge or by positive reinforcement	

Decision	
Symptomatic treatment (e.g., behavior therapy)	Thematic treatment (e.g., insight therapy)

(Cont.)

TABLE 5-1   *(Continued)*

Motivational Distress

Low emotional arousal/distress	High emotional arousal/distress
Low symptom distress	High symptom distress
Low investment in treatment	Difficulty with concentration
Low energy	Hypervigilance
Blunted or constricted affect	Intense feelings

Decision

Activating techniques (e.g., experiential therapy)	Calming techniques (e.g., relaxation training, specific techniques in cognitive therapy)

Coping Style

Internalization	Denial
Self-punishing	Intellectualization
Emotional overcontrol or constriction	Ambivalence
Unrecognized wishes and desires	Projection
Social withdrawal	Paranoid reactions
Somatization (autonomic nervous system symptoms)	Stimulation seeking
Externalization	Blaming (others and self)
Acting out	Somatization (seeks secondary gain from symptoms)

Decision

Work to increase awareness	Change behavior

Resistance Potential

Has history of interpersonal conflicts	Has intense need for autonomy
Seeks direction	Refuses interpretations
Complies with therapist directions	Interventions have paradoxical effects
Displays tolerance for events out of client's control	Does not complete homework assignments
Completes homework assignments	
Is open to experience	

Decision

Nondirective aproaches (e.g., client-centered therapy or paradoxical techniques)	Directive approaches (e.g., guidance, interpretation)

Adapted from Beutler, Consoli, & Williams (1995).

Assessment and Diagnosis

Another area of concern is the lack of relationship between diagnosis and treatment. Beutler (1989) pointed out:

> The descriptive dimensions embodied in the current diagnostic system bear little relationship to the selection of the mode or frequency of psychosocial interventions . . . [W]hile it would be unthinkable in any practice of medicine for the mode of treatment to be independent of client diagnosis, this is precisely the case in the assignment of psychotherapy modes and formats. (p. 272).

It also is clear that the various therapies and procedures from the diverse schools of psychotherapy are applied differently across diagnostic groupings of clients. "[The] rapid growth of integrative approaches to mental health treatment in recent years attests to the readiness of therapists to accept comprehensive theories of intervention which cut across disciplines, theoretical systems, and diagnostic labels to provide a comprehensive system for selectively assigning different treatment protocols" (Beutler, 1989, p. 273). Citing the work of Cole and Magnussen (1966) and the more recent work on "operational diagnosis" by Cummings and VandenBos (1979), Beutler calls for basing diagnostic and assessment decisions on a more disposition-focused assessment. Decisions about client care need to rest on a foundation of empirically derived relationships between client characteristics, available environmental systems, and therapeutic effects. Such a focus on disposition, rather than merely focusing on symptoms, would keep the orientation on the "primary mission of enhancing the efficacy of care" (Beutler, 1989, p. 273). Beutler (1989) concludes that this method of selectively applying treatments to clients

> represents a compromise between the intense matching of individual clients and therapists and the more global effort to match type of therapy to client diagnosis. While still in its infancy, this approach to the problem of treatment selection is represented in the so-called technical eclectic psychotherapy movement [Lazarus, 1981; Norcross, 1986]. . . . Dispositional assessment proposes that diagnosis is a dynamic process that delineates the probability that an identified problem will respond to a given treatment or setting. An assessment procedure such as this will entail a sequential multistepped process of defining treatment propensities, needs, settings, enabling factors, and social contexts through which effective treatment occurs.(pp. 275–276)

Overview of Theoretical Orientations

So how do we choose among the different orientations for each specific client? What do the research findings tell us about choosing among the various forms of therapy? We will first briefly discuss family and individual therapies (format). Two individual approaches, interpersonal and cognitive-based therapies, will be described, and then a comparison of these therapies through meta-analysis will be presented. The considerations related to the two case studies of Sandra and Clare will illustrate the decision-making process.

Family Therapies

Family therapy emerged out of systems communication work (Bateson, 1979). Bateson hypothesized that linear causality was inadequate for the description of family interactions; causality is seen as a series of circular feedback processes in which everyone's actions affect everyone else and no first cause can be identified. For example, we cannot find a specific cause to the following interaction: The mother nags the child because the child doesn't do as the mother says, or does the child refuse to act because the mother nags? The behaviors of the family are seen as mutually reinforcing; stable patterns of interaction emerge and are perpetuated.

The focus of treatment is on the family as a whole. Pathology is therefore not seen as existing in any one individual. Symptoms are seen as adaptations to stress that stabilize the family and are maintained by the interactions of the other members. If a symptomatic family member starts to get better in individual therapy, family systems theory predicts that the family will tend to exert pressure on the member to resume the symptomatic way of behaving—even if the symptoms are disturbing for the rest of the family. Thus, it is not uncommon to see children pulled out of therapy by their parents when they start to improve (Haley, 1991). Family therapy approaches promote an adaptive change in the family system as a whole.

There are a wide range of family therapies based on behavioral, psychodynamic, experiential, constructivist, and communication principles. The specific goals and techniques differ but in general, the focus of therapy is on communication patterns and the family structure, or power relationships rather than individual perception (Haley, 1971). Recent meta-analyses (Hazelrig, Cooper, & Borduin, 1987; Shadish et al., 1993) indicate that family therapy is at least as successful as alternative treatment modalities.

Family therapists have been in the forefront of advocating greater use of one-way mirrors and videotaping for teamwork and supervision (Haley, 1987; Madanes, 1984; Minuchin & Fishman, 1981). This is seen as a method for learning to track the significant processes in the interactions of several family members in the therapy as well as the greater anxiety many beginning therapists experience when they initially work with multiple individuals.

The family therapist certainly needs to be more active than the individual therapist (Haley, 1991). Minuchin, and Fishman, (1981) have found that learning new skills sometimes disorganizes beginning therapists. It takes time for a set of techniques to coalesce into a coherent therapeutic style. They believe the objective of training is to achieve a level of internalization at which therapists are no longer preoccupied with how to execute a technique so they can spontaneously engage the family. Minuchin and Fishman (1981) state that the first task of therapists is to find a way to engage or join the family. Different therapists will find different ways of doing this; some therapists may encourage the family to teach them the family's way of doing things, others may assume the role of an expert, and still others will move from individual to individual attempting to achieve an alliance.

While some family systems theorists have stressed the epistemological differences between individual and family therapy (Sluzki, 1978; Watzlawick, Beavin, & Jackson, 1967), there has been recently been a trend toward eclecticism and hybrid forms of therapy (Alexander, Holtzworth-Munroe, & Jameson, 1994). In contemporary psychological practice it is no longer unusual to explain symptoms in terms of interaction patterns among intimates. Turgay (1989) presents another dimension to family therapy; "integrative therapy combines various therapeutic strategies and modalities." For example, family therapy or support can be integrated with individual child or adolescent psychotherapy (Bongar & Harmatz, 1989).

Turgay presents three levels of integration. The first integration level is the theoretical orientation. Therapists may use a combination of different schools of family therapy because the needs and characteristics of clients vary greatly. The second integration level is the "target system for the interventions" (Turgay, 1989, p. 975). At this level the therapist may focus on the family as opposed to the child's individual therapy. The third integration level deals with primary, secondary, and tertiary prevention. For such prevention the therapist must also consider genetic and familial aspects of the clinical psychiatric syndromes. Thus, a therapist who is integratively oriented may move from individual outclient child therapy to pharmacotherapy incorporated into an inpatient milieu, simultaneously providing the family with strong support so that their ability to care for the suicidal client increases. In integrative therapy the target intervention systems include the client, family, friends, school, health care systems, and society (Turgay, 1989).

Interpersonal Therapies

Interpersonal therapies are based on the theories of psychoanalysis, object relations, ego psychology, and interpersonal theory (see reviews by Henry et al., 1994; Karon & Widener, 1995). Interpersonal theory (Anchin & Kiesler, 1982) is based on the premise that present-day relationships are based, in large part, on relationships of the past, especially with significant others. The characteristics of these past relationships have become internalized as "maps" or "schemas" that guide interactions. The repertoire of schemas, which generally were adaptive in the past, becomes less functional in the present and are associated with conflict and maladjustment. The concept of interpersonal complementarity, or the reciprocal interactions based on input by both parties, helps us think about the interactions between the client and therapist. What are (1) the qualities of relationship that the client transfers (transference) onto the therapist based on his or her schemas and (2) the qualities that the therapist unwittingly matches in terms of the transference? The therapy occurs when the therapist is able to step outside this active and compelling dance to provide a new relationship for the client. The qualities of this relationship, with its particular boundaries (two people in a room, the regular 50-minute hour, the lack of contact outside the hour, the goals of the relationship clarified), is conceptualized as one way in which the client can come to a new understanding of his or her nonfunctional patterns of interaction as well as experience new patterns of interactions with another person who will be neutral, not judgmental (Levenson & Shiang, 1995). Barkham, Stiles, and Shapiro (1993) use four parameters to describe the course of change in the subjective intensity of personal problems during psychotherapy: (1) the problems' initial severity (problems were grouped by category: symptom, mood, relationships, self-esteem, specific performance), (2) the rate of change of the problems, (3) its day-to-day instability, and (4) the rate of change over the course of therapy.

How do these therapies conceptualize the process of change? Barber and Crits-Christoph (1991) suggest that the following guidelines be used:

1. Maintain focus, generally related to interpersonal problems.
2. Attempt to relieve the client's distressing and current symptoms.
3. Make the link between present problems and core conflicts, especially as these patterns relate to affective dynamics. Find ways to challenge old beliefs/feelings about how the client construes self and others.
4. Assess current strengths, coping skills, etc.
5. Fulfill a modeling function: Learning from and identifying with the therapist in vivo allows the construal of clients' interpersonal patterns to be available for modification.

There are many therapies that use interpersonal theories but relatively few systematically delineate a psychodynamic formulation that serves as a guide for determining a client's schemas, help create more adaptive schemas, and allow their methods to be empirically studied. It is essential to conduct studies in order to make sense of the complicated and too often confusing vicissitudes of the relationship. While we believe that the relationship of therapist to client can be curative, we also want to establish that the factors we believe are important are in fact empirically shown to be important in our specific cases.

Luborsky (1977), using a method to extract what he called the *core conflctual relationship theme (CCRT)*, showed that the CCRT could be determined reliably and validated with issues related to transference. Other methods include Weiss and Sampson's (1986) plan diagnosis, Benjamin's (1982) structural analysis of social behavior, M. Horowitz and colleagues' (1984) configurational analysis, L. Horowitz and colleagues' (1989) consensual response formulation, Kiesler's (1983, 1987) impact message inventory and Checklist of Interpersonal and Psychotherapy Transactions—Revised (CLOIT-R and CLOPT-R), Perry, Augusto, and Cooper's (1989) idiographic conflict summary, Klerman and colleagues' (1984) interpersonal therapy of depression, and Strupp and Binder's (1984) case formulation. Each of these approaches has developed technical aspects of the therapy that are consonant with their psychodynamic formulations. Each has standard selection and exclusion criteria. Consideration of both inclusion as well as exclusion criteria are important as factors that contribute to the probability of "successful" client outcomes. Theoretically, this involves an assessment of the characteristics of the client's personality and an initial presentation that includes the types of problems that can best be served by the practitioner's therapeutic approach. Adherence to these criteria is thought to be necessary because the limited time frame requires a concentration on specific issues that are amenable to change. We will not attempt to summarize in detail all the studies or issues on each of these areas; they have been discussed extensively elsewhere (e.g., Bergin & Garfield, 1994).

Cognitive Therapy

Cognitive therapies focus on schemas in the here and now. This approach was pioneered by Beck (1967) and Ellis (1962). Beck's form of cognitive therapy has been extensively studied using empirical methods. The basis of the approach is that people suffer from mental illnesses, such as depression or anxiety, because of the cognitive attributions they make about events in their lives (Beck et al., 1979). For example, a client may have a primary assumption that, "If I'm nice, bad things won't happen to me." The client might believe "If I suffer for others or take care of all their needs, then divorce and other bad things won't happen to me." This can lead to a secondary assumption, "It is my fault when bad things happen (because I wasn't nice)." Then, in the course of daily living, when something that is perceived as bad actually occurs, the client will have an automatic thought such as "Bad things happen because I 'm not nice." It has been shown that changing the automatic thoughts will ameliorate the depressive feelings.

In the treatment of depression the therapist works with the client to identify situations that trigger depressive or anxious feelings. The intensity of the distressing feelings is given a subjective numeric rating. The automatic thoughts and underlying assumptions are brought into awareness and tested for their rationality. The client and therapist also generate more accurate alternative attributions. The client is taught to identify the situations in which the automatic thoughts are triggered so she or he can internally challenge them with the alternative attributions. In the cognitive approach the therapist is seen as an instructor. Beck uses a collaborative empirical approach, whereas Ellis uses a Socratic method of dispute in his *rational emotive therapy*.

From the beginning, cognitive therapy has striven for empirical validity (Beck, 1967). Assessment instruments are administered to establish a baseline and to monitor progress. Homework assignments, such as monitoring and charting automatic thoughts and changes in affect, are used to monitor progress. The individual sessions are highly structured.

Constructivism is having an impact on developments in cognitive therapies (Mahoney, 1991; Neimeyer, 1993). It is argued that there is no one correct or rational way of formulating reality. It is believed that irrational beliefs, such as hope in a rationally hopeless situation, can actually serve the individual in adaptive ways. Constructivists argue that the criteria for ideas should be their functionality and coherence within the client's frame of reference. This requires a greater understanding of the whole person and the narratives the client constructs about his or her life. Part of this trend is an increased focus on the client's organizing metaphors (Lakoff & Johnson, 1980; Meichenbaum, 1994).

The efficacy of cognitive therapy for the treatment of unipolar depression has been studied and has been found to be equally as effective as antidepressive medications in numerous studies (Blackburn et al., 1981; Dobson, 1989; Hollon, 1990; Robinson, Berman, & Neimeyer, 1990; Simons et al., 1986). However, differential effects have also been shown (Blackburn, Eunson, & Bishop, 1986); assessments of clients over time show that at 6-month and 2-year follow-up, subjects who had been treated with cognitive therapy showed significantly fewer relapses than subjects treated with anti-depressive medications. The same findings were replicated in several other studies with subject pools suffering from acute depression (Kovacs et al., 1981).

Comparison of Approaches—Meta-Analytic Studies
Two relatively recent studies can help us with the issue of which therapy is most efficacious. They both make use of a method of statistical analysis, called meta-analysis, to compare relatively similar studies based on a corrected treatment effect size. The first study, by Svartberg and Stiles (1991) review several different brief therapy approaches. They chose nineteen clinically relevant studies that met specific criteria to compare (1) short-term psychodynamic psychotherapies (STPP); (2) alternative therapies (AP) such as cognitive-supportive therapies, cognitive-behavioral therapies, experiential therapies, and

attendance at self-help groups; (3) and no treatment (NT) controls. They concluded the following: (1) STPP were superior to NT at post-treatment but inferior to AP both at posttreatment and at 1-year follow-up; and (2) STPP treatments were found to be less successful for treating depression, especially major depression; but (3) STPP and AP were equally successful for mixed neurotic clients. Svartberg and Stiles (1991), in discussing their results, point to the need to differentiate among different STPP approaches. For example, the research designs using STPP differed in their formulation of a focus, in the application of techniques, and in the use of experienced or inexperienced therapists.

Another meta-analysis was conducted by Crits-Christoph (1992), who a reviewed comparable studies of brief therapies based on a psychodynamic orientation. Eleven studies met the criteria for inclusion: (1) use of specific short-term dynamic psychotherapy (twelve sessions minimum) guided by a treatment manual or manual-like guide, (2) use of experienced psychotherapists trained in the modality being offered, (3) use of a client group (not analog), (4) comparison with a control group, and (5) reported data that allowed for the calculation of effect sizes based on Cohen's d statistic (1977). These criteria are now increasingly being used to define high-quality research. Results indicated that brief dynamic therapy demonstrates large effects when compared with waiting list conditions but was only slightly superior to nonpsychiatric treatments. The largest effect size was found for the alleviation of target symptoms; 62% of the psychodynamically treated clients were more improved than nonpsychiatric comparison groups. However, comparisons across approaches showed that all psychiatric treatments and medications were equally effective. It is clear that the specific profile of the client must guide treatment decisions and not the orientation of a therapist who has been trained only in one form of therapy.

Application to Case Examples

Let us assume that both case example clients are motivated to make some changes. Sandra, who states she would like to be "independent," would benefit from a course of one-on-one psychotherapy. We also know that cognitive therapies have been found to be efficacious for alleviating depression. If, for example, she says, "I just keep thinking that nothing is going to get better, that I'm just no good because everyone rejects me," then she may be a good candidate for cognitive therapy—optimally one-to-one. If, on the other hand, she presents her problems within the context of how they are related to her past relationships, especially with her parents, then she may be a good candidate for some form of interpersonal therapy. In both cases the goal of therapy would be to improve the interpersonal functioning of the client.

Let us now consider Clare, the young Chinese American woman. After meeting several times with Clare, it becomes clear that she is really worried about leaving town to take a new job in a distant city largely because she is worried about her parents and the problems in their relationship. The problem is now defined as systemic; the therapist will want to explore the possibility of bringing the whole family in for a course of family therapy. The initial goal of the therapy might be to clarify each person's contribution to the problem in order to determine what are viable options for Clare in terms of her relationship to her family. It may be possible that Clare would benefit from a course of individual therapy after family issues have been addressed.

INTERACTING WITH CLIENTS

Interactions: Qualities of the Therapeutic Alliance

We start our discussion of interacting with clients by considering the characteristics of the therapeutic alliance—the reciprocal interactions between the client and therapist. This unique interaction has been found to be a key ingredient in successful therapeutic outcome. Each person in the dyad brings his or her specific and personal way of being to the relationship.

The therapeutic alliance has been put forward by clinicians and researchers as the bedrock indicator of the client's willingness to seek help and sustenance through personal relationships. So important are the therapeutic alliance skills that London (1986) suggests that it is wise to consider training novice psychologists in the fundamental skill of establishing good interpersonal relationships as a prerequisite to the later development of specialized and advanced therapeutic proficiencies. The first step in this process involves learning basic rules and procedures related to interviewing and listening (see also Chapter 4). Exercises that can foster growth in this area are taking the role of the patient, practicing how to react to hostile and challenging statements, peer review of videotapes, exploration of one's reactions to patients in the context of supervision, and one's own personal therapy.

In the interpersonal approaches an "active ingredient" of the therapy is the building of the therapeutic alliance, which Koss & Shiang (1994) define as the emotional bond and reciprocal involvement that develops between client and therapist during the course of therapy. Among the best of all possible therapeutic outcomes is that the quality of this relationship serves as a source of support for the client even after the client leaves the therapy. While therapy is ongoing the therapist must monitor and interpret selected aspects of the transference relationship to the client. Gaston (1990) differentiated four independent aspects of the therapeutic alliance: (1) the therapeutic alliance, or the client's affective relationship to the therapist; (2) the working alliance, or the client's capacity to purposefully work in therapy; (3) the therapist's empathic understanding and involvement; and (4) the client–therapist agreement on the goals and tasks of treatment. Although different definitions of the therapeutic alliance have been used in the past, these four categories have been repeatedly identified in empirical studies (Gomes-Schwartz, 1978; Hartley & Strupp, 1983; Marmar, Weiss, & Gaston, 1989).

Kiesler and Watkins (1989) argue that the client and therapist must be considered in their reciprocal dyadic context rather than as two subjects following separate linear paths. Within two dimensions, people interact in complementary ways. On the affiliation dimension, people act in correspondence with each other (hostility pulls for hostility, etc.), whereas on the control dimension, people act reciprocally manner with each other (dominance pulls for submission, etc.).

The use of sequential analyses is exemplified in the work of McCullough and colleagues (1991), who tracked the emotional responses, positive and negative, of clients and found that emotional responses predicted a positive outcome. On the other hand, defensive responses, or "shutting down," predicted a poor outcome. As a therapist it is important to monitor the quality of the client's responses. Intellectual insights alone are unlikely to produce significant change. An affective component can mobilize the entire person. With most clients it's not likely that an affective arousal will occur until a strong bond of trust is established such that the client feels safe enough to risk revealing his or her world.

When working with painful or shameful experiences, some comments and interpretations can elicit defensive client responses. Finding the line between optimum affective arousal and defensiveness is a skill that is refined over time. Furthermore, defensive responses will often produce emotional reactions in the therapist, who may in turn respond defensively or try to convince the client of the correctness of the interpretation. When a client has a defensive response, it is usually best to shift the focus of the therapy to discussing the quality of the therapist–client relationship, exploring what the client's experience was when the therapist made the statement that elicited the defensive response, and working out a common understanding of how this happened. Implicitly, the message is conveyed that this is a "trip wire" for both client and therapist.

In the McCullough et al. (1991) study, two forms of brief therapy were provided: *short-term dynamic psychotherapy and brief adaption-oriented psychotherapy*. The interaction sequences of sixteen client–therapist cases were reviewed using a process coding system. Emotional responses that followed interventions were found to be significantly related to outcome; the frequency of clients' affective and defensive responses after a therapist's intervention accounted for 66% of the outcome variance. An interpretation of the therapist followed within 3 minutes by an affective response on the part of the client was related to improvement at termination, whereas a therapist interpretation followed by a defensive response by the client was linked to negative outcome. These findings are based on a small sample, and there are inherent problems with the use of self-reports as measures of outcome. Nevertheless, sequential analysis holds promise for understanding the interactional process that contributes to successful outcome.

The stages of brief psychotherapy have also been addressed from a systems perspective (Tracey, 1985; Tracey & Ray, 1984). Here the change process is seen as a movement out of an initial stage of homeostasis into a state of flux and terminating in a new point of homeostasis. These stages have been explored by comparing the sequence of client–therapist topic initiation and topic continuation among successful and unsuccessful therapy dyads. Results revealed a pattern of high-low-high complementarity in topic initiation/topic following among successful therapy cases. Therapists in successful dyads were found to initiate more topics during the middle or "conflict" stage of therapy. This finding suggests that in cases with successful outcomes the middle phase of therapy consisted of the therapist directing attention to issues the client did not necessarily want to address. Agreement over the focus then gradually emerged in the final stage of therapy. Where outcome was unsuccessful, clear-cut changes were not seen in complementarity. Weiss (1993) notes that clients often seem to lose sight of their goals and decrease in their insight during the middle stage of therapy. Many beginning therapists find it difficult to negotiate clear goals with their clients, but setting clear goals and keeping the therapy on track during the middle stage of treatment will improve treatment. In order to do this, therapists need to learn how to effectively confront clients. Most importantly, beginning therapists must understand their own reactions to confrontations, the possible range of emotions that may surface, and then learn to effectively monitor these emotions and use them in the service of the clients' needs.

Client and Therapist Variables

Let us now consider client and therapist variables that have been shown by research to contribute to the development of the therapeutic alliance and positive outcomes. Once again, it important to emphasize that it is the interaction, not merely the individual contributions, that has the greatest impact on the development of the therapeutic alliance. Given our space limitations, we will only be able to discuss two of the more salient client variables—expectations of outcome and dispositional qualities—that have been related to successful therapeutic outcomes. (The reader is referred to Bergin and Garfield [1994] for a more extensive discussion of these and other client and therapist variables).

Client Expectations of Outcome

The influence of client expectations on positive therapeutic outcome has been recognized as an important factor to consider in determining whether or not therapy will help produce positive change, in making interventions, and in analyzing research projects on psychotherapy. Clients who believe they are receiving some form of help even though contact is minimal generally show greater improvement than comparison clients who receive no contact (e.g., Cross, Sheehan, & Kahn, 1982; Frank, 1974; Sloane et al., 1975). Frank (1974) asserts that early psychotherapeutic gains and placebo effects are both due to mobilization of hope. In this case the use of placebo, rather than being considered "useless," can be considered as part of the mobilization toward more adaptive functioning. Later in therapy symptomatic changes due to relearning may appear.

Expectation of change and of receiving help are important considerations for any type of psychotherapy, but perhaps especially so for brief therapy, since the time constraints require that treatment sessions be fast moving and goal-oriented. Client readiness to change has been studied in therapies with limited goals, such as relieving problems related to medical illnesses or job-related distress. The assumption underlying this work is that clients enter therapy in different states of readiness and that specific techniques that correspond to these states of readiness will provide clients with more successful outcomes. For example, DiClemente and Prochaska (1982) studied specific behavioral changes; their results may be applicable to attempts to change many types of behaviors. In the DiClemente and Prochaska study, clients who were attempting to stop smoking were studied in two settings: those engaged in therapy and those attempting to quit on their own. They examined clients' readiness to change and developed a four level classification system: Precontemplation, Contemplation, Action, and Maintenance. They have recommended therapeutic techniques depending upon the stage of readiness. For example, behavioral techniques such as counterconditioning and contingency control were found to be best suited for phobic clients who were in the Action stage (Prochaska, 1991). The match of technique to stage of readiness was found to facilitate the greatest gains in alleviating the clients' presenting problem. These types of studies point to the need to assess the expectations of the client in several areas (does the client expect immediate symptomatic changes; is the client thinking about change but not yet able to change behaviors; does the client recognize his or her responsibility in engaging in the process of change).

Dispositional Qualities of the Client

Studies that focus on dispositional qualities of the client address issues related to the formation and maintenance of the therapeutic relationship. For example, Beutler and colleagues (1991) attempted to optimally match clients with therapy according to variations in clients' defensiveness (resistance potential) and coping styles (externalization). The results suggested that client dispositional characteristics can be used to maximize response to psychotherapy. For example, clients with externalizing coping styles reacted most positively to behavioral/symptom-focused procedures of cognitive therapy. In contrast, evidence also suggested that clients who were self-punitive and depressed benefited from an internally focused and reflective treatment. Therapy approaches that emphasize more authority-directed interventions were found to yield poor results among individuals who were prone to be resistant to therapy.

A study by Alpher and colleagues (1990) assessed clients' developmental level of object representation. They found that the variables that predicted a higher level of client change were the measures of object relatedness such as "differentiation" and "articulation" (using the Rorschach) and not the clinical interpersonal interview. They did discover some evidence of a relationship between the Rorschach and the capacity to engage in short-term dynamic psychotherapy as assessed through an interview. Another study that considered dispositional characteristics was done by Pilkonis and colleagues (1991). They hypothesized that the dropout rate from psychotherapy is related to therapists' and clients' levels of attachment and their personality styles. Using the theoretical framework of Bowlby (1979) and measures such as the Checklist of Interpersonal Transactions (Kiesler, 1987), the study examined differences in the attachment security and personality styles of clients and therapists via the Interpersonal Relations Assessment. Pairing of insecurely attached clients with less securely attached therapists was associated with a high dropout rate, as was pairing dependent clients with autonomous therapists.

Therapist Variables

Beutler, Machado, and Neufeldt (1994) suggest that therapist characteristics can be organized along two dimensions. The first dimension spans the difference between objective characteristics and subjective characteristics. The second dimension relates to characteristics that are defined as situation/context-specific or as general qualities that exist in all situations/contexts. When the two dimensions are compared, therapist characteristics can lie in one of four quadrants (e.g., high on objective and cross situational). A review of these dimensions showed that the objective variables in the therapy-specific states (level of training, use of manuals, therapist styles and interventions) appear to make the greatest contribution to successful outcome.

Maintenance of Focus

In the clinical literature there is general agreement that maintenance of focus within the therapy is an essential aspect to promoting a successful outcome.

The cognitive-behavioral therapies generally use detailed cognitive and behavioral assessment tools that help define the agreed upon focus of the therapy. Interpersonal therapies such as time-limited dynamic therapy create a focus based on interpersonal patterns, which guide therapists in their own minute-to-minute behavior in sessions as well as providing a framework for overall interventions.

Negative Actions

Research studies have shown that psychotherapy can have negative effects (Henry et al., 1994). Hostile and controlling therapist behaviors have been found to be related to negative outcomes. The Vanderbilt Negative Indicators Scale (Suh, Strupp, & O'Malley, 1986) was developed to measure such behaviors. It consists of five subscales that reflect issues such as patient negative attitudes, therapist exploitative tendencies, errors in technique, problems in the therapeutic relationship, and ineffectiveness. In therapies in which there is not a good match between the therapist and the client, many more instances of these actions have been found to occur. The beginning therapist can, with the aid of the supervisor, focus on reviewing those actions that are considered hostile and controlling. Why does the therapist consider these acts hostile? Does the client actually experience them as hostile? What appears to be their effect on the course of the session? Exploring these types of questions can provide a rich source of learning and self-development for the therapist.

Application to Case Examples

In order to apply these ideas to our case material, we will construct the cases to illustrate our points. Both clients are motivated to change and expect the therapist to help them.

In terms of expectations, Sandra has had therapy once before and reports that it was beneficial. On Prochaska's scale she is at the Action stage. In terms of disposition, Sandra attributes her problems to her beliefs that (1) people reject her and (2) this makes her think of herself as "no good." Her first reaction to a situation is that others will reject her. She tends to interprets body language (e.g., a turning of the shoulder, a less than enthusiastic smile), negatively and convinces herself that the other person doesn't like her. She is unaware of the signals she sends to others—her hesitancy, her lack of eye contact. Beutler would categorize these types of reactions as externalizing. Working within the frame of Beutler's systemic treatment model, we would recommend a behavioral/symptom-focused therapy.

Clare has never had therapy before, expresses hesitancy, and says she is not sure what psychotherapy is all about. Thus, the first several sessions will require that the therapist take a stance to educate Clare about what might be achieved through therapy, who might be included in the family session, and the possibility that a home visit might facilitate communication between the institution and the client. The therapist must also take a learning stance in order to determine how best to facilitate building a therapeutic alliance with the client and any others who might be involved in the therapy. Once this phase is completed, Clare will have more realistic expectations about what might be achieved in therapy and be willing to actively engage. Let us say that this phase is successfully negotiated, that a home visit facilitated Clare's parents' willingness to engage in a brief course of family therapy, and that the issues regarding Clare's place in the family and their need for her physical proximity are clarified. It becomes apparent that Clare herself would benefit from a course of individual therapy.

In terms of disposition, Clare, as would be true of many other Chinese Americans, would be an "internalizer" (Beutler & Clarkin, 1990) She believes that if she changes her behavior, things will get better. She blames herself for the present situation. According to Beutler and Clarkin, Clare would benefit from an insight-oriented course of therapy . To enhance the possibility of success, the therapist would need to learn from Clare more about the specific "cultural" rules (e.g., issues of identity, role expectations, marriage expectations) that impact her behaviors.

Termination

Why consider termination as part of initial decision making? It may seem odd to discuss the topic of termination and setting the length of therapy as part of the initial phase of therapy, but a determination of the overall length (and intensity) of a therapy for a specific client will help the therapist decide on manageable goals. In the present-day climate of HMOs and third-party providers, most therapies will be time-limited.

Terminations of relationships occur every day—we meet a friend and say good-bye, we send a relative to catch her airplane after a holiday celebration. How the therapist helps to find an ending to the therapy is dependent upon many different factors, including the therapist's own beliefs about endings as well as what issues the ending of this relationship raises for the client. Mann (1973) developed a form of brief therapy in which termination is a central issue. The client starts therapy knowing that he or she will meet for a set period of time (twelve weekly sessions) and a date for the final session is set. Because a central issue in the therapy is resolving feelings related to the process of ending relationships, the therapist must strictly adhere to the time line. In this form of therapy it has been found that clients become engaged in conflicts that are thought to be universal: independence versus dependence, activity versus passivity, adequate versus lowered self-esteem, and unresolved or delayed grief. The issues that arise from the client's transference with the therapist, the client's current problems, and recurrent interpersonal problems that are based in the past all create a situation of heightened anxiety that can lead to change. The course of therapy follows a rather predictable sequence of interactional stances: the client experiences a honeymoon phase, then a feeling of betrayal, often relapses, and then may move to resolve the conflicts induced by the inevitability of the termination. A mature resolution of the separation between client and therapist (incorporating both positive and negative aspects) is viewed as a way of internalizing the more positive aspects of the therapist.

Generally, the therapist gently "reminds" the client that therapy will be ending, approximately three or four sessions before the actual date of termination. This allows the client to consider what the ending might mean to him or her. The client's reactions to this information can range from "What? I don't remember that and I won't address it at all" to "This reminds me of when my father died." The therapist must also check his or her own reactions to terminations and try to ensure that these feelings do not impede the way the client wants to end the therapy. Providing the client with a framework in which to say "goodbye" is especially important in the present climate of providing care, as many clients will engage in intermittent therapy—coming into several sessions of therapy a number of times over a number of years. Termination is not a final goodbye to the person or institution, but a stopping point in a larger journey.

CONCLUSIONS

There is no easy formula to follow to become a competent psychotherapist. We wish there were. Human interactions are complicated and various. It is fully understandable for beginning therapists to be anxious and bewildered by the many issues that confront them. Gaining competency requires, first of all, self-observation, self-knowledge, and the ability to reflect on one's own attitudes and behaviors. If, for example, a therapist has the ability to observe himself or herself feeling or acting with hostility, the therapist is more able to make changes that take into account the needs of the client. If, on the other hand, the therapist is unaware of his or her own feelings and actions, cannot monitor them, and thus cannot change them, he or she will unwittingly provide less than a successful course of therapy (See Chapter 3 for ideas on working with supervisors to overcome such deficits).

Not all therapies will be successful to the same degree. The success of therapy will largely depend on the development of the therapist's level of competence, the ability to use specific techniques, and the integration of book learning with the genuine use of the self.

REFERENCES

Alexander, J. F., Holtzworth-Munroe, & Jameson (1994). The process and outcome of marital and family therapy: Research review and evaluation. In A. Bergin & S. L. Garfield (Eds.), *Handbook of psychotherapy and behavior change* (pp. 595–630). New York: Wiley.

Alpher, V. S., Perfetto, G. A., Henry, W. P., & Strupp, H. H. (1990). Dynamic factors in patient assessment and prediction of change in short-term dynamic psychotherapy. *Psychotherapy, 27*, 350–361.

American Psychiatric Association. (1994). *Diagnostic and statistical manual of mental disorders* (4th ed.). Washington, DC.: Author.

Anchin, J. C., & Kiesler, D. J. (Eds.) (1982). *Handbook of interpersonal psychotherapy.* New York: Pergamon Press.

Barber, J. P., & Crits-Christoph, P. (1991). Comparison of the brief dynamic psychotherapies. In P. Crits-Christoph & J. P. Barber (Eds.), *Handbook of short-term dynamic psychotherapy* (pp. 323–355). New York: Basic Books.

Barkham, M., Stiles, W. B., & Shapiro, D. A. (1993). The shape of change in psychotherapy: Longitudinal assessment of personal problems. *Journal of Consulting and Clinical Psychology. 61*, 667–677.

Basch, M. F. (1980). *Doing psychotherapy.* New York: Basic Books.

Bateson, G. (1979). *Mind and nature.* New York: Dutton.

Beck, A. T. (1967). *Depression: Causes and treatment.* Philadelphia: University of Pennsylvania Press.

Beck, A. T., Shaw, A. J., Rush, B. F., & Emery, G. (1979). *Cognitive therapy of depression.* New York: Guilford Press.

Benjamin, L. S. (1982). Use of structural analysis of social behavior (SASB) to guide interventions in therapy. In J. Anchin & D. Keisler (Eds.), *Handbook of interpersonal psychotherapy* (pp. 190–212). New York: Pergamon Press.

Bergin, A. E., & Garfield, S. L.(Eds.) (1994). *Handbook of psychotherapy and behavior change.* New York: Wiley.

Beutler, L. E. (1989). Differential treatment selection: The role of diagnosis in psychotherapy. *Psychotherapy, 26*, 271–281.

Beutler, L. E., & Clarkin, J. F. (1990). *Systematic treatment selection toward targeted therapeutic interventions.* New York: Brunner/Mazel.

Beutler, L. E., Consoli, A. J., & Williams, R. E. (1995). Integrative and eclectic therapies in practice. In B. Bongar & L. E. Beutler (Eds.), *Comprehensive textbook of psychotherapy* (pp. 274–292). New York: Oxford University Press.

Beutler, L. E., Engle, D., Mohr, D., Daldrup, R. J., Bergan, J., Meredith, K., & Merry, W. (1991). Predictors of differential response to cognitive, experiential, and self-directed psychotherapeutic procedures. *Journal of Consulting and Clinical Psychology, 59*, 333–340.

Beutler, L. E., Machado, P. P. P., & Newfeldt, S. A. (1994). Therapist variables. In A. Bergin and S. L. Garfield (Eds.), *Handbook of psychotherapy and behavior change* (pp. 664–700). New York: Wiley.

Blackburn, I. M., Bishop, S., Glen, A. I. M., Whalley, L. J., & Christie, J. E. (1981). The efficacy of cognitive therapy in depression: A treatment trial using cognitive therapy and pharmacotherapy, each alone and in combination. British Journal of Psychiatry, 139, 181–189.

Blackburn, I. M., Eunson, K. M., & Bishop, S. (1986). A two-year naturalistic follow-up of 38 depressed patients treated with cognitive therapy, pharmacotherapy and a combination of both. *Journal of Affective Disorders, 10,* 67–75.

Bongar, B., & Harmatz, S. (1989). The management of the suicidal patient: Clinical assessment of the suicidal patient. Colloquium presented to the Clinical Psychology Program of the Department of Psychology, University of Massachusetts at Amherst.

Bowlby, J. (1979). Psychoanalysis as art and science. *International Review of Psychoanalysis, 6,* 3–14.

Bruch, H. (1974). *Learning psychotherapy: Rationale and ground rules.* Cambridge, MA: Harvard University Press.

Chessick, R. D. (1969). *How psychotherapy heals: The process of intensive psychotherapy.* New York: Science House.

Cohen, J. (1977). *Statistical power analysis for the behavioral sciences.* New York: Academic Press.

Cole, J. K., & Magnussen, M. (1966). Where the action is. *Journal of Consulting and Clinical Psychology. 30,* 539–545.

Crits-Christoph, P. (1992). The efficacy of brief dynamic psychotherapy: A meta-analysis. *American Journal of Psychiatry, 149,* 151–158.

Cross, D.G., Sheehan, P. W., & Kahn, J. A. (1982). Short amd long term follow-up of clients receiving insight-oriented therapy and behavior therapy. *Journal of Consulting and Clinical Psychology, 50,* 103–112.

Cummings, N. A., & Vandenbos, G. (1979). The general practice of psychology. *Professional Psychology: Research and Practice, 10,* 430–440.

Dewald, P. (1964). *Psychotherapy: A dynamic approach* (2d ed.). New York: Basic Books.

DiClemente, C. C., & Prochaska, J. O. (1982). Self-change and therapy change of smoking behavior: A comparison of processes of change in cessation and maintenance. *Addictive Behaviors, 7,* 133–142.

Dobson, K. (1989). A meta analysis of the efficacy of cognitive therapy for depression. *Journal of Consulting and Clinical Psychology, 57,* 414–419.

Ekstein, R., & Wallerstein, R. S. (1972). *The teaching and learning of psychotherapy* (2d ed.). New York, International Universities Press.

Ellis, A. (1962). *Reason and emotion in psychotherapy.* New York: Stuart.

Frank, J. D. (1974). Therapeutic components of psychotherapy: A 25-year progress report of research. *Journal of Nervous and Mental Disease, 159,* 325–342.

Garfield, S. L. (1978). Research on client variables in psychotherapy. In S. L. Garfield & A. E. Bergin (Eds.), *Handbook of psychotherapy and behavior change* (rev. ed., pp. 191–232). New York: Wiley.

Garfield, S. L. (1986). Research on client variables in psychotherapy. In S. L. Garfield & A. E. Bergin (Eds.), *Handbook of psychotherapy and behavior change* (3d ed., pp. 213–256). New York: Wiley.

Gaston, L. (1990). The concept of the alliance and its role in psychotherapy: Theoretical and emperical considerations. *Psychotherapy, 27,* 143–153.

Gilligan, C. (1982). *In a different voice.* Cambridge, MA: Harvard University Press.

Gomes-Schwartz, B. (1978). Effective ingredients in psychotherapy: Prediction of outcome from process variables. *Journal of Consulting and Clinical Psychology, 46,* 1023–1035.

Green, H. (1964). *I never promised Yyu a rose garden.* New York: Signet.

Haley, J. (1971). Family therapy: A radical change. In J. Haley (Ed.), *Changing families: A family therapy reader* (pp.272–284). New York: Grune & Stratton.

Haley, J. (1991). *Problem-solving therapy.* San Francisco: Jossey-Bass.

Hartley, D., & Strupp, H. (1983). The therapeutic alliance: Its relationship to outcome in brief psychotherapy. In J. Masling (Ed.), *Empirical studies of psychoanalytic theories,* (vol. 1, pp. 1–27). Hillsdale, N.J.: Analytic Press.

Hazelrig, M. D., Cooper, H. M., & Borduin, C. M. (1987). Evaluating the effectiveness of family therapies: An integrative review and analysis. *Psychological Bulletin, 101,* 428–442.

Henry, W. P., Strupp, H. H., Schact, T. E., & Gaston, L. (1994). Psychodynamic approaches. In A. E. Bergin & S. L. Garfield (Eds.), *Handbook of psychotherapy and behavior change,* (pp. 467–508). New York: Wiley.

Hollon, S. D. (1990). Cognitive therapy and pharmacotherapy for depression. *Psychiatric Annals, 20,* 249–258.

Horowitz, L. M., Rosenberg, S. E., Ureno, G., & Kalehzan, B. M. (1989). Psychodynamic formulation, consensual response method, and interpersonal problems. *Journal of Consulting and Clinical Psychology. 57,* 599–606.

Horowitz, M., Marmar, C., Krupnick, J., Wilner, N., Kaltreider, N., & Wallerstein, R. (1984). *Personality styles and brief psychotherapy.* New York: Basic Books.

Karon, B. P., & Widener, A. J. (1995). Psychodynamic therapies in practice. In B. Bongar & L. E. Beutler (Eds.), *Comprehensive textbook of psychotherapy* (pp. 24–47). New York: Oxford University Press.

Kiesler, D. J. (1987a). The 1982 interpersonal circle: A taxonomy for complementarity in human interactions. *Psychological Review. 90,* 185–214.

Kiesler, D. J. (1987b). *Revised version of the Checklist of Interpersonal Transactions,* Richmond, VA: Commonwealth University.

Kiesler, D. J., & Watkins, L. M. (1989). Interpersonal complementarity and the therapeutic alliance: A study of relationship in psychotherapy. *Psychotherapy, 26,* 183–194.

Kitayama, S., & Markus, H. R. (1994). *Emotion and culture: Empirical studies of mutual influence.* Washington DC: American Psychological Association.

Kleinman, A., & Kleinman, J. (1985). Somatization: The interconnections in Chinese society among culture, depressive experiences, and the meaning of pain. In A. Kleinman & B. Good (Eds.), *Culture and depression: Studies in the anthropology and cross-cultural psychiatry of affect and disorder* (pp. 429–490). Berkeley: University of California Press.

Klerman, G. L., Weissman, M. M., Rounsaville, B. J., & Chevron, E. S. (1984). *Interpersonal psychotherapy of depression.* New York: Basic Books.

Koss, M., & Shiang, J. (1994). Research on brief psychotherapy. In A. Bergin & S. L. Garfield (Eds.), *Handbook of psychotherapy and behavior change* (pp. 664–700). New York: Wiley.

Kovacs, M., Rush, A. J., Beck, A. T., & Hollon, S. D. (1981). Depressed outpatients treated with cognitive therapy or pharmacotherapy. *Archives of General Psychiatry, 38,* 33–39.

Lakoff, G., & Johnson, M. (1980). *Metaphors we live by.* Chicago: University of Chicago Press.

Lambert, M. J., Shapiro, D. A., & Bergin, A. E. (1986). The effectiveness of psychotherapy. In S. L. Garfield & A. E. Bergin (Eds.), *Handbook of psychotherapy and behavior change* (pp. 157–212). New York: Wiley.

Lazarus, A. A. (1981). *The practice of multimodal therapy.* New York: McGraw-Hill.

Levenson, & Shiang, J. (1995). Case formulation in time-limited dynamic psychotherapy. *In Session, 1,* 19–34.

Lindner, R. (1982). *The fifty minute hour: A collection of true psychoanalytic tales.* Northvale, NJ: Aronson.

London, P. (1986). Exploration of psychotherapy integration. *International Journal of Eclectic Psychology. 5,* 211–216.

Luborsky, L. (1977). Measuring a pervasive psychic structure in psychotherapy: The core conflictual relationship theme. In N. Freedman and S. Grand (Eds.), *Communicative structures and psychic structures* (pp. 367–395. New York: Plenum.

Madanes, C. (1984). *Behind the one-way mirror.* San Francisco: Jossey-Bass.

Mahoney, M. J. (1991). *Human change process.* New York: Basic Books.

Mann, J. (1973). *Time-limited psychotherapy.* Cambridge, MA: Harvard University Press.

Marmar, C. R., Weiss, D. S., & Gaston, L. (1989). Towards the validation of the California Therapeutic Alliance Rating System. *Journal of Consulting and Clinical Psychology, 1,* 46–52.

McCullough, L., Winston, A., Farber, B. A., Porter, F., Pollack, J., Laikin, M., Vingiano, W., & Trujillo, M. (1991). The relationship of patient–therapist interaction to outcome in brief psychotherapy. *Psychotherapy, 28,* 525–533.

Meichenbaum, D. (1994). *A clinical handbook/practical therapist manual for assessing and treating adults with post-traumatic stress disorder (PTSD).* Waterloo, Ontario: Institute Press.

Minuchin, S., & Fishman, H.C. (1981). *Family therapy techniques.* Cambridge, MA: Harvard University Press.

Neimeyer, R. A. (1993). An appraisal of constructivist psychotherapies. *Journal of Consulting and Clinical Psychology. 61,* 221–234.

Norcross, J. C. (1986). Eclectic psychotherapy: An introduction and overview. In J. C. Norcross (Ed.), *Handobook of eclectic psychotherapy* (pp. 3–24). New York: Brunner/Mazel.

Perry, J. C., Augusto, F., & Cooper, S. H. (1989). Assessing psychodynamic conflicts: I. Reliability of the Idiographic Conflict Formulation method. *Psychiatry, 52,* 289–301.

Pilkonis, P. A., Heape, C. L., Ruddy, J., & Serrao, P. (1991). Validity in the diagnosis of personality disorders: The use of the LEAD standard. *Psychological Assessment, 3,* 46–54.

Prochaska, J. O. (1991). Prescribing to the stage and level of phobic patients. *Psychotherapy, 28,* 463–468.

Robinson, L. A., Berman, J. S., & Neimeyer, R. A. (1990). Psychotherapy for the treatment of depression: A comprehensive review of controlled outcome research. *Psychological Bulletin, 108,* 30–49.

Shadish, W. R., Montgomery, L. M., Wilson, P., Wilson, M. R., Bright, I., & Okwumabua, T. (1993). The effects of family and marital psychotherapies. *Journal of Consulting and Clinical Psychology. 61,* 992–1002.

Siddall, L. B., Haffey, N. A., & Feinman, J. A. (1988). Intermittent brief psychotherapy in an HMO setting. *American Journal of Psychotherapy, 62,* 96–106.

Simons, A. D., Murphy, G. E., Levine, J. L., & Wetzel, R. D. (1986). Cognitive therapy and pharmacotherapy for depression. *Archives of General Psychiatry, 43,* 43–48.

Sloane, R. B., Staples, F. R., Cristol, A. H., Yorkston, N. J., & Whipple, K. (1975). Short-term analytically oriented psychotherapy versus behavior therapy. *American Journal of Psychiatry, 132,* 373–377.

Sluzki, C. E. (1978). Marital therapy from a systems theory perspective. In T. J. Paolino & B. S. McCrady (Eds.), *Marriage and marital therapy: Psychoanalytic, behavioral and systems theory perspectives.* New York: Brunner/Mazel.

Storr, A. (1980). *The art of psychotherapy.* New York: Methuen.

Strupp, H. H., & Binder, J. L. (1984). *Psychotherapy in a new key: A guide to time-limited dynamic psychotherapy.* New York: Basic Books.

Suh, C. S., Strupp, H. H., & O'Malley, S. S. (1986). The Vanderbilt process measures: The psychotherapy process scale (VPPS) and the negative indicators scale (VNIS). In L. S. Greenberg & W. M. Pinsof (Eds.), *The psychotherapy process: A research handbook.* (pp. 285–324. New York: Guilford Press.

Svartberg, M., & Stiles, T. C. (1991). Comparative effects of short-term psychodynamic psychotherapy: A meta-analysis. *Journal of Consulting and Clinical Psychology, 59,* 704–714.

Tracey, T. J. (1985). Dominance and outcome: A sequential examination. *Journal of Counseling Psychology, 32,* 119–122.

Tracey, T. J., & Ray. P. B. (1984). Stages of successful time-limited counseling: An interactional examination. *Journal of Counseling Psychology, 31,* 13–27.

Turgay, A. (1989). An integrative treatment approach to child and adolescent suicidal behavior. *Psychiatric Clinics of North America, 12,* 971–985

Watzlawick, P., Beavin, J. H., & Jackson, D. D. (1967). *Pragmatics of human communication.* New York: Norton.

Weinberg, G. (1990). *The Taboo Scarf and other tales.* New York: St. Martin's Press.

Weiss, J. (1993). *How psychotherapy works: Process and technique.* New York: Guilford Press.

Weiss, J. & Sampson, H. (1986). *The psychoanalytic process.* New York: Guilford Press.

Whitaker, C., & Malone, T. (1953). *The roots of psychotherapy.* Philadelphia, Blakiston.

Wolberg, L. (1954). *The technique of psychotherapy.* New York: Grune & Stratton.

▶ 6

Psychological Screening

LEE H. MATTHEWS

There are a variety of situations in which a screening assessment of one type or another can aid in the diagnosis, referral, treatment, or termination of therapy for an individual whether as a client (outpatient) or patient (inpatient). This chapter will deal primarily with specific screening devices for the assessment of adults, although several general references for children's assessments will also be listed. The chapter is organized into broad categories of screening measures.

Screenings have grown in popularity with changes in the mental health care delivery systems in this country as managed care has become a dominant force in both practice and training (Cummings, 1995). The increased reliance on managed care, for example, has resulted in significant decreases in length of stay for inpatient facilities. Decreased funds available for psychological assessments and the need for "pre-certification" of evaluations potentially shorten the length of time in which a psychological evaluation can be accomplished. In community mental health centers increasing patient load along with decreasing numbers of staff members also calls for more rapid assessment.

Psychological screening, in contrast to more comprehensive evaluations, has a highly specific point of focus. That is, there may be a more specific referring question, rather than a broad-based request for an evaluation of an individual's cognitive and personality structure. In broad based evaluations the aim may be to assess a variety of the individual's behaviors in situations that are structured, semistructured, and unstructured. Screening techniques, with the exception of clinical interviews, tend to use highly structured formats in which the individual is asked to respond in a relatively restrictive range to questions presented in either verbal or written form.

There are some risks obviously inherent in any screening evaluation. These risks include the issue of decreased reliability due to a small number of test items being administered. Reliability in this case refers to the instrument's consistency. Will the same test or procedure produce essentially the same score for the same person when reexamined on different occasions? This limitation can be partially overcome by focusing on highly specific referral questions and/or by having sufficient clinical knowledge (or access to reference material) about specific measures so that appropriate samples of behavior can be obtained with a limited number of items in a relatively short period of time.

In addition to the issue of reliability, the question of validity needs to be considered. Reliability is concerned with whether or not the same person tested with the same test will get essentially the same score. Validity has to do with what that score means. The *validity* of a test concerns what the test measures and how well it does so. All methods for determining test validity basically are concerned with the relationship between a person's performance on a test and other independently observable facts about the behavior characteristics under consideration. With cognitive screening measures there is a tendency to overestimate the actual level of intellectual functioning. On the other hand, use of too short a personality screening measure or neuropsychological evaluation may lead to underestimating the degree of pathology. Careful selection of instruments can greatly decrease these types of errors.

GENERAL SCREENING APPROACHES

There are a variety of psychological screening assessment resources. These include such traditional texts as Anastasi (1988), Butcher (1994), Goldstein and Hersen (1984), Hersen and Turner (1994), Sattler (1992), and Wechsler (1981) for general screening purposes. Maruish (1994) provides information on psychological testing for treatment planning and outcome assessment. Hartlage, Asken, and Hornsby (1987), as well as Lezak (1995), are excellent references for many of the norms for neuropsychological screening measures. Books by Berg and his associates provide information about the major screening measures for cognitive dysfunction, which are extremely broad-based and cover a variety of assessment areas. Although originally conceptualized as resources for neuropsychological evaluation, they have broad implications for the clinician. These books include the assessment of adults (Berg, Franzen, & Wedding, 1994) and children (Franzen & Berg, 1989). In their book on neuropsychological tests, Spreen and Strauss (1991) also include information about a variety of measures that can be used to screen language and academic functioning. The publication by Reeves and Wedding (1994) of an overview of the assessment of memory provides a single location for a comprehensive review of most memory functions.

The specific screening measures reviewed in this chapter represent the clinical bias of the author. Thus, readers should discuss these measures in detail and obtain approval for their use from their supervisor before using any of the techniques or instruments outlined here.

INTERVIEWING

The interview is the most widely employed tool in clinical psychology (Watkins et al., 1995). The interview plays a prominent role in both treatment and assessment. In basic terms, an interview is a conversation with a purpose or goal (Matarazzo, 1965). Interviewing is a skill that requires practice and careful supervision to learn. There are a number of excellent sources available as to the structure of the interview (Cormier & Cormier, 1979; Hersen & Turner, 1994; Siassi, 1984). Chapter 4 of this book covers the basic elements in diagnostic interviewing and provides a more in-depth analysis of the issues involved in conducting a clinical interview, so these areas will be briefly reviewed but not covered in detail in this chapter.

The most common form of clinical interview is an initial assessment. When a client or patient comes to the clinician because of some problem in daily functioning, the interviewer is often asked for a classification or diagnosis of the problem (Wiens & Matarazzo, 1983). Hersen and Turner (1994) note that interviews designed to classify client problems are most common in mental health settings where a diagnosis is required. Patterned after the question-and-answer format used in traditional medical history taking, such psychological or psychiatric interviews are usually structured according to a sequence of important topics. Interviews focusing on describing clients and their problems in more comprehensive terms usually occur within the context of a full-scale clinical exploration that precedes treatment (Helzer, 1983).

Although there are many guides to conducting a structured psychiatric and mental status examination, a typical outline of topic areas has been recommended by Siassi (1984). Such a system includes emphasis on *general appearance and behavior,* including the client's level of activity, dress, and grooming; *speech and thought,* including the presence of any delusions; *consciousness,* or whether or not the person's *sensorium* is clear or cloudy; *mood and affect,* including evidence of depression, anxiety, and restlessness as well as having affect appropriate to the situation; *perception,* that is, does the individual exhibit any distortions of perception such as evidence of depersonalization, auditory or visual hallucinations; specific concerns such as *obsessions and compulsions* including the nature and quality of such symptoms; and *general orientation* regarding person, place, time, and situation. Other aspects that might be considered include *attention* and *concentration*, which is frequently determined by asking the client to start at 100 and count backward by 7s. The client's *general fund of information* can be assessed with questions such as "Who is the President." The *level of intellectual functioning* is frequently based on past educational achievement, or on the person's ability to engage in abstract reasoning. An assessment of *insight and judgment* (i.e., does the individual understand the probable outcome of his or her behavior?) needs to be included. In addition, *higher cognitive functioning* (i.e., can the person deal with abstract abilities such as correctly interpreting proverbs?) is frequently assessed.

In addition to these formal aspects, many of which focus on verbal behavior, the interviewer should be attuned to nonverbal communication. This includes body language, ease of interacting with the examiner, and other behaviors that build rapport (Goldstein, 1976; Harper, Wiens, & Matarazzo, 1978).

In recent years the major developments in psychological interviewing have focused on structured and semistructured interviews. This trend can be traced to several sources including the increased reliance on diagnostic procedures using operationally defined criteria for making psychiatric diagnoses. Such techniques, originally developed to gain epidemiological information, involve having the interviewer ask specific questions that can be replicated by other interviewers. Structured interviews do not eliminate open-ended questions, nor do they prevent interviewers from asking their own additional questions to clarify responses. However, they do provide detailed rules, sometimes called "decision trees," for telling the interviewer what to do in the event of certain responses. For example, if a client answers "No" to a basic question about some class of feelings or behaviors associated with anxiety, rather than continue with such a list the examiner would move on to another problem area, such as questions on depression. There are a variety of these methods; one of the more widely used is the Structured Clinical Interview (SCID) for *DSM-IV*, which was initially developed by Spitzer and colleagues (1988). The SCID is organized into several different modalities, with each modality devoted to a major class of disturbances such as mood disorders, anxiety disorders, or adjustment disorders. An advantage of this approach to assessment is that the SCID can be customized for specific research purposes or for clinical use. A drawback is that it is very time-consuming to administer.

One of the oldest screening instruments is still widely used by many mental health disciplines. This is the Mini-Mental Status (MMS) Examination by Folstein, Folstein, and McHugh (1975). The MMS is a thirty-item test that assesses orientation, recall, short-term memory, serial subtractions, mental registration, and language in approximately 10 minutes. The test items involve both paper-and-pencil tasks and responding to verbal commands. Points are awarded for each correct response. These are totaled and compared to cut-off scores indicating the level of cognitive functioning of the individual. Cut-off scores are provided with the MMS to differentiate levels of cognitive functioning in comparison to normal populations, demented populations, and psychiatric populations. The MMS has significant positive correlations with Wechsler Intelligence Scale IQ scores. The major advantages of this assessment tool are ease of administration and scoring. In addition, functional levels differentiate between nonimpaired functioning, mild impairment, and moderate impairment. The major disadvantage is a heavy reliance on verbal and auditory comprehension. Thus, in an elderly population with minimal formal writing and reading education or with a history of English as a second language scores may be lower than the actual level of day-to-day impairment. Individuals with sensory deficits, such as decreased hearing or vision, may also be unable to accomplish some tasks, not due to cognitive impairment but to incomplete understanding of the task requirements.

The Neurobehavioral Cognitive Status Examination (NCSE), more recently renamed the Cognistat, was designed to assess intellectual functioning in five basic ability areas (Kiernan et al., 1987). These areas are Language, Construction, Memory, Calculations, and Reasoning. Measures of Attention, Level of Consciousness, and Orientation are assessed independently. The NCSE also divides language functioning into Spontaneous Speech, Comprehension, Repetition, and Naming. While there is no score for Spontaneous Speech, subjective scoring can be obtained. In addition, the Reasoning subtest has two sections, Similarities and Judgment. An additional advantage of the NCSE is that, with the exception of the Memory section, all subtests can be administered in a "screen" and "metric" paradigm. That is, the patient is first presented with a screen item, which is the most demanding test item under that section. If the individual passes that item, it is not necessary to administer the metric, which is a series of test items of increasing difficulty. Time of administration can be as little as 10 minutes, if the individual passes all of the screen items; although clinically, the average time is usually about 20 minutes. Scores are plotted on a profile that illustrates the overall pattern of abilities and disabilities. The normative sample includes normal subjects in two separate groups from age 20- to 39 and 40- to 66. Geriatric population norms are available on a group of 70- to 92-year-olds, as well as a sample of neurosurgical patients with documented brain lesions. The NCSE does not assess reading, writing or spelling and thus individuals with such deficits would not be detected unless associated with aphasia. The NCSE has been used to assess patients with dementias. Examples of profiles for individuals with Alzheimer's, Korsakoff's amnestic syndrome, cerebral infarct with aphasia, and encephalitis with psychotic features are presented in the manual.

The Mattis Dementia Rating Scale (MDRS) was developed by Mattis (1976) to quantify the mental status of elderly persons with profound cognitive impairment. Items on this test are similar to those employed by neurologists in bedside mental status examinations. The items are arranged hierarchically so that adequate performance on an initial item allows the examiner to discontinue testing within that section and assume that credit can be given for adequate performance on subsequent tests. The subtests include measures of intelligence, initiation and perseveration, construction, conceptualizations, and verbal as well as nonverbal short-term memory. The average time required is approximately 10 to 15 minutes for normal elderly subjects. With a demented patient, administration may take up to a half-hour.

The Cognitive Capacity Screening Exam (CCSE) is also a thirty-item questionnaire (Jacobs et al., 1977). The CCSE assesses orientation, immediate recall, short-term memory, serial subtractions, synonyms and antonyms and registration. The scoring is similar to the MMS. A score of less than 20 suggests impaired cognition. There is a significant correlation between the diagnosis of organic brain syndrome and a score of less than 20 in several studies reported by Jacobs et al. (1977). Several advantages accrue to the CCSE as a screening tool for dementia. One advantage is the inclusion of the individual's educational level, occupation, and medical diagnosis in the scoring procedure, since these variables have been shown to influence scores. One disadvantage of this instrument is that it does not differentiate between mild and significant cognitive impairment. Another negative aspect of this measure is the 5-minute time limit for administration. Since older adults do not optimally perform on tests with time constraints, this administration format can negatively influence results.

The Short Portable Mental Status Questionnaire (SPMSQ) is much shorter than the two previous instruments since it only has ten items. This tool assesses orientation, short-term memory, long-term memory, serial subtractions, and information on current events. This measure, developed by Pfeiffer (1975), is scored on the basis of the number of errors rather than the number of correct responses. The tallied scores are compared to a scale similar to that used on the MMS, reflecting the functioning level of the individual. A major benefit of this measure is its shortness; and, like the MMS, it is untimed. A disadvantage is its reliance on verbal and auditory comprehension. In addition, the incorporation of multipart questions places elderly individuals in an unfavorable position since all the parts of the entire question must be answered correctly in order to avoid receiving a point for an incorrect response.

The Mental Status Examination by Strub and Black (1985) is a much more extensive and detailed mental status examination than the previously described procedures. The record form includes places for behavioral observation, levels of consciousness, and attentional aspects. Language functions, both in terms of spontaneous speech and verbal fluency, are calculated. Language skills are further assessed using comprehension subtests requiring the patient to make appropriate verbal responses as well as answering a series of "yes" and "no" questions such as "Is it raining today?" Repetition and naming skills, as well as word-finding tests, are also included, as is identification of clothing and objects that are commonly found in clinic or hospital rooms. Reading, writing, and spelling are assessed. Memory functions include general orientation, historical facts, and a new learning ability task, based on remembering four unrelated words and being able to recall them at 5-, 10-, and 30-minute intervals. There is a verbal story for immediate recall and a visual memory task for hidden objects. This assessment also has a paired associate learning task that includes items that have both high and low association ratings. The patient is also asked to copy a variety of drawings beginning with relatively simple drawings, proceeding to three-dimensional tasks, and drawing a series of pictures on verbal command without a visual prompt. Higher cortical functions are assessed by fund of information, calculations, proverb interpretation, similarities, conceptual series, and comprehension tasks. Other tasks assess related cortical dysfunctions of apraxia (inability to perform complex motor sequences, such as combing hair or brushing teeth), agraphia (inability to write), acalculia (inability to perform math operations) right-left disorientation, finger agnosia (inability to name, with the eyes closed, the fingers on either hand when they are being touched), and Gerstmann's syndrome (the presence in a person of all four symptoms of finger agnosia, right-left confusion, agraphia, and acalculia). Geographic orientation tasks are included, as well as items to assess denial, visual neglect, and frontal lobe dysfunction.

INTELLECTUAL/COGNITIVE SCREENING

The most "traditional" cognitive screening measures have been short forms of the Wechsler Adult Intelligence Scale—Revised (Wechsler, 1981). Abbreviated versions of the WAIS-R fall into two general categories: those methods that involve administering a selected number of subtests, and those methods that involve administering selected items from each of the eleven subtests. Selected subtest short forms usually consist of two or more WAIS-R subtests that are used as brief screening devices to estimate the Full Scale IQ (Kaufman, 1990). In contrast, the selected item method of Satz and Mogel (1962) involves various reductions in the number of items administered on most of the eleven subtests, such as using only the odd-numbered items. Because all subtests are given in this technique, such screenings are meant to serve as a replacement not only for the Full Scale IQ, but to provide estimates of Verbal and Performance IQ scores. Paolo and Ryan (1993) recently compared these two types of administrations in samples of nonimpaired and neurologically impaired elderly persons 75 years and older. Both of the short forms were highly similar in administration times, correlation with WAIS-R IQs, and estimate of average IQ scores. Finally, both the short forms correctly estimated significant Verbal–Performance IQ discrepancies about 75% of the time. Thus, both these screening techniques appear to have good clinical utility in estimating overall intellectual functioning.

Ward (1990) proposed a somewhat longer, seven-subtest short form using the subtests with the shortest administration times. Recent comparisons of several short-form measures in psychiatric inpatients (Benedict, Schretlen, & Bobholz, 1992) indicated that errors in predicted IQ were smallest for this seven-subtest short form. In addition, the longer seven-subtest version provided better predictive validity than the two- and four-subtest methods.

Sattler (1992) has tables in the appendix of his book on the ten best short-form combinations of two, three, four, and five WAIS-R subtests. One of the most clinically popular is a two-subtest combination consisting of Vocabulary and Block Design. Although this method may overestimate the average Full Scale IQ of clinical samples, most of the research strongly suggests that it does so by less than 3 points. Another technique reviewed by Sattler uses the subtest intercorrelations as constant values, allowing conversion of selected Wechsler age-corrected subtest scores into Deviation IQs. The advantage of this method is that any combination of subtests (up to a total of five) can be selected, depending upon the specific referral question or focus of the screening. For example, if one wished to assess an individual's verbal skills regarding social situations and abstract categorization skills, it would be possible to calculate a Verbal IQ score focusing on just these skills, using the Comprehension and Similarities subtests.

Kaufman, Ishikuma, and Kaufman-Packer (1991) formulated three short forms of the WAIS-R that gave attention to both the factor structure of the WAIS-R and to the ways in which selected subtests relative to the full evaluation. These short forms have been shown to have high reliability and validity based on the standardization sample, and in a recent study (McCusker, 1994) the short form was found to display the same excellent psychometric properties with respect to a psychiatric population as had been originally indicated with the normative sample. As always, an important caution should be given regarding the reporting of estimated IQs obtained from short forms. In general, four-subtest estimated IQs result in misclassification of approximately 25% of individuals (McCusker, 1994). Even with this risk, however, short forms may serve as a useful component to assess cognitive levels as part of a personality or memory assessment.

The Kaufman Brief Intelligence Test (K-BIT) was developed by Kaufman and Kaufman (1990). This is an individually administered brief measure of verbal and nonverbal intelligence with an age range of 4 to 90 years. It is used for educational screening or to obtain an estimate of intelligence as part of a personality evaluation (a variety of other uses are outlined in the manual). The test takes approximately 15 to 30 minutes to administer. Standard scores are based on the same norms as numerous intelligence and achievement tests, permitting direct comparison with a variety of measures such as the WAIS-R (Wechsler, 1981).

There are two K-BIT subtests, Vocabulary and Matrices. The authors indicate that Vocabulary primarily measures verbal, school-related skills, and crystallized thinking (acquired skills and knowledge such as the ability to recall previously learned material). Matrices primarily measures fluid intelligence (nonverbal thinking, figural analysis, and the ability to combine information to solve new problems).

The K-BIT Vocabulary subtest includes both Expressive Vocabulary, in which the individual is required to provide the name of a pictured object such as a lamp or a calendar, and Definitions. Under Definitions the person has to produce the word that best fits two clues, a phrase description and a partial spelling of the word. For example, the phrase might be "a bright color" and a partial word spelling might be R _ D.

The K-BIT Matrices subtest is a forty-eight–item nonverbal measure comprising of several types of items involving visual stimuli that are both meaningful and abstract forms that do not use words. All of the items require understanding the relationships among the stimuli. The ability to solve visual analogs, especially those with abstract stimuli, has been shown to be an excellent measure of general intelligence, simultaneous processing, nonverbal reasoning, and fluid thinking.

The Shipley Institute of Living Scale (SIL) consists of two brief subtests requiring about 20 minutes to administer. There is a forty-item Vocabulary test that requires the patient to choose which of four listed words means the same thing or nearly the same thing as a target word. The second test, a twenty-item abstract thinking task, requires the individual to fill in numbers or letters that logically complete a given sequence, such as a word or number list. Summary scores are provided for Vocabulary, Abstraction, and a Total. It is also possible to calculate a Conceptual Quotient (CQ), which is an index of impairment based on a comparison of the vocabulary to abstraction scores, and an Abstraction Quotient, which the CQ score adjusted for age. Estimates for Full Scale WAIS and WAIS-R IQ scores can also be obtained (Shipley, 1987).

The Slosson Intelligence Test—Revised (SIT-R) is a restandardization of the original test that provides a quick index of intellectual ability in approximately 10 to 15 minutes. Test items include tasks measuring general information, comprehension, math, vocabulary, auditory memory, and similarities (Slosson, Nicholson & Hibpshman, 1991).

ACHIEVEMENT/VERBAL SCREENING

The Wide Range Achievement Test—Third Edition (WRAT3) is the most recent development of a test originally designed in the 1930s by Joseph Jastak (Wilkinson, 1993). This newest edition of the WRAT has returned to a single-level format for all individuals ages 5 to 75. Two alternative test forms (Blue and Tan) provide the three subtests of Reading, Spelling, and Arithmetic. Each of these forms takes 15 to 30 minutes to administer. With alternate forms a test-retest can be accomplished relatively easily. This test assesses single word reading, spelling, and a variety of math problem-solving tasks. The test provides age-corrected norms and in the newest edition uses Absolute scores, so that computations can be made not only for standard scores but also for more accurate grade-level assignment. The advantage of this achievement test is that it provides assessment of skills in a manner similar to those presented in most classroom settings. The normative sample for the WRAT3 was nationally stratified and controlled for age, regional residence, gender, ethnicity, and socioeconomic level.

The Woodcock-Johnson Revised: Tests of Achievement (Woodcock & Mather, 1989) are a series of achievement tests assessing Reading, Mathematics, Written language, and Knowledge Skills. The normative sample includes adults through the age of 90 and thus may be of assistance in assessing achievement and daily functional level in older individuals.

The Peabody Picture Vocabulary Test—Revised (PPVT-R) (Dunn & Dunn, 1981) is a nonverbal, multiple-choice test designed to evaluate the receptive vocabulary knowledge of children and adults. The PPVT-R also correlates significantly with measures of reading, language, and general achievement.

Verbal fluency measures have also been used to assess vocabulary skills. These include tests such as Word Naming, Control Word Association Test, and the Set Test (Berg, Franzen, & Wedding, 1994). For a review of more academic achievement assessments, see Chapter 7.

VISUAL-MOTOR SCREENING

The Bender Visual-Motor Gestalt test (BG) is certainly one of the oldest and most widely used tests of visual functioning (Watkins et al., 1995). However, while its popularity is based in part on its sensitivity in representing complex spatial functions in both cerebral hemispheres, its clinical sensitivity as a general index of brain dysfunction is often greatly overestimated. Unfortunately, the BG is frequently misused as the sole indicator for the presence or absence of brain damage, making it the most misused test for assessment of organicity. Several studies have reported negative results when attempting differential diagnoses between brain-impaired and psychiatric populations (Berg, Franzen, & Wedding, 1994). Other widely known visual-motor tests such as the Beery Developmental test of Visual-Motor Integration and the Draw-A-Person test are specifically normed for children and thus are not reviewed here. (These measures are described in Chapter 7.)

The Rey-Osteriech Complex Figure Test can be used to assess visual-spatial construction ability and visual memory (Spreen & Strauss, 1991). This single, complex drawing task permits the examiner to watch not only how well the individual can draw the shape, but also how he or she approaches the task. An Accuracy score based on the scoring of a number of different elements is obtained. In addition, a memory trial can be administered, including immediate and delayed recall of the design. Normative information is available on a large cross-section of population including healthier elderly people.

PERSONALITY/EMOTIONAL SCREENING

The screening instruments covered in this section are, in general, very short, often single-scale tests, most taking less than 20 minutes to complete. The emphasis here is on depression (often described as the common cold of mental health) and anxiety measures, as these are among the most frequent disorders seen in general clinical practice.

The Beck Depression Inventory (BDI) (Beck, 1987) is the most widely used instrument for assessing the intensity of depressive symptomatology. The BDI ranks in the top ten assessment instruments used by clinical psychologists. The twenty-one items are each rated on a 4-point scale reflecting the severity of symptoms. This test takes less than 5 minutes for most individuals to complete. It measures cognitive, affective, somatic, and performance symptoms of depression. A diagnostic range statement as to overall depression severity is also provided.

The Hamilton Depression Inventory (HDI), a self-report measure, was developed by Reynolds and Kobak (1995) based on the original structured interview technique of the Hamilton Depression Rating Scale (HDRS). The twenty-three–item HDI is written at a fifth-grade reading level and takes approximately 10 to 15 minutes to administer and score. Several shorter versions, including a seventeen-item form consistent with the HDRSs, are also available.

The Suicide Probability Scale (SPS) (Cull & Gill, 1988) provides for the rapid assessment of suicide risk. The thirty-six items, each rated on a 4-point scale, generate a total score, four subtest measures, and the Suicide Probability Score. The four subscales are Hopelessness, Suicide Ideation, Negative Self-Evaluation, and Hostility. Administration time is approximately 10 minutes. The total score can be compared to low-, moderate-, or high-risk populations drawn from both inpatient and outpatient settings to calculate the Suicide Probability Score, making the SPS diagnostically useful in a variety of situations.

The Cognitive Checklist (CCL) is used to investigate differences in automatic thoughts or cognitions characteristic of anxiety and depression. The CCL items are rated on a 5-point frequency scale, with fourteen items reflecting negative thoughts about oneself, past experience, and future expectations. These make up the Depression Cognition subscale, while the remaining twelve items represent thoughts about physical and personal danger and constitute the Anxious Cognition subscale. In a recent study, Steer and colleagues (1994) noted this instrument's ability to differentiate between an outpatient clinical population and a group of first-year undergraduates.

The State-Trait Anxiety Inventory (Spielberger, 1983) comprises two separate twenty-item, self-report rating scales for measuring state and trait anxiety. Each item is rated for intensity of feeling on a 4-point scale. While the State scale is a sensitive indicator of changes in transitory anxiety, the Trait scale has proven useful in identifying persons with high levels of neurotic anxiety. Consistently strong correlations between A-State and A-Trait scale scores with MMPI Depression and Psychasthenia scales, as well as the Beck Depression Inventory, provide supportive evidence for good validity of this measure in white, black, and Hispanic populations (Novy et al., 1993).

The Beck Anxiety Inventory (BAI) (Beck et al., 1988) measures symptoms of anxiety in older adolescents and adults. The BAI consists of twenty-one items, each descriptive of some anxiety feature such as subjective distress and somatic or panic-related symptoms. Each item is rated on a 4-point scale of severity. The score on the test can be compared to individuals diagnosed with a variety of anxiety and panic disorders.

The Trauma Symptom Inventory (TSI) is an easy-to-use test of post-traumatic stress and dysfunction developed by Briere (1995). Testing time is approximately 20 minutes. This one hundred–item test includes ten clinical scales that measure the extent to which the individual endorses trauma-related symptoms. These are subsumed under four broad categories of stress including post-traumatic stress, dysphoric mood, sexual difficulties, and self-dysfunction. There are three validity scales that assess the individual's tendency to either deny symptoms that others commonly endorse or to overendorse symptoms. Separate norms are presented for males and females ages 18 to 54 and those over 54 years. The test correlates well with individuals diagnosed with borderline personality disorder.

Somewhat longer than the previously mentioned measures, the Symptom Checklist-90—Revised is a ninety-item, multidimensional inventory on which each of the items is rated on a 5-point severity scale. The SCL-90-R takes approximately 15 minutes to complete. It measures nine primary symptom dimensions in mental health including problems such as depression, anxiety, somatization, obsessive-compulsivity, hostility, psychoticism, phobic anxiety, and paranoid ideation. It also provides three global indices of distress including a Global Severity Index and a Positive Symptoms Distress Index (Derogatis, 1992). A shorter version of this test, the Brief Symptom Inventory (BSI), consists of only fifty-three items and measures the same nine primary symptom dimensions as assessed on the parent instrument.

ATTENTION/MEMORY SCREENING

The abilities for attending to information and remembering data and how to accomplish tasks are necessary for daily functioning. The Digit Span subtest of the WAIS-R (Wechsler, 1981) is perhaps the most widely used method for assessing immediate attention and verbal memory. Since the test includes both Digits Forward and Digits Backwards, and standard scores can be readily obtained from the manual, it is a excellent way to assess not only immediate memory, but also a person's capacity to process and manipulate information mentally by being able to reverse sequences effectively. Digits Backwards requires that the individual both keep the initial numbers in memory and operate simultaneously on them (Hartlage, Asken, & Hornsby, 1987). Because of these memory, attention, and mental processing aspects, Digit Span is one of the tests on the WAIS-R most sensitive to the effects of brain dysfunction. A difference of 3 or more points between Digits Forward and Digits Backwards reflects a concentration deficit that is probably of organic origin (Berg, Franzen, & Wedding, 1994).

The WAIS-R Digit Symbol subtest (Wechsler, 1981) is a task requiring matching numbers with symbols. It is a motor performance test that requires sustained attention, motor speed, visual-motor coordination, and persistence. Although it is very sensitive to brain dysfunction, emotional problems (especially depression) can also affect performance on this task (Hartlage, Asken, & Hornsby, 1987).

The Trail Making test (Reitan & Wolfson, 1993) can be used as a test of attention as well as of more complex cognitive functioning. It consists of two parts. Part A, a visual search task, consists of circled numbers randomly scattered over a page. The instructions call for connecting the numbers in order. Part B includes circled numbers and letters, and the task involves alternating between numbers and letters to connect them serially. This part of the test assesses visual search, attention, mental flexibility, and visual-motor functions. Norms are available based on age and level of education (Berg, Franzen, & Wedding, 1994).

It is not within the scope of this chapter to provide a comprehensive review of all available memory assessment instruments. In recent years, however, there has been a marked growth in clinical tests developed to assess both specific areas of memory function, such as visual or verbal, as well as a number of test batteries that have been updated to provide a more in-depth assessment of memory processes. Examples of such batteries include the Wechsler Memory Scale—Revised (Wechsler, 1987), the Memory Assessment Scales (Williams, 1991), and the Randt Memory Test (Randt, Brown, & Osborne, 1980).

The Luria-Nebraska Neuropsychological Battery (LNNB) developed by Golden (Golden, Hammeke, & Purisch, 1980) is available in two forms. Form I (Golden, Purisch, & Hammeke, 1985) can be hand scored, which allows an examiner to administer any of the eleven subtests as a screening measure. The Memory subtest measures short-term memory for both verbal and nonverbal information. Both interference and noninterference tasks are included in this subtest. Paired-associate learning, both to words and to pictures, and the ability to recall the main idea of a paragraph are among the memory functions that can be assessed using this relatively brief scale.

The Memory Assessment Scale (MAS) by Williams (1991) is designed for ages 18 through 90 years and takes approximately 40 minutes to administer. The MAS consists of a series of subtests based on memory functioning that tap verbal span, list learning, prose memory, visual span, visual recognition, visual reproduction, and names-faces. Comparisons can be made between the Global Memory Scale score and WAIS-R scores. Norms are based on adults grouped by age decade, age and educational level, and adults matching the U.S. census on the basis of age, education, and gender. Validity data indicate that MAS scores distinguish nonimpaired from neurologically impaired subjects and provide expected profiles for criterion groups for individuals with neurological disorders such as dementia, closed head injury, and left and right hemisphere lesions.

Another relatively short memory test is the Randt (Randt, Brown, & Osborne, 1980). This memory test, although not widely known, has a number of advantages. The instrument not only provides assessment of initial memory functions, but also provides a means to measure recall with interference of a variety of tasks. The test consists of a series of separate subtests including general information, list-learning tasks, repeating numbers, paired associate, learning, and short story recall. The interference component is one in which the individual, for example, learns a serial list of five items. Another subtest, such as repeating digits, is given, and then the individual is asked to recall those five items. Thus, this is a measure more closely approaching daily memory tasks, in which interference may occur between initial learning and later recall. There is also an incidental memory component to the test that assesses the ability to remember information when one is not told one will be asked to recall it later. Another advantage of the Randt is that it has a 24-hour recall component. The individual is told at the time of initial evaluation that he or she will be contacted about this information. In an inpatient setting this would normally be done by a face-to-face meeting with the individual. However, in outpatient settings or in other facilities, the bulk of the 24-hour delay recall can be obtained by telephone. Raw scores are converted to standard scores for easy reference to other assessment instruments.

NEUROPSYCHOLOGICAL SCREENING

Although the ideal patient seen for psychological services is someone who has already had a physical evaluation or work-up, in fact, in some settings a very small number of clients will have had a physical examination and a number of those may well have disorders presenting with psychological symptoms. Thus, one of the most important aspects for a clinician is recognizing brain dysfunction and determining when screening or referral for neuropsychological assessment is needed. The chapter on organic disorders (Chapter 11) provides a broad review of neuropsychology issues and describes conditions for which a comprehensive neuropsychological evaluation might be needed. Holmes (1992) has produced a guide describing techniques to help a mental health practitioner identify and refer potential organic problems for medical and neuropsychological assessment.

There have been attempts over the years to identify a single test that differentiates brain-impaired individuals from nonimpaired individuals. Most attempts at such an evaluation have failed. While there is general agreement that assessments with a single test are not possible due to the variety of deficits that may be present, the one test that does seem to best estimate overall organic dysfunction is the Halstead Category Test (Parsons, 1986; Reitan & Wolfson, 1985). However, several short screening batteries have been utilized with success.

An excellent reference for neuropsychological screening to identify brain impairment is the manual by Berg, Franzen, and Wedding (1994). This volume presents an overview of adult screening; the companion volume by Franzen and Berg (1989) describes screening for children. Lezak (1995) also provides a broad overview of neuropsychological measures.

As noted earlier, the Category Test was originally designed by Halstead to measure an individual's ability to profit from experience and new learning information. The Short Category Test, Booklet Format (SCT), was developed by Wetzel and Boll (1987) to reduce the length and complexity of the original Category Test while retaining its desirable psychometric and diagnostic properties. The SCT is short, using fewer than half the items on the original test, and is in a booklet format consisting of five booklets, one for each subtest, with twenty cards per subtest. The number of errors on each subtest are added up to provide raw error scores. These raw scores are then converted to normalized T-scores and percentile rank equivalents. Normative and standardization samples include a wide range of socioeconomic and educational levels that encompass individuals with both psychiatric and neurological diagnoses in the clinical sample. The age range includes individuals up through the age of 79 and as low as 20. The SCT shows correlations with Full Scale IQs and other measures of cognitive functioning similar to those reported for the original Category Test.

The Luria-Nebraska Screening Test is made up of fifty items taken from the Luria-Nebraska Neuropsychological Battery (Golden, 1987). The purpose of this screening test is to predict overall performance on the respective full-length battery. This test is available in forms for both adults and children. It should be noted that this measure is not intended to classify patients as organic or nonorganic but rather to predict the severity of overall LNNB performance. In contrast to the scoring used on more familiar instruments such as the WAIS-R, on which the best or most rapid response earns the highest score (an incorrect answer is 0 points while 2 or more points are awarded for the best performance), on the Luria-Nebraska, points are earned for poorer performances, resulting in higher scores (a correct answer results in 0 points, with the most incorrect answer earning 2 points). This scoring system is based on the medical concept of "absence" of symptoms indicating normal functioning. The screening is discontinued when 8 or more points are achieved in a running total. Thus, all of the items in the screening test do not need to be administered, as once a total error score of 8 is exceeded, the individual should be referred or given a more complete neuropsychological evaluation.

The Kaufman Short Neuropsychological Assessment Procedure (K-SNAP) is a recently developed screening device by Kaufman and Kaufman (1994). This test measures an individual's ability to demonstrate intact mental functioning in three levels of cognitive complexity from Attention Orientation tasks through simple Memory and Perceptual Skills to the most complex Reasoning and Planning Ability items. The K-SNAP is intended for ages 11 to over 65. Raw scores are converted into scale scores based on age groupings that include conversions for older individuals in their 70s. The four subtests include Mental Status, Number Recall, Gestalt Closure, and Four-Letter Word subtests. The two middle-level subtests, Number Recall and Gestalt Closure, are combined to provide a Recakll/Closure Composite score. The medium- and high-level subtests are combined to yield a Composite score. The Mental Status subtest requires answering simple questions that assess memory and orientation. The Number Recall test is a standard Digit Span task. Gestalt Closure consists of a series of objects or scenes printed in a partially completed "ink blot" drawing. That is, the individual has to fill in the missing details and name the object. The Four-Letter Word subtest involves the examinee having to figure out "secret" words by studying several different lists of four letters, each list having some of the letters that make up the target word. The task is to generate hypotheses and pick the correct word from a list. Materials for all four subtests are included in one easy-to-use format. Administration time is approximately 25 minutes. In addition to the standardization sample, the clinical samples normed with this test include individuals with a variety of neurological deficits, reading disabilities, clinical depression, and mental retardation. Interpretation of the scores is based on descriptive categories for the Mental Status exam. In addition, a standard score with a mean of 100 and a standard deviation of 15 can be calculated for the Composite score. An 8-point Impairment Index can be used to identify individuals who are likely to need further diagnostic testing.

Abbreviated versions of the Halstead-Reitan Neuropsychological Battery (Reitan & Wolfson, 1985) have been used for screening. Golden (1976) described a version requiring 1 hour of administration and consisting of nine tests. Erickson, Calsyn, and Scheupback (1978) report on a version consisting of four tests. These include Trail-Making, Aphasia Screening, as well as the Block Design and Digit Symbol subtests from the Wechsler Adult Intelligence Scale—Revised. Berg, Franzen, and Wedding (1994) have reviewed most of these procedures.

CONCLUSIONS

Screening instruments have always had a place within the field of clinical psychology. The application of highly focused measures can help identify and diagnose potential problem areas for therapeutic investigation; assess the severity of specific symptoms; assist with differential diagnosis; or help rule out cognitive, learning, or personality patterns that can impede the process of treatment. Given the trend for shorter lengths of treatment and more focused treatment in both psychiatric and medical facilities, the need for rapid, focused psychological assessment is increasing in importance. There is also an increased interest in outcome studies addressing the effectiveness of individual, group, partial, and day treatment programs and therapies. Such a trend is likely to produce a greater demand for short, repeatable screening instruments to assess therapeutic progress in such areas.

REFERENCES

Anastasi, A. (1988). *Psychological testing* (6th ed.). New York: Macmillan.
Beck, A. T. (1987). *Beck Depression Inventory manual.* San Antonio, TX: Psychological Corporation.

Beck, A. T., Epstein, N., Brown, G., & Steer, R. A. (1988). An inventory for measuring clinical anxiety: Psychometric properties. *Journal of Consulting and Clinical Psychology, 56*, 893–897.

Benedict, R. H., Schretlen, D., & Bobholz, J. H. (1992). Concurrent validity of three WAIS-R short forms in psychiatric inpatients. *Psychological Assessment, 4*, 322–328.

Berg, R., Franzen, M., & Wedding, D. (1994). *Screening for brain impairment: A manual for mental health practice* (2d ed.). New York: Springer.

Briere, J. (1995). *Trauma Symptom Inventory professional manual.* Odessa, FL: Psychological Assessment Resources.

Butcher, J. N. (Ed.) (1994). *Clinical personality assessment: Practical approaches.* New York: Oxford University Press.

Cormier, W. H., & Cormier, L. S. (1979). *Interviewing strategies for helpers: A guide to assessment, treatment, and evaluation.* Monterey, CA: Brooks/Cole.

Cull, J. G., & Gill, W. S. (1988). *Suicide Probability Scale (SPS) manual.* Los Angeles: Western Psychological Services.

Cummings, N. A. (1995). Impact of managed care on employment and training: A primer for survival. *Professional Psychology: Research and Practice, 26*(1), 10–15.

Derogatis, L. R. (1992). *Symptom Checklist-90—Revised manual.* Minneapolis, MN: National Computer Systems.

Dunn, L. M., & Dunn, L. M. (1981). *Peabody Picture Vocabulary Test—Revised manual.* Circle Pines, MN: American Guidance Service.

Erickson, R. C., Calsyn, D. A., & Scheupbach, C. S. (1978). Abbreviating the Halstead-Reitan Neuropsychological Test Battery, *Journal of Clinical Psychology, 34*, 922–926.

Folstein, M. F., Folstein, S. E., & McHugh, P. R. (1975). "Mini-Mental State": A practical method for grading the cognitive state of patients for the clinician. *Journal of Psychiatric Research, 12*, 189–198.

Franzen, M., & Berg, R. (1989). *Screening children for brain impairment.* New York: Springer.

Golden, C. J. (1976). The identification of brain damage by an abbreviated form of the Halstead-Reitan Neuropsychological Battery. *Journal of Clinical Psychology, 32*, 821–826.

Golden, C. J. (1978). *Stroop color and word test.* Chicago: Stoelting.

Golden, C. J. (1981). *Diagnosis and rehabilitation in clinical neuropsychology* (2d ed.). Springfield, IL: Thomas.

Golden, C. J. (1987). *Screening test for the Luria-Nebraska Neuropsychological Battery: Adult and children's forms.* Los Angeles: Western Psychological Services.

Golden, C. J., Hammeke, T. A., & Purisch, A. D. (1980). *Manual for the Luria-Nebraska Neuropsychological Battery.* Los Angeles: Western Psychological Services.

Golden, C. J., Purisch, A. D., & Hammeke, T. A. (1985). *Luria-Nebraska Neuropsychological Battery: Forms I and II manual.* Los Angeles: Western Psychological Services.

Goldstein, A. P. (1976). Relationship-enhancement methods. In F. H. Kanfer & A. P. Goldstein (Eds.), *Helping people change* (pp. 15–49). New York: Pergamon Press.

Goldstein, G., & Hersen, M. (Eds.) (1984). *Handbook of psychological assessment.* New York: Pergamon Pr.ess.

Harper, R. G., Wiens, A. N., & Matarazzo, J. D. (1978). *Nonverbal communication: The state of the art.* New York: Wiley.

Hartlage, L. C., Asken, M. J., & Hornsby, J. L. (Eds.) (1987). *Essentials of neuropsychological assessment.* New York: Springer.

Helzer, J. E. (1983). Standardized interviews in psychiatry. *Psychiatry Developments, 2,* 161–178.

Hersen, M., & Turner, S. M. (Eds.) (1994). *Diagnostic interviewing* (2d ed.). New York: Plenum.

Holmes, C. B. (1992). *Recognizing brain dysfunction: A guide for mental health professionals.* Brandon, VT: Clinical Psychology.

Jacobs, J. W., Bernard, M. R., Delgado, A., & Strain, J. J. (1977). Screening for organic mental syndromes in the medically ill. *Annals of Internal Medicine, 86,* 40–46.

Kaufman, A. S. (1990). *Assessing adolescent and adult intelligence.* Needham Heights, MA: Allyn & Bacon.

Kaufman, A. S., Ishikuma, T., & Kaufman-Packer, J. L. (1991). Amazingly short forms of the WAIS-R. *Journal of Psychoeducational Assessment, 9,* 4–15.

Kaufman, A. S., & Kaufman, N. L. (1990). *Kaufman Brief Intelligence Test.* Circle Pines, MN: American Guidance Service.

Kaufman, A. S., & Kaufman, N. L. (1994). *Kaufman Short Neuropsychological Assessment Procedure.* Circle Pines, MN: American Guidance Service.

Kiernan, R. J., Mueller, J., Langston, J. W., & Van Dyke, C. (1987). The Neurobehavioral Cognitive Status Examination: A brief but differentiated approach to assessment. *Annals of Internal Medicine, 107,* 481–485.

Lezak, M. D. (1995). *Neuropsychological assessment* (3d ed.). New York: Oxford University Press.

Maruish, M. E. (Ed.) (1994). *The use of psychological testing for treatment planning and outcome assessment.* Hillsdale, NJ: Erlbaum.

Matarazzo, J. D. (1965). The interview. In B. B. Wolman (Ed.), *Handbook of clinical psychology* (pp. 403–450). New York: McGraw-Hill.

Mattis, S. (1976). Mental status examination for organic mental syndrome in the elderly patient. In L. Bellak & T. B. Karasu (Eds.), *Geriatric psychiatry.* New York: Grune & Stratton.

McCusker, P. J. (1994). Validation of Kaufman, Ishikuma, and Kaufman-Packer's Wechsler Adult Intelligence Scale—Revised short forms on a clinical sample. *Psychological Assessment, 6*(3), 246–248.

Novy, D. M., Nelson, D. V., Goodwin, J., & Rowzee, R. D. (1993). Psychometric comparability of the State-Trait Anxiety Inventory for different ethnic subpopulations. *Psychological Assessment, 5*(3), 343–349.

Paolo, A. M., & Ryan, J. J. (1993). WAIS-R abbreviated forms in the elderly: A comparison of the Satz-Mogel with a seven-subtest short form. *Psychological Assessment, 5*(4), 425–429.

Parsons, O. A. (1986). Overview of the Halstead-Reitan Battery. In T. Incagnoli, G. Goldstein, & C. J. Golden (Eds.), *Clinical applications of neuropsychological test batteries.* New York: Plenum.

Pfeiffer, E. (1975). A short portable mental status questionnaire for the assessment of organic brain deficit in elderly patients. *Journal of the American Geriatric Society, 23,* 433–441.

Randt, C. T., Brown, E. R., & Osborne, D. P. (1980). A memory test for longitudinal measurement of mild to moderate deficits. *Clinical Neuropsychology, 2,* 184–194.

Reeves, D., & Wedding, D. (1994). *The clinical assessment of memory.* New York: Springer.

Reitan, R. M., & Wolfson, D. (1993). *The Halstead-Reitan Neuropsychological Test Battery: Theory and clinical interpretation* (2d ed.). Tucson, AZ: Neuropsychology Press.

Reynolds, W. M., & Kobak, K. A. (1995). *Hamilton Depression Inventory professional manual.* Odessa, FL: Psychological Assessment REesources.

Sattler, J. (1992). *Assessment of children: Revised and updated third edition.* San Diego, CA: Author.

Satz, P., & Mogel, S. (1962). An abbreviation of the WAIS for clinical use. *Journal of Clinical Psychology, 18,* 77–79.

Shipley, W. C. (1967). *Manual: Shipley Institute of Living Scale.* Los Angeles: Western Psychological Services.

Siassi, I. (1984). Psychiatric interviews and mental status examinations. In G. Goldstein & M. Hersen (Eds.), *Handbook of psychological assessment* (pp. 259–275). New York: Pergamon Press.

Slosson, R. L., Nicholson, C. L., & Hibpshman, T. H. (1991). *Slosson Intelligence Test—Revised manual.* Los Angeles: Western Psychological Services.

Spielberger, C. D. (1983). *Manual for the State-Trait Anxiety Inventory (Form Y).* Palo Alto, CA: Consulting Psychologists Press.

Spitzer, R. L., Williams, J. B., Gibbon, M., & First, M. B. (1988). *Instruction manual for the Structured Clinical Interview for DSM-III-R (SCID), 6/1/88 revision).* New York: Biometrics Research Department, New York State Psychiatric Institute.

Spreen, O., & Strauss, E. (1991). *A compendium of neuropsychological tests.* New York: Oxford University Press.

Steer, R. A., Beck, A. T., Clark, D. A., & Beck, J. S. (1994). Psychometric properties of the Cognition Checklist with psychiatric outpatients and university students. *Psychological Assessment, 6*(1), 67–70.

Strub, R. L., & Black, F. W. (1985). *The mental status exam in neurology* (2d ed.). Philadelphia: Davis.

Ward, L. C. (1990). Prediction of Verbal, Performance and Full Scale IQs from seven subtests of the WAIS-R. *Journal of Clinical Psychology, 46,* 436–440.

Watkins, C. E., Campbell, V. L., Nieberding, R., & Hallmark, R. (1995). Contemporary practice of psychological assessment by clinical psychologists. *Professional Psychology: Research and Practice, 26*(2), 54–60.

Wechsler, D. A. (1981). *Manual for the Wechsler Adult Intelligence Scale—Revised.* New York: Psychological Corporation.

Wechsler, D. (1987). *Wechsler Memory Scale—Revised.* New York: Psychological Corporation.

Wetzel, L., & Boll, T. J. (1987). *Short Category Test, Booklet Format manual.* Los Angeles: Western Psychological Services.

Wiens, A. N., & Matarazzo, J. D. (1983). Diagnostic interviewing. In M. Herzen, A. E. Kazdin, & A. S. Bellack (Eds.), *The clinical psychology handbook* (pp. 309–328). New York: Pergamon Press.

Wilkinson, G. S. (1993). *Wide Range Achievement Test administration manual* (1993 ed.). Wilmington, DE: Wide Range.

Williams, J. M. (1991). *Memory Assessment Scales administration manual.* Odessa, FL: Psychological Assessment Resources.

Woodcock, R. W., & Mather, N. (1989). *Woodcock-Johnson Tests of Achievement.* Allen, TX: DLM Teaching Resources.

▶ 7

Psychological Testing

KEVIN R. KRULL

Psychological testing is a multistep process of obtaining relevant information about the patient, interpretation of this information in light of the patient's personal and social history, and disposition of the patient based on the results of the testing process. The evaluation begins with a referral from other professionals, parents, or the patients themselves and typically ends with feedback of the results to the patients and/or referral sources. In many cases, patients are followed through the beginning phases of treatment. Testing should lead to differential treatment suggested by the implications of the test results.

Psychological testing may encompass a very broad range of observation and testing procedures. Common assessment devices include tests of intellectual ability, tests of academic functioning, and tests of emotional functioning and personality development. In certain cases more detailed assessment may be required, including neuropsychological evaluation or structured behavioral observations. Neuropsychological evaluations typically include assessment of intellectual ability and academic achievement, as well as specific processes such as attention and concentration, memory, language, visual perception, gross and fine motor skills, sensory and perceptual functions, mental flexibility, and problem solving. Structured behavioral observations may be conducted in an artificial laboratory/clinic setting or real world settings such as classroom or home environments.

This chapter will review the basic steps in general psychological testing procedures, beginning with the referral process and ending with case disposition. It will also address specific assessment devices. The focus will be on the process of psychological assessment. Many existing texts provide an exhaustive review of major assessment instruments (Lezak, 1995; Sattler, 1992; Spreen & Strauss, 1991), and this type of review will not be attempted here.

THE REFERRAL

Referrals for psychological testing come from a variety of sources and occur at different stages in the patient's contact with mental health professionals. Many referrals come from medical professionals such as primary care physicians. Frequently educational institutions refer patients for assessment. With child referrals from public school systems it is common to have intellectual and academic testing done by a school psychologist working with the school district. Thus, these referrals typically are for assessment of emotional or personality functioning or for more specialized forms of assessment such as neuropsychological testing. Referrals from private school systems are somewhat different since many do not employ school psychologists. In these cases no previous assessment of the child may have occurred. In either case, at the time of the referral it is important to determine whether previous testing has occurred. If so, results should be obtained prior to the evaluation so that an appropriate plan of action can be developed. In most cases one should not repeat testing within 12 months at the risk of practice effects leading to artificially inflated scores.

As with all procedures in clinical psychology, the psychologist has the right—and in some circumstances the ethical responsibility—to refuse to accept a referral. Such a decision should be based on whether the referree is appropriate for testing, whether the psychologist is properly trained to conduct such testing, and whether the testing can be accomplished in a reasonable amount of time. In some instances it is obvious at the time of the referral that psychological testing would not be appropriate for the patient at that particular time. For example, a referral for intellectual testing in an untreated patient with obvious psychotic symptoms would best be delayed until treatment of the symptoms. Otherwise, testing is likely not to be a valid measure of true ability.

A psychologist should accept a referral only if properly trained to conduct the type of testing requested or required. Assessment of children requires the use of different testing instruments and administration procedures. A psychologist who is not accustomed to working with children or who is not knowledgeable in the specific testing procedures or interpretations should not conduct evaluations with children. Another clear example is neuropsychological testing. With the increase in popularity of "neuropsychological evaluations," many psychologists have begun administering specific neuropsychological tests without receiving proper training or supervision. Due to its complexity, the current recommendations for training to conduct neuropsychological evaluations include the equivalent of 2 years of post-doctoral training combined with specific courses during graduate education (Reports of the INS, 1987). Without such training one should not engage in the administration and interpretation of such tests. Some psychologists have attempted to circumvent the training guidelines by conducting "neuropsychological screening" in which they administer a shortened battery of tests. This procedure is also troublesome. If the tests are not administered properly, they will not be valid. Furthermore, repeat testing may not be possible due to the patient's recent exposure to the test items. An additional concern is that the patient or another professional may accept this invalid assessment as an accurate portrayal of the patient's functioning. Thus, in these situations the psychologist has a responsibility to the patient, profession, and society to decline the referral and suggest another psychologist trained in that particular area.

Being able to conduct testing within a responsible amount of time following the referral is also a factor that should determine acceptance of a referral. A practice or service cannot operate without a steady flow of patients, and thus a waiting list is often necessary. However, the waiting list should not be allowed to grow to unreasonable lengths. A 4- or 5-month waiting list is undesirable and likely unnecessary. Most individuals referred for assessment will present much differently 4 or 5 months after a referral. In such cases, patients should be given the option of waiting for the appointment or accepting a recommendation from the psychologist for another professional who can conduct the testing sooner.

Once the nature of the referral is deemed appropriate and a decision is made to accept the patient, the referral question(s) should be clarified. Many sources who are not accustomed to referring patients to psychologists may simply request "psychological testing." These individuals may or may not have a specific question in mind. Psychological testing may mean an IQ test to one physician and a personality assessment to another. If a psychologist does not clarify exactly what type of information is needed, the question may go unanswered and result in a disservice to the patient and present the psychologist and the field of psychology in a negative light. It is also unlikely that that referral source will continue to refer patients to the psychologist.

RECORD GATHERING

The first step in the actual evaluation of a patient is the gathering of medical, academic, and vocational records and previous evaluations. Release-of-information forms should be obtained from the patient, parent, or legal guardian. Medical and educational records should be requested directly from the respective institutions if possible. Ideally, this information would be obtained prior to beginning the testing with the patient, because the contents of the records frequently influence the testing process. For example, if the patient had recently received a partial evaluation through the school or another institution, selection of standard test devices may have to be modified. Patients, parents, and/or significant others may not recall the specifics of previous evaluations, including which tests were given. Additionally, the content of medical records may influence the interpretation of test results. For example, a diagnosis of thyroid dysfunction in a child with hyperactive behavior would likely rule out the presence of an Attention Deficit Hyperactivity Disorder.

Rating forms and history packages should be mailed prior to the scheduled evaluation. For children, behavioral rating forms should be sent to the teachers far enough in advance to allow them to complete the rating and return them in time for the evaluation. Parents, spouses, and the patient can also complete some of the forms before testing or on the day of the evaluation. Comprehensive history forms will generally be completed in more detail by the patient or parents if they are allowed to review records at home or spend time recalling the information. A good history form should include questions about development, education, vocation, medical and psychological experiences, and family make-up. Examples of history forms can be obtained from Barkley (1990). It is important to have much of this material before the evaluation is completed, so that you can be sure all relevant problem areas are assessed. For example, the patient or significant others may complain of only emotional and behavioral problems observed in the home, whereas a teacher may report that the child lags behind in the development of reading skills or displays poor peer relations, while an employer may be more likely to report changes in work productivity. Focusing your evaluation only on the report of behaviors in the home (e.g., assessing only behavioral and emotional functioning), may miss a primary cause of the behavioral problems (e.g., low academic achievement and subsequent low self-esteem).

TESTING SESSION

The testing session should be viewed as a multistage process. Observations and interviews can be more telling than actual test results. Observations should be collected not only during interactions with other family members and/or the test examiner, but also during completion of test questions or breaks between test instruments. Symptoms may wax or wane over the course of testing or in different situations and may present differently across various environments.

Observations

Observations should be conducted of the patient and relevant family members. With children, parent–child interactive observations are often very useful. Barkley (1990) and Forehand and McMahon (1981) have outlined procedures for structured interactions that provide data on parental as well as child behavior. Interactions between spouses or significant others can be obtained during the interview session. Additionally, observations should include behaviors which are inconsistent with presenting complaints. Observations conducted as part of an evaluation of an adult with chronic low back pain, for example, should include the consistency of apparent physical discomfort in the waiting room, during testing, and during the interview when the patient's attention is focused on the condition. Another example of observations being inconsistent with other data would include the patient who reports significant memory problems and gives unusually poor responses during IQ testing, such as the shape of a ball being square, but manages to arrive for the session unescorted and on time after three transfers on the public bus system.

Although the degree to which specific behavioral observations are important will depend on the presenting problem, Table 7-1 presents some of the more common areas that should receive attention.

Interviews

Interviews should be conducted with the patient as well as all significant others. Who the significant others are often depends on the nature of the presenting problem and the age of the patient. With children, significant others include parents and teachers, whereas with adults, spouses and employers may provide more relevant information. Medical professionals and counselors or therapists who have had recent contact with the patient should also be questioned, or at least their records should be obtained. As with all communication, the clinician must obtain signed releases from the patient, if over 17, or a parent or legal guardian before contacting these other professionals, including referral sources. A release is also necessary for wards of the state. In these cases the case manager can often sign a release. One should not assume that all adult patients are capable of giving permission for contacts. An adult who has been determined to be incompetent or who has a legal guardian will not be able to provide consent, although assent should still be obtained.

TABLE 7-1   Behavioral Observations Relevant to Psychological Testing

A. Appearance
    1. Age—facial features and size related to the age of the patient
    2. Physical presentation—dress, grooming, and hygiene
B. Affect
    1. Prevalent—typical affect of the patient and significant others
    2. Range—range of emotional expression
C. Emotional State
    1. Consistent—consistent with displayed affect
    2. Type—apparent mood of patient
    3. Level—intensity of apparent mood
D. Motivation
    1. Effort—put forth during administration of test material
    2. Interest—in test materials and/or results of process
    3. Cooperation—degree and consistency in cooperation with demands
    4. Reinforcement—frequency and intensity of reinforcement required
E. Motor
    1. Level—activity level of patient during testing
    2. Range—variability of activity or stamina of patient
    3. Gross—gait, weakness, and balance
    4. Fine—dexterity, laterality, and speed
F. Cognitive
    1. General—cognitive control or impulsiveness
    2. Attention—sustained, selective, and divided
    3. Language—communication skills
    4. Memory—immediate and delayed, verbal and visual
G. Bizarre or Unusual Behaviors

Collection and review of relevant records and clinical interviews should be performed before the evaluation of the patient. In many cases this may not be possible. Still, an attempt to contact parents/spouses, teachers/employers, and referring physicians should occur prior to the testing session. Without such contact, informed decisions about which tests should be administered cannot be made. For example, one would not want to administer one of the Wechsler Intelligence Scales as part of an assessment battery if it had recently been administered as part of an educational or vocational evaluation.

Interviews often focus on variables relevant to the patient's symptoms. Often this process can be quite time-consuming, spreading across multiple sessions. When used with a history form completed by the patient or parent in advance, an interview can be conducted very efficiently and comprehensively. Under such circumstances a brief review of the completed forms can lead to an interview focusing on areas that require further elaboration rather than covering all psychosociobiological data.

Test Administration

Prior to testing, attempts should be made to make the patient at ease and as comfortable as possible. Although it is important to adhere to test administration procedures, it is equally important to obtain the subject's best performance during the testing session. To ensure this, the examiner must maintain adequate motivation, reduce physical and emotional distractions as much as possible, and present the instructions and material in a way suitable to the individual's perceptual abilities.

Motivation is maintained by presenting adequate reinforcers for participation in the testing procedure. Some patients arrive for the session with motivation arising from internal factors, while others may require external incentives. With adults and older children or adolescents these incentives typically involve verbal praise or acknowledgment for effort. Younger children may require physical reinforcers, such as stickers or small trinkets. Edible reinforcers are not advised unless approved by parents before the session. As with any behavioral schedule, these reinforcers should be applied sparingly so as not to satiate the patient. Additionally, in order to comply with standard administration tangible reinforcers should be withheld until after the particular test is completed.

Testing can be compromised by a variety of physical and mental distractions. Patients who are excessively anxious or depressed will not perform to their true potential on measures of intellectual functioning, although the anxiety or distraction is useful to observe. Testing in distracting environmental situations or conditions will also be associated with artificially reduced performance. Thus, care should be taken to reduce extraneous noises and interruptions. Whenever possible, testing should occur in a room with little visual stimulation such as books, posters, or puzzles unrelated to the test itself. Only items needed for the actual test should be visible to the patient. Tests that are not currently being administered and items needed for other subtests should be hidden from the patient's view. Care should be taken to ensure that the test room is adequately lighted and at a reasonable temperature.

The physical condition of the patient should be considered before and during testing. Young children should be tested around their daily routine. If a child frequently takes an afternoon nap, he or she should be tested in the morning. Similarly, most individuals will not perform to their true potential if tested in the late afternoon or evening. As a general rule, the testing should be interrupted if the patient becomes fatigued. Fatigue may occur in unexpected situations, for example, testing a young adult early in the morning after a late night out. Even patients who arrive full of energy may become fatigued during a full day of testing. Comprehensive testing of an older child or an adult may take place on a single day over a span of 6 to 8 hours. Most individuals will become fatigued at some time during such a battery of tests. If it is not feasible to split testing into multiple sessions, the order of testing should be considered to place tests most sensitive to fatigue early in the day or following a lengthy break (e.g., lunch). For example, tests of memory or attention should occur early in the day, not at the end of it. Often these tests are not part of a planned battery but arise due to patterns of performance observed earlier in the day. Patients referred for a learning disability assessment may show patterns suggestive of an attention deficit disorder while being given an intelligence test and a measure of academic functioning. Too frequently, a continuous performance task may be administered at this point. This test order will place the patient at a disadvantage over a patient referred for an attention deficit disorder evaluation who is administered the continuous performance measure first. That is, the individual who is administered the measure of attention, the continuous performance test, at the end of a test battery will be more fatigued and be more likely to respond poorly.

Occasionally testing is required for patients with physical disabilities. Patients who have a hearing or visual impairment require modified administration instructions in order to ensure their comprehension of the test demands. In these cases one cannot simply assume that the patient comprehends the test instructions. An example would be a deaf patient who also has a speech delay. Such a patient will not only have difficulty understanding the verbal test instructions, but may also not be able to adequately communicate understanding or misunderstanding to the examiner. Sattler (1991) outlines useful procedures for testing children with physical disabilities.

Test Instruments

Care should be taken in selecting test instruments. Many different versions of tests exist, some of which do not have research or data supporting their use for specific populations. A test should not be assumed to have adequate validity or reliability simply because it is marketed by a reputable company. The examiner is responsible not only for knowing how to administer and score the test, but also for knowing its strengths and weaknesses for specific populations. One should examine the reported data on the standardization sample to determine its applicability to a specific patient. Table 7-2 lists commonly used tests and briefly describes their application.

Some instruments overlap in the age range for which they have been designed. For example, the Wechsler Intelligence Scale for Children—Third Edition (WISC-III) has an applicable age range of 6 to 17 years (Wechsler, 1991), while the Wechsler Adult Intelligence Scale—Revised (WAIS-R) has

TABLE 7-2   Common Instruments Employed in Psychological Testing

I. Intellectual
   A. Wechsler Preschool and Primary Scales of Intelligence—Revised (WPPSI-R) (Wechsler, 1989)
      1. Ages: 3–7 years
      2. Application: The WPPSI-R is a measure of general intellectual functioning. It consists of a Verbal and Performance scale, each comprising several subtests. The Verbal scales are used to examine expressive and receptive functions such as word knowledge, verbal problem solving, general information, verbal abstraction, and auditory attention and recall. The Performance scales assess nonverbal functions such as visual perception and sequencing, nonverbal problem solving, spatial organization and integration, and visual-motor speed and coordination.
   B. Wechsler Intelligence Scale for Children—Third Edition (WISC-III) (Wechsler, 1991).
      1. Ages: 6–17 years
      2. Application: *See I.A., WPPSI-R.*
   C. Wechsler Adult Intelligence Scale—Revised (WAIS-R)
      1. Ages: 16–74 years
      2. Application: *See I.A., WPPSI-R.*
   D. Differential Ability Scales (DAS) (Elliott, 1990)
      1. Ages: 2.5 to 17 years
      2. Application: The DAS is a measure of cognitive ability and academic achievement. It includes a measure of General Conceptual Ability for all age levels, measures of Verbal and Nonverbal Abilities for children 3 to 17 years, and a measure of Spatial Abilities for children 6.0 to 17 years.
   E. Stanford-Binet Intelligence Scale: Fourth Edition (SB-IV) (Thorndike, Hagen, & Sattler, 1986)
      1. Ages: 2.0 years to adult
      2. Application: The Stanford-Binet IV includes four content areas: Verbal Reasoning, Quantitative Reasoning, Abstract/Visual Reasoning, and Short Term Memry. A composite score, which is taken as a total IQ, can be derived from the combination of these areas.
   F. Kaufman Assessment Battery for Children (K-ABC) (Kaufman & Kaufman, 1983)
      1. Ages: 2.5 to 12.5 years
      2. Application: The K-ABC is a collection of ability and achievement measures that produce four scaled scores: Sequential Processing, Simultaneous Processing, Achievement, and Nonverbal. A composite score, which is similar to a total IQ, can be derived from the combination of the Sequential and Simultaneous measures.
   G. McCarthy Scales of Children's Abilities (McCarthy, 1972)
      1. Ages: 2.5 to 8.5 years
      2. Application: The McCarthy includes measures of verbal and nonverbal subtests with five subscales: Verbal, Perceptual-Performance, Quantita-

(Cont.)

TABLE 7-2   *(Continued)*

tive, Memory, and Motor. The first three subscales can be combined to obtain a General Cognitive Index, with a distribution similar to a total IQ score.

H. Leiter International Performance Scale (Leiter, 1948)
  1. Ages: 2 years to adult
  2. Application: The Leiter is a nonverbal measure of general cognitive ability that requires no verbal instructions. Since mental ages are obtained, IQs can be estimated at the lower end of the normal distribution.

I. Woodcock-Johnson Revised: Tests of Cognitive Ability (Woodcock & Johnson, 1989)
  1. Ages: 2 years to adult
  2. Application: The cognitive subtests of the WJ-R are divided into seven subscale clusters: Long-Term Retrieval, Short-Term Memory, Processing Speed, Auditory Processing, Visual Processing, Comprehension-Knowledge, and Fluid Reasoning.

II. Achievement

A. Wide Range Achievement Test—Third Edition (WRAT-3) (Wilkinson, 1993)
  1. Ages: 5–75 years
  2. Application: The WRAT-3 is a measure of basic reading, spelling, and arithmetic skills.

B. Woodcock-Johnson Revised: Tests of Achievement (Woodcock & Johnson, 1989)
  1. Ages: 2–90 years
  2. Application: The achievement subtests from the WJ-R are divided into five subscale clusters: Reading, Mathematics, Written Language, Knowledge, and Skills.

C. Wechsler Individual Achievement Test (WIAT) (The Psychological Corporation, 1992)
  1. Ages: 5–19 years
  2. Application: The WIAT is a series of subtests designed to measure academic achievement skills across four areas: Reading, Mathematics, Language, and Writing. It was normed on the same sample as the WISC-III and can therefore be used to calculate difference scores between predicted and actual achievement levels.

D. Peabody Individual Achievement Test—Revised (PIAT-R) (Markwardt, 1989)
  1. Ages: 5–18 years
  2. Application: The PIAT-R measures academic achievement in the areas of Mathematics, Reading, Recognition, Reading Comprehension, Spelling, Written Expression, and General Information.

III. Language

A. Test of Language Development—Second Edition (TOLD-2) (Newcomer & Hammill, 1991)
  1. Ages: 4–12 years
  2. Application: The TOLD provides measures of receptive and expressive

TABLE 7-2 *(Continued)*

language skills. It employs measures of phonology, syntax, morphology, and semantics.

B. Clinical Evaluation of Language Fundamentals—Revised (CELF-R) (Semel, Wiig, & Secord, 1987)
   1. Ages: 5–16 years
   2. Application: The CELF-R provides measures of receptive and expressive language skills. Measures of verbal fluency and auditory comprehension are also available.

C. Peabody Picture Vocabulary Test—Revised (PPVT-R) (Dunn & Dunn, 1981)
   1. Ages: 2.5 to 40 years
   2. Application: The PPVT-R is a test of receptive one-word picture vocabulary.

D. Expressive One-Word Picture Vocabulary Test (EOWPVT) (Gardner, 1990)
   1. Ages: 2.5 to adult
   2. Application: The EOWPVT is a test of receptive one-word picture vocabulary.

E. Receptive One-Word Picture Vocabulary Test (ROWPVT) (Gardner, 1985)
   1. Ages: 2.5 to adult
   2. Application: The ROWPVT is a test of expressive picture-naming ability.

IV. Visual/Spatial
A. Beery Developmental Test of Visual Motor Integration (VMI) (Beery, 1989)
   1. Ages: 2–18 years
   2. Application: The VMI is a paper-and-pencil test of visual-motor integration. It requires the reproduction of geometric designs within a structured format.

B. Bender Visual-Motor Gestalt Test (Bender, 1938)
   1. Ages: 5 to adult
   2. Application: The Bender-Gestalt is a paper-and-pencil test of visual-motor integration. It requires the reproduction of geometric designs within a free copy format.

C. Test of Visual Perceptual Skills (TVPS) (Gardner, 1982)
   1. Ages: 4–10 years
   2. Application: The TVPS is a test of visual/spatial perception that requires very little motor response.

V. Attention and Memory
A. Continuous Performance Test (CPT) (Conners, 1992)
   1. Ages: 4 years to adult
   2. Application: The CPT is a computerized measure of sustained attention. It requires attention to visually presented verbal stimuli with the identification of a predetermined target. The CPT requires a response for each nontarget stimulus.

B. Gordon Diagnostic System (Gordon, 1983)
   1. Ages: 4 years to adult
   2. Application: The Gordon is a computerized measure of sustained attention. It requires attention to visually presented verbal stimuli with

(Cont.)

TABLE 7-2   *(Continued)*

the identification of a predetermined target sequence. The Gordon requires a response for each target sequence.

C. Test of Memory and Learning (TOMAL) (Reynolds & Bigler, 1994)
 1. Ages: 5–19 years
 2. Application: The TOMAL is a comprehensive battery for the assessment of immediate and delayed verbal and nonverbal memory.

D. Wide Range Assessment of Memory and Learning (WRAML) (Sheslow & Adams, 1990)
 1. Ages: 5–17 years
 2. Application: The WRAML is a battery of tests for the assessment of learning and memory.

E. Wechsler Memory Scale—Revised (WMS-R) (Wechsler, 1987)
 1. Ages: 20–75 years
 2. Application: The WMS-R is a battery of tests for the assessment of verbal and nonverbal memory that also measures attention and delayed recall.

VI. Behavioral Measures

A. Vineland Adaptive Behavior Scales (Sparrow, Balla & Cicchetti, 1984)
 1. Ages: Birth to 18 years
 2. Application: The Vineland is a structured interview of parents or a person familiar with the patient. It assesses behavior in four areas: Communication, Daily Living Skills, Socialization, and Motor Skills.

B. Conners Rating Scales (Goyette, Conners & Ulrich, 1978)
 1. Ages: 3–17 years
 2. Application: The Conners Rating Scales include checklists completed by parents and teachers to identify disruptive behavior at home and in the classroom.

C. Child Behavior Checklist (CBCL) (Achenbach & Edelbrock, 1983)
 1. Ages: 4–18 years
 2. Application: The CBCL includes checklists completed by parents and teachers to identify disruptive behavior at home and in the classroom.

D. Beck Depression Inventory (BDI) (Beck et al., 1961)
 1. Ages: Adults
 2. Application: The BDI is a self-report measure of depressive symptomatology.

E. Reynolds Depression Scales (RD) (Reynolds, 1986, 1988)
 1. Ages: 8–17 years
 2. Application: The RDS is a self-report measure of childhood and adolescent depression.

F. Revised Children's Manifest Anxiety Scale (R-SMAS) (Reynolds & Richmond, 1985)
 1. Ages: 6–17 years
 2. Application: The R-CMAS is a self-report measure of anxiety in children, comprising four scales: Physiological Anxiety, Worry/ Oversensitivity, Social Concerns/Concentration, and Lie.

TABLE 7-2 *(Continued)*

G. Minnesota Multiphasic Personality Inventory—Second Edition (MMPI-2) (Butcher et al., 1989)
  1. Ages: 18 years to adult
  2. Application: The MMPI-2 is a self-report measure of psychopathology that includes scales of clinical symptoms and test validity.
H. Minnesota Multiphasic Personality Inventory—Adolescent Version (MMPI-A) (Butcher et al., 1992)
  1. Ages: 14–18 years)
  2. Application: The MMPI-A is a self-report measure of psychopathology that includes scales of clinical symptoms and test validity.

an applicable range of 16 to 75 years (Wechsler, 1981). The determination of which of these tests to use must be based on a variety of factors. A follow-up assessment of a 16-year-old who had taken the WISC-III at the age of 13 years might best be accomplished by repeating the same test so that a direct comparison of change can be made. However, an initial evaluation of a 16-year-old who is expected to be reevaluated in 24 months following a therapeutic intervention would best be accomplished by administering the WAIS-R so that the same test can be given to the patient at 18 years of age. Assessment of patients who fall in the age range where the tests overlap and who appear to be in either the lower or upper range of general ability also require special consideration. Sixteen-year-olds who appear to be functioning in the borderline or mental retardation range are best assessed with the WISC-III to avoid a significant floor effect, while 16-year-olds who appear unusually bright or gifted are best assessed with the WAIS-R to avoid a significant ceiling effect.

TEST RESULTS

Results of psychological testing are the basis of interpretations and recommendations that influence the education and treatment of the patient and thus need to be error-free. Until the examiner is quite proficient with the specific tests, results should be rechecked for errors in scoring or addition. Results that suggest functioning that is at odds with general appearance or previous test results should routinely be rechecked for errors as well.

All results should be examined in regard to overall levels as well as for relative and overall strengths and weaknesses. Overall levels can be examined on the basis of standardized or scaled scores. Strengths and weaknesses are determined by comparing scores to one another. Overall strengths and weaknesses are scores falling above or below the average range, respectively.

Relative strengths and weaknesses are scores falling significantly above or below the mean performance level of the individual patient. That is, a WAIS-R subtest score of 6 on Vocabulary is an overall weakness for the patient but may be a relative strength if all other subtests scores are 3 or below.

To facilitate comparison of the patient's abilities, test results should be transformed into uniform scaled scores. Any scaled score with which the examiner is comfortable working is acceptable, although certain tests present results in a standard score format (i.e., mean of 100 and standard deviation of 15), and transformation of scores into this format is advised. The only major difficulty arises when scores are calculated in a variety of formats, which makes comparisons between tests difficult. For example, the determination of strengths and weaknesses in an individual with an IQ of 80, a continuous performance attention measure at a T score of 37, a visual-motor integration score at the 9th percentile, and language measures falling at a Z score of −1.33 may be quite difficult. If all these scores are placed on the same scale, one would find them to be entirely equivalent. All scaled or standard scores can be transformed into any other scale by using the following formula:

$$ SS_n = \left[\left[\left[\frac{(X - \mu_1)}{\sigma_1} \right] \bullet \sigma_2 \right] + \mu_2 \right] $$

where

SS_n = the new standard score.
X = the raw score or the unconverted standard score for the patient.
μ_1 = the mean for the patient's demographic group or the original standard score distribution.
μ_2 = the mean of the new standard score distribution.
σ_1 = the standard deviation of the original standard score distribution.
σ_2 = the standard deviation of the new standard score distribution.

For example, suppose one wanted to convert the results of a continuous performance test with a T score of 59 to the same distribution as the WISC-III. Using the formula, one would find:

$$ 113.5 = \left[\left(\frac{59 - 50}{10} \right) \bullet 15 \right] + 100 $$

This procedure works for all measures of correct performance or time on task. For error measures (e.g., number incorrect, time to achieve correct response, reaction time) a slight modification of the formula is required in order to maintain consistency in the direction of the standard score (e.g., a high number indicates a good performance). This modification is as follows:

$$SS_n = \left[\left[\left[\frac{(\mu_1 - X)}{\sigma_1} \right] \bullet \sigma_2 \right] + \mu_2 \right]$$

Presentation of scores to other professionals, the patient, parents, or significant others is another consideration in the use of test results. Many individuals may not be familiar with the shape or range of a distribution of standard scores. Often the presentation of scores in percentiles will be comprehended by a wider range of audiences. With young children, presentation of results in developmental levels (e.g., Receptive Language at the 2.5 year level) may be comprehended better by parents.

Interpretation

Test results must not be interpreted in isolation. Data should be viewed in light of behavioral observations, medical tests, and previous psychological test findings. The degree of motivation and effort put forth on testing can greatly influence the interpretation of results. Under conditions of low motivation, patients' abilities will be vastly underestimated and thus lead to unjustified recommendations if interpreted blindly.

The overall level of performance as well as variability of test data should be examined. For example, performance on standard measures of intelligence must include examination of Full Scale, Verbal, and Performance IQs. However, an examination of the individual's performance across subtests is often more telling in the identification of pathology. Although an individual's overall IQ score may be well within the average range, impairment on select subtests can cause significant problems.

Report Writing

Reports are written for a variety of purposes and to a variety of individuals. The purpose of the report and the audience to whom it is written will determine the style and content. Traditional outpatient evaluations of cognitive and/or emotional/personality functioning should be of a different style and length than inpatient evaluations or consultations to primary care physicians.

Traditional outpatient evaluations should include at least several report sections. These sections include but are not limited to: Presenting Problems, Background Information, Behavioral Observations, Tests Administered, Test Interpretation, and Implications and Recommendations.

The section on Presenting Problems will include at least one paragraph reviewing the circumstances leading up to the evaluation. The section on Background Information or History can often be quite long and typically is broken into subsections. These subsections include a further description of the nature and history of the present condition, medical history, birth history, developmental history, academic history, vocational history (if appropriate), family history, and a history of peer and/or social interactions. Behavioral Observations can include comprehensive or brief descriptions of relevant abnormalities. Behavioral Observations should include discussion of the relevant findings in the categories outlined in Table 7-1.

Due to the need for quick turnaround, typically within 24 hours, inpatient assessment reports are usually much more brief and direct. In medical settings these reports will usually be one to two pages in length and focus on test interpretation and recommendations. For further discussion on the evaluation of inpatients see Chapter 6.

The reporting of test results poses other issues. Test results can be presented in either tabular or narrative format. When presented to busy professionals, such as pediatricians or internal medicine physicians, the presentation of results in narrative format may be overlooked or misinterpreted. Additionally, if not already provided in the report, school officials will request the actual test data. For these reasons, it is suggested that major data be presented in a table, with summarization for major processes rather than long narratives. These summaries will draw attention to major conclusions without losing other professionals or laypeople.

Test findings can be organized by presenting information by test or by process. Although discussion of findings by test is often easier to do, tests often overlap or require comparison to make valid and accurate conclusions. Thus, rather than presenting separate paragraphs for each individual test, organization of tests and subtests into processes is advised. For example, the Test Interpretation section of the report could include the following subsections: Intellectual Abilities, Academic Functioning, Language and Communication, Visual Motor Integration, and Emotional and Behavioral Functioning.

The Implications and Recommendations section of the report will be the one the majority of readers paid most attention to, and thus should be a focus of the report. All too often, reports are written with an in-depth coverage of background information, test results, and interpretations but end weakly due to a lack of sufficient conclusions and recommendations. The purpose of the psychological testing should be to provide data that suggest differential treatment. The Implementations and Recommendations section should include at least one paragraph that pulls together the presenting problem and the major test results. It should not simply summarize what is reported in previous sections, but instead should make conclusions that explain the patient's problems based on observations, test data, and knowledge of psychological disorders.

Following these conclusions, specific, realistic recommendations should be made. Recommendations are frequently recalled and implemented better if laid out clearly and specifically, for example in a numbered list or outline. Recommendations should be presented in order of importance and sequentially if contingent upon one another. For example, a recommendation that the patient should have a physical examination should come before a recommendation of beginning an exercise program and a recommendation for a neurological exam to rule out seizure activity should precede a recommendation for a medication management program for stimulant therapy.

Recommendations presented in a report can be viewed as a "recipe" for the patient. The following samples illustrate inappropriate and appropriate types of recommendations.

Samuel should be referred to a therapist for psychological treatment of his behavioral problem. *(inappropriate)*

OR

Based upon current research findings, it is recommended that Samuel begin a behavioral management program in the home and school environments to address his aggressive and oppositional behavior. Such a program will require parental and teacher participation through the employment of a structured schedule of consequences for appropriate and inappropriate behaviors. This program can be initiated by contacting Dr. Julia Smith at 555-4949 or Dr. Peter Jones at 555-6234. *(appropriate)*

Feedback

Feedback should differ according to the recipient. In most circumstances the written report should not take the place of an individual feedback session. It is the examiner's responsibility to ensure the material is comprehended by the recipient. To this end, presentation of data to parents, patients, referring physicians, or school or vocational systems will differ appropriately. Feedback to individuals who are emotionally tied to the patient (e.g., relatives or the patients themselves) should be presented more sensitively. Often such information is best presented in terms of relative strengths and weaknesses. Presenting parents or the patient with scientifically descriptive terminology is useless in most cases and often offensive. Rather than reporting to parents that their child's IQ falls in the Mild range of mental retardation, one will impart more information with a statement like the following: "Your child's general cognitive functioning falls at the 2nd percentile. Sam's strengths appear to be in the area of general word knowledge and visual-spatial organization, while he seems to be having difficulty with abstract reasoning and problem solving." Such statements are not likely to offend people. For the patient's sake, it is important not to antagonize the patient or the parents, or the specific recommendations are less likely to be followed. Ending feedback sessions with positive information, such as discussions of strengths, will lead to a higher degree of compliance.

School systems often require more specific information to implement services. Although federal guidelines exist specifying categories of services, criteria for specific disabilities are defined by the individual school districts. Some districts will base decisions for learning disability (LD) placement on significant grade level discrepancies (e.g., 1.5 to 2.5 grades below current grade placement), while other districts will define LD as a significant ability–achievement discrepancy (e.g., Standard scores on achievement tests > 18 points below general intelligence). Districts will at times refuse to accept certain measures of intellectual or academic functioning, which is another reason to contact officials prior to test administration. Before presenting test results to a school counselor at an individual educational planning (IEP) meeting, one should contact the local school board to get a copy of the specific criteria used in that district. Presentation of test data to the IEP using the district's terminology will result in a more effective course of action for getting services for the patient.

Feedback to adult patients should be conducted prior to discussing results with others involved in the case. Again, this feedback should be presented in a manner sensitive to the patients' feelings. Although all relevant results need to be discussed with patients, terminology should be selected wisely to avoid offending them. Ideally, the patient should be left informed and with realistic expectations of treatments or interventions available to them. Feedback to individuals in vocational or educational systems that is requested by the patient should also be discussed with the patient prior to this feedback being given. The patient should be aware of what will be made available to the other recipients, although this should in no way dictate the interpretations of the results.

Psychological assessment is a time-consuming process that often results in a major impact on a patient's life, both in determination of financial and educational services as well as self-esteem. The process needs to receive the utmost attention to detail and procedural control, so that it produces an accurate portrayal of the individual that will lead to the provision of any help needed.

REFERENCES

Achenbach, T., & Edelbrock, C. (1983). *Manual for the Child Behavior Checklist and Revised Child Behavior Profile.* Burlington: University of Vermont.

Barkley, R. (1990). *Attention-deficit hyperactivity disorder: A handbook for diagnosis and treatment.* New York: Guilford Press.

Beck, A., Ward, C., Mendelson, M., Mock, J., & Erbaugh, J. (1961). An inventory for measuring depression. *Archives of General Psychiatry, 4,* 561–571.

Beery, K. (1989). *The Developmental Test of Visual-Motor Integration: Administration, scoring, and teaching manual* (3d rev.). Cleveland, OH: Modern Curriculum Press.

Bender, L. (1938). *A visual motor Gestalt test and its clinical use.* New York: American Orthopsychiatric Association.

Butcher, J., Dahlstrom, W., Graham, J., Tellegen, A., & Kaemmer, B. (1989). *MMPI-2: Manual for administration and scoring.* Minneapolis: University of Minnesota Press.

Butcher, J., Williams, C., Graham, J., Archer, R., Tellegen, A., Ben-Porath, Y., & Kaemmer, B. (1992). *MMPI-A: Manual for administration, scoring, and interpretation.* Minneapolis: University of Minnesota Press.

Conners, C. (1992). *Continuous Performance test computer program.* North Tonawanda, NY: Multi-Health Systems.

Dunn, L., & Dunn, L. (1981). *Peabody Picture Vocabulary Test—Revised manual.* Circle Pines, MN: American Guidance Service.

Elliott, C. (1990). *Differential Abilities Scale: Administration and scoring manual.* San Antonio, TX: The Psychological Corporation.

Forehand, R., & McMahon, R. (1981). *Helping the noncompliant child: A clinician's Guide to Parent Training.* New York: Guilford Press.

Gardner, M. (1982). *Test of Visual-Perceptual Skills (non-motor): Manual.* Los Angeles: Western Psychological Services.

Gardner, M. (1985). *Receptive One-Word Picture Vocabulary Test: Manual and form.* Novato, CA: Academic Therapy.

Gardner, M. (1990). *Expressive One-Word Picture Vocabulary Test—Revised: Manual and form.* Novato, CA: Academic Therapy.

Gordon, M. (1983). *The Gordon diagnostic system.* Dewitt, NY: Gordon Systems.

Goyette, C., Conners, C., & Ulrich, R. (1978). Normative data on Revised Conners Parent and Teacher Rating Scales. *Journal of Abnormal Child Psychology, 6,* 221–236.

Kaufman, A., & Kaufman, N. (1983). *Kaufman assessment battery for children.* Circle Pines, MN: American Guidance Service.

Leiter, R. (1948). *Leiter international performance scale.* Chicago: Stoelting.

Lezak, M. (1995). *Neuropsychological assessment* (3d Ed.). New York: Oxford University Press.

Markwardt, F. (1989). *Peabody individual achievement test—revised.* Circle Pines, MN: American Guidance Service.

McCarthy, D. (1972). *Manual for the McCarthy Scales of Children's Abilities.* San Antonio, TX: The Psychological Corporation.

Newcomer, P. & Hammill, D. (1991). *Test of language development—second edition.* Austin, TX: Pro-Ed.

Reports of the INS-Division 40 Task Force on Education, Accreditation, and Credentialing (1987). *The Clinical Neuropsychologist, 1,* 29–34.

Reynolds, C., & Bigler, E. (1994). *The test of memory and learning.* Austin, TX: Pro-Ed.

Reynolds, C., & Richmond, B. (1985). *What I think and feel (RCMAS).* Los Angeles: Western Psychological Services.

Reynolds, W. (1986). *Reynolds adolescent depression scale.* Odessa, FL: Psychological Assessment Resources.

Reynolds, W. (1988). *Reynolds child depression scale.* Odessa, FL: Psychological Assessment Resources.

Sattler, J. (1992). Assessment of children: Revised and updated third edition. San Diego, CA: Author.

Semel, E., Wiig, E., & Secord W. (1987). *Clinical Evaluation of Language Fundamentals— Revised: Examiner's manual.* San Antonio, TX: The Psychological Corporation.

Sheslow, D., & Adams, W. (1990). *Wide range assessment of memory and learning.* Wilmington, DE: Jastak Associates.

Sparrow, S., Balla, D., & Cicchetti, D. (1984). *Vineland adaptive behavior scale.* Circle Pines, MN: American Guidance Service.

Spreen, O., & Strauss, E. (1991). *A Compendium of neuropsychological tests: Asministration, norms, and commentary.* New York: Oxford University Press.

Thorndike, R. L., Hagen, E.P ., & Sattler, J. M. (1986). *The Stanford-Binet Intelligence Scale: Fourth Edition. Guide for Administering and Scoring* (2d Ed.). Chicago: Riverside.

Wechsler, D. (1981). *Wechsler adult intelligence scale—revised.* San Antonio, TX: The Psychological Corporation.

Wechsler, D. (1987). *Wechsler Memory Scale—Revised: Manual.* San Antonio, TX: The Psychological Corporation.

Wechsler, D. (1989). *Wechsler preschool and primary scale of intelligence—revised.* San Antonio, TX: The Psychological Corporation.

Wechsler, D. (1991). *Wechsler intelligence scale for children—third edition.* San Antonio, TX: The Psychological Corporation.

Wilkinson, G. (1993). *The Wide Range Achievement Test: Administration manual.* Wilmington, DE: Wide Range.

Woodcock, R., & Johnson, M. (1989). *Woodcock-Johnson revised psychoeducational battery.* Allen, TX: DLM Teaching Resources.

▶ 8

Record Keeping

LEON VANDECREEK   SAMUEL KNAPP

Records play an important role in patient care today. Trainees will learn quickly that their field placement settings place strong emphasis on record-keeping requirements, both in terms of content and timeliness of record entries. Most agencies will have a records department or a person designated to oversee all clinical records, although teaching about record keeping may occur at the departmental or unit level.

In years past, record keeping by psychologists was variable in quality and quantity, varying largely by requirements of their institutional settings. In private practice settings, records were even more inconsistent, with some psychologists reportedly keeping no records at all. A survey of the American Psychological Association's (APA) Division 29 (Psychotherapy) members showed that 12% of the respondents typically limited treatment documentation to the patient's name, date of service, and fee (Pope, Tabachnick, & Keith-Spiegel, 1987).

In recent years, especially as insurance companies, governmental agencies, and other entities have become key players in patient care, psychologists have needed to give more attention to their record-keeping practices. Nonetheless, psychology as a health care discipline does not have a single record keeping format to which all practitioners adhere.

At least in part to strengthen the record-keeping practices of psychologists and to gain at least some consensus on record keeping, the APA Committee on Professional Practice and Standards (COPPS) developed, and the

---

*The views expressed here do not necessarily represent those of the Pennsylvania Psychological Association.

APA Council of Representatives approved, the document entitled *Record Keeping Guidelines* (1993). The *Guidelines* provides only general assistance with record keeping, however, recognizing that records will be governed extensively by agency and funding requirements and by state laws and regulations.

This chapter provides an overview of the purposes of records, common rules of thumb about the content of records, guidelines for record retention and destruction, access to records, release of records, record ownership, and confidentiality of records.

PURPOSES OF RECORD KEEPING

A record is any information (including that stored in a computer) that concerns the professional treatment of patients. Records serve several purposes, including chronicling the care of the patient, refreshing the psychologist's memory if the patient returns to treatment after a period of time, conveying information to other or future treatment providers, documenting or justifying treatment for third-party payers such as insurance companies or accrediting and review bodies, building archival databases that can be used for outcome research, and providing a means of defense in the event of an allegation of professional negligence. Each of these functions will be described in more detail here.

Psychologists use the record to document the presenting complaints, assessment, and ongoing care of patients. The record should provide a clear "paper trail" of the patient's care to anyone who might review it. As part of the treatment process, record keeping also forces the psychologist to give serious thought to the treatment plan and progress of the patient.

If patients discontinue treatment and return at some later date, the record documents the clinical issues and treatment progress. Psychologists should not rely on their memories alone or the self-report of their former patients for a thorough account of what transpired months or years earlier. Records also inform new treatment providers about the patient's earlier symptoms, diagnoses, treatment plans, success of treatment, and other clinical data.

Insurance companies and other payers for psychological services typically require providers to keep records. They may have specific record keeping requirements beyond those of practitioners. Furthermore, third-party payers increasingly require copies of records or summaries of records as a precondition for reimbursement for services. The frequency of review of records by payers has increased substantially with the proliferation of managed care systems.

Most provider agencies are accredited or licensed by state or federal bodies, which enables the agencies to provide services and receive reimbursement for care. These credentialing and reimbursement bodies have record keeping requirements that are unique and may be enforced by periodic site visits.

Records can be used as a source of outcome data on patients. Although the average psychologist will not be conducting outcome research of the quality that appears in a peer reviewed journal, many psychologists and agencies gather data such as basic screening information, length of treatment, level of patient satisfaction, and so forth as a means of self-evaluation or for marketing of services. Third-party payers, especially managed care companies, increasingly request data on patient satisfaction and length of treatment as part of the application to become a provider.

Finally, records are crucial as a defense in cases of alleged negligence. An axiom of risk management is "If it is not documented, it did not occur." Very often court decisions come down to the credibility of persons who give contradictory statements of what did or did not occur. Good documentation (the paper trail) provides substantial support for practitioners. Lack of documentation or inadequate documentation can make the difference between a successful or unsuccessful outcome of a lawsuit. In other instances, records can influence the decision about whether a case goes to court at all (Soisson, VandeCreek, & Knapp, 1987). Because the plaintiff's attorneys will have access to the records, they may elect not to proceed with the case if the record fails to give evidence of substandard care (Woody, 1988). On the other hand, poor records have been a major factor in determining that mental health professionals provided inadequate treatment (e.g., *Abille v. United States*, 1980).

RULES GOVERNING RECORD KEEPING

The rules governing record keeping, data storage, and release of patient information are determined by a combination of laws, regulations, case law (court cases), and ethics codes (those of the APA and those included in state licensure laws). Except for the APA *Ethics Code* (1992) these regulations vary considerably from state to state and, within states, according to the facility in which treatment is provided. In addition, as previously noted, institutions such as hospitals, schools, drug and alcohol treatment facilities, and public mental health centers typically have record-keeping requirements beyond those mandated by ethics codes and licensure boards.

Despite the variations in requirements, there is some uniformity in rules. Psychologists who belong to the APA are bound by the APA *Ethical Principles of Psychologists and Code of Conduct* (APA, 1992; hereafter referred to as the *Ethics Code*). Furthermore, this code or similar codes are part of the regulations upheld by many state licensure boards for psychologists. As already noted, the APA has adopted record-keeping guidelines (1993) that, like the code of ethics, may be binding on psychologists through the actions of their state licensure boards.

CONTENTS OF RECORDS

One of the most vexing questions about records is what should be included. Some general guidance comes from the APA *Ethics Code* (1992) and the *Record Keeping Guidelines* (1993). The *Ethics Code* states that "[P]sychologists appropriately document their professional and scientific work in order to facilitate provision of services later by them or by other professionals, to ensure accountability, and to meet other requirements of institutions or the law" (1992, section 1.23 (a)).

Good records are

- Comprehensive
- Objective
- Consistent
- Retrievable
- Secure
- Current.

Failure in any of these characteristics may create difficulties for psychologists sometime in the future.

Comprehensive

The APA's *Record Keeping Guidelines* (1993) states that records should include at least: "(a) identifying data, (b) dates of services, (c) types of services, (d) fees, (e) any assessment, plan for intervention, consultation, summary reports, and/or testing reports and supporting data as may be appropriate, and (f) any release of information obtained" (p. 3). The authors recommend that records include additional information such as the diagnosis or presenting problem; factual basis for the diagnosis; dates and substance of treatment; correspondence with the patient; intake sheets (if any); notations of phone calls and all other therapeutic contacts; and collateral contacts with physicians, attorneys, family members, and others. Custody arrangements of children should also be included.

Client productions such as letters, cards, poems, or diaries should be placed in the record. It is advisable to obtain permission from patients about the eventual disposition of these materials, as some patients may value their productions and want them returned.

Records should include a discharge summary or final note for the patient that reviews the course of treatment and relates the diagnosis to the way the treatment plan was implemented.

Many practitioners anticipate questions from their patients by developing service brochures, or descriptions of the fees, billing arrangements, office hours, and other office policies. It is desirable to give the service brochure to the patient and note this fact in the record.

Any special financial arrangements, such as waiving copayments (which is permissible on a case-by-case basis; see Knapp & VandeCreek, 1993) or providing services at a reduced or pro bono rate, should be noted in the record.

Psychotherapists should document high-risk situations very carefully. Situations such as suspected child abuse, threats of violence toward self and others, or transference problems are often the basis of allegations of negligence. Mental health providers are usually not found liable for negligence only because an unfortunate event occurred (e.g., suicide, homocide). That is, the fact of a negative outcome is not by itself proof of negligence. If a court concludes that negligence occurred, the finding will be based on a failure to adequately assess or treat the patient, not on the outcome alone. The best way to document adequacy of treatment is through the use of well-kept records. Ideally, agencies have standardized procedures for assessing and documenting such high-risk clinical situations.

Other high-risk situations that should be noted clearly in the record are extreme resistance to the treatment plan, noncompliance with portions of the treatment, cancelled or missed appointments, or arriving under the influence of alcohol or other drugs.

The need for comprehensive records is especially important in situations in which psychologists believe their professional services will be used in legal proceedings. In these situations the APA *Ethics Code* states that psychologists "have a responsibility to create and maintain documentation in the kind of detail and quality that would be consistent with reasonable scrutiny in an adjudicative forum" (APA, 1992, section 1.23 (b)).

Records for group therapy should be individualized for each patient. The names of other group members should not appear in individual patient records. Some group therapists develop a "process" file for the group as a whole, but such a file does not include individual client names.

Family therapy raises special issues for record keeping. A single record for family therapy is appropriate when the focus of treatment is on the family. In contrast, the record should identify an individual as the recipient of treatment when that individual is the central focus of care, even if other family members sometimes participate in the therapy. The decisive issue here is the specification of the "identified patient." When a single person is the patient, the record should be kept in the individual patient's name; when the "patient" is the family, the record should be listed under the family name.

There will likely be insurance reimbursement implications for record keeping with families as well in light of the fact that many insurance policies will not reimburse for family therapy, although they may reimburse for individual therapy when other family members attend sessions to benefit the individual's treatment.

Psychologists need to obtain special permission from patients, with documentation in the record, for audio or visual recordings of sessions. Patients should understand the reason for the recording and what will be done with the recording. Patients have a right to be fully informed about matters such as whether the recording will be destroyed after review, used for training purposes, shown to general audiences at other sites, etcetera. When there are unusual issues dealing with confidentiality of the record, psychologists should note the discussion and conclusion about them in the record.

Objective

As much as possible, the treatment record should be objective. The psychotherapeutic process is inherently subjective. Psychologists necessarily relate to their patients as human beings with feelings. Nevertheless, statements in the chart should be as objective as possible. Psychotherapists should use behavioral descriptions whenever possible and avoid vague statements such as "He has control problems." Something more behavioral is preferred, such as "He was upset when his secretary went away on her vacation and he put his fist through the wall of his office." Direct quotes from patients may be helpful in creating an objective record.

Psychotherapists record only material relevant to the care of the patient. Embarrassing facts should be included only if they are relevant to treatment. Tentative conclusions and impressions should be identified as such.

Psychotherapists write all records as if the patient will read them. Although the record belongs to the provider, the patient has a "property interest" in it, and as will be discussed later, state and federal regulations and the courts have increasingly granted patients the right to review their records. Pejorative comments seen by the patient may evoke anger and create a perception of the therapist as insensitive and uncaring.

Consistent

Conscientious psychologists look for consistency in their treatment records. The treatment plan created when the patient entered therapy should be consistent with the diagnosis used months later. If there is a difference, the reason for the change in the diagnosis or the treatment plan should be documented.

Under no circumstances should a psychotherapist alter or delete sections of a record. Rather, if a correction or addition to a record is needed, the new material is added to the current section of the record with a note indicating that this entry clarifies or corrects an earlier entry.

Retrievable

Although it is not unethical to be inefficient, competent practitioners try to keep records easily retrievable. Handwritten notes are acceptable, although it is important that they be legible so others can read them. An efficient filing system saves time. This means more than just placing the charts in a file in alphabetical order in a file cabinet; it also means having a specific location (or specific color) in the chart for intake forms, release of information forms, treatment notes, and other information. Each entry is properly dated and signed. If records are kept on computer files and security codes are used, at least one person in addition to the person doing the entry must know the code so that the records can be accessed if the recorder leaves employment or dies.

Secure

Records are kept in a secure place. According to the APA *Ethics Code* (1992), "[P]sychologists maintain appropriate confidentiality in creating, storing, accessing, transferring, and disposing of records under their control, whether these are written, automated, or in any other medium (APA, 1992, section 5.04). It is inappropriate to leave records in full view of patients (patients' names can be decifered from the file tab) or in piles on a desk where janitorial staff or others can read them. Generally, it is ill advised to take records home to work on them, although supervisors may be willing to make exceptions for trainees to complete assessment reports or other entries off site.

Current

Records should be kept current so that the resignation or death of a therapist does not jeopardize patient care. Ideally record entries should be made regularly, either after every session of care or after some specified number of sessions. Agencies typically have guidelines on both the preferred frequency of entries and their timeliness.

FORMATTING THE RECORD

The content of the record can be placed in many formats. Each agency and practitioner will have preferences or requirements that students will be expected to follow.

Progress and Process Notes

One distinction in note taking is made between process notes and progress notes. Process notes typically are written during or after each session and may include anything that comes to the therapist's mind about the patient. The notes may be written in private shorthand or personal style. Their function is to document the therapist's reactions, ideas, hypotheses, etcetera, regarding the patient.

Progress notes, on the other hand, describe treatment procedures, observations, and progress of the patient in more factual and descriptive fashion. The purpose of progress notes is to document treatment planning and services, and they are often written periodically rather than at each session. A standard format may be required. Some psychologists may use process notes as a source for making progress notes.

Some authors have recommended keeping both sets of notes, and we recommend this for training purposes. Because keeping both types of notes is cumbersome and time-consuming, however, most therapists and agencies do not do so on a regular basis.

It is important to note that both types of notes are discoverable by subpoena, so if process notes are kept, the writer is advised to keep in mind that the patient and the court may someday view them.

Major Record Formats

The three major formats for patient records are source-oriented, problem-oriented, and goal-oriented. Source-oriented records are most often used in settings where members of several disciplines must make entries in the record. Members of each discipline write their own notes in separate sections of the file. Each section of the source-focused record is kept chronologically.

In the problem-oriented record the treatment team or individual therapist makes a list of all relevant problems reported by the patient. Then all treatment decisions are based upon that list with the goal of alleviating the problems focused on in treatment. As a problem is addressed, the date is placed next to that problem on the list. The problem is never erased from the list, and new problems can be added to the list at any time. All entries in the record are explained and evaluated based on the identified and listed problems (Sturm, 1987).

The goal-oriented record is similar to the problem-oriented record in that the treatment team or individual therapist creates a list of goals from the intake and assessment information. All treatment decisions are aimed at reaching these goals, and all entries into the record are then evaluated based upon these treatment goals. Treatment ends when the goals have been met.

Many clinicians have contended that these formats for records are too cumbersome for everyday use. Variations have been proposed. For example,

Levenstein (1994) described the Problem-Intervention- Resistance-Change (PIRC) format. In this system therapeutic events are divided into four basic categories: problem or goal (P), intervention or plan (I), resistance or obstacle (R), and change indicators (C).

Computerized versions of record keeping systems are also available and are marketed extensively to private practices and small agencies.

PATIENT ACCESS TO RECORDS

According to the APA *Ethics Code* (1992), "[p]sychologists take reasonable and lawful steps so that records and data remain available to the extent needed to serve the best interests of patients, individual or organizational clients, research participants, or appropriate others" (section 5.10).

Generally speaking, patients have a right to obtain a copy of their medical records. Although the physical paper upon which the records appears belongs to the practitioner or health care facility, the patient has a right to possess or inspect a copy of the record. One of the exceptions to this rule, however, involves psychological or psychiatric records. In numerous states, laws or regulations permit psychotherapists to withhold limited amounts of information if it is in the best interest of the patient.

Occasionally patients' requests to see their records are a way of raising clinical issues such as "What does my therapist think of me?" or "What is wrong with me?" Usually it is sufficient to address these issues directly within psychotherapy without showing patients their records. In some instances, when the provider does not believe the patient should view the record, the patient will be satisfied or reassured if the provider prepares a summary of the record or an overview of the kinds of material that are contained in the record.

On other occasions, however, patients may insist on seeing or possessing a copy of their records. In these situations, psychologists need to understand the legal issues surrounding this request. The laws addressing patient access to psychological records vary from state to state and may even vary within the same state depending on the facility. Commonly, the laws allow mental health practitioners to withhold the records, or portions of the record, if it is believed that the patient will suffer harm from viewing them. A record may, for example, accurately record the diagnosis of a serious mental illness that would upset the patient if he or she were to read it. Agency policies will dictate how to proceed when portions of a record are withheld. In any case, the patient has a right to know that portions of the record have been withheld, and the patient may have the right to enjoin legal proceedings to obtain the full record. Each step in the process of patient access should be documented in the record.

If a decision is made to show the record to the patient, then the psychologist or someone else very familiar with the patient's care should be present to review the record with the patient. Patients seldom understand the technical terms used and may misconstrue the record unless someone is there to interpret. Sometimes it is possible to use the record review to refocus the patient on the treatment procedures and goals.

LIMITS TO CONFIDENTIALITY OF RECORDS

Confidentiality refers to the laws or rules of professional ethics that regulate the disclosure of information obtained in therapy. A related term, and one that is sometimes incorrectly used interchangeably, is *privileged communication*. Privileged communication is a narrower term than confidentiality, referring only to the legal right that protects patients, under certain circumstances, from having their communications revealed in court without their permission (Knapp & VandeCreek, 1987). Both concepts will be discussed in this section as they pertain to record keeping.

Few psychotherapists would make the error of gossiping about their patients. However, it is more common for inadvertent breaches of confidentiality to occur through quiet conversations in hallways, bathrooms, and elevators and through phone conversations with patients in the presence or within hearing of other patients in the office or waiting room. Care should be taken to prevent these disclosures from occurring.

Patients also expect their communications to their therapists and the records of their treatment to be kept confidential. Nonetheless, there are many exceptions to the principle of confidentiality, and patients have a right to be told of these relevant exceptions or limits as early in their treatment as possible. [See Chapter 1.]

The APA *Ethics Code* specifies:

> (a) Psychologists . . . discuss with persons and organizations with whom they establish a scientific or professional relationship (including, to the extent feasible, minors and their legal representatives) (1) the relevant limitations on confidentiality, including limitations where applicable in group, marital, and family therapy or in organizational consulting, and (2) the foreseeable uses of the information generated through their services. (b) Unless it is not feasible or is contraindicated, the discussion of confidentiality occurs at the outset of the relationship and thereafter as new circumstances may warrant" (APA, 1992, section 5.01)

It should be noted that the *Ethics Code* requires discussing with the patient only the relevant limitations to confidentiality. Psychologists are not required to recite a laundry list of remotely possible exceptions. On the other hand, the experiences of many psychotherapists have taught us that it is not possible to predict with accuracy where the content of therapy will lead, and it may be devastating to patients to learn that their admissions of child abuse, for example, must be reported to authorities in spite of expectations of confidentiality. Consequently, many agencies and private practitioners provide to new patients a service brochure that alerts readers to the fact that exceptions to confidentiality exist, along with some examples. More detailed discussions of the limitations can be held with the patient as the need arises.

Confidentiality with Family Members

Some of the most difficult questions concerning confidentiality occur when family members of patients inquire about treatment or volunteer information about the patient. Family members who feel uninformed or who do not understand the principle of confidentiality may be angered by the rules that prohibit them from discussing the status of their relatives in treatment. Psychotherapists can anticipate these problems and address them at the beginning of psychotherapy. Patients can be encouraged to sign release-of-information forms for certain family members. The best solution is to have family members involved in the therapy on a periodic basis to keep them informed or to have the patient regularly provide updates to family members. Another solution is to ask the patient to permit the therapist to discuss relevant issues with family members.

For the most part, parents control the access of their children to mental health treatment (some states have created narrow exceptions to this general rule). Consequently, parents have the right to access all information on their children. This right may create a conflict with some children, especially adolescents, in that the parents may have legitimate questions concerning high-risk behaviors such as alcohol and drug use or sexual activity. Open disclosure to parents about such information, however, may discourage adolescent patients from confiding in their psychotherapists and undercut the effectiveness of therapy.

Psychotherapists are wise to address these confidentiality issues with minors and their parents before treatment begins. It is wise to inform the parents of the need for confidentiality in the therapeutic process and to come to agreement about what types of disclosures, if any, will be made to them about their child's treatment. Some therapists who specialize in work with families and adolescents recommend that therapists agree at the outset to disclose to parents information about any behaviors that place the adolescent or another person in immediate physical danger. Regardless of the scope of the agreement on disclosure to parents, psychotherapists are responsible for setting the ground rules at the outset of treatment for both the parents and child and to summarize this agreement in the record.

Consensual Release of Information

Except in unusual situations, psychotherapists may not release information about patients without their consent. Although the APA *Ethics Code* (1992) does not specify that patient signatures are required for all requests to release information, prudent practitioners obtain signatures on all release-of-information forms. These signed forms provide irrefutable proof that the patient consented to the release. Surprisingly, Handelsman and colleagues (1986) found that only about one-third of psychologists in private practice use release-of-information forms, preferring to rely on oral agreements. The content of release of information forms varies according to state law. However, most states require at least the name of the patient; name of the psychologist permitted to make the disclosure; name of the person or organization sending and receiving the information; the specific information requested (e.g., progress notes, assessment report); dated signature of the patient (or patient's guardian); dated signature of a witness; and the date or circumstance under which the consent will expire, if it is not revoked earlier. Rarely would an entire record be sent. Copies of the release should be offered to the patient and a permanent copy should be placed in the patient's file.

Information received from a prior source should not be released. The release-of-information authorization applies only to the records that were generated by the setting releasing the information and not to records created elsewhere. Because each health care provider has a property interest in the records it has created, each provider should control, with the patient's consent, the dissemination of its records (Woody, 1988).

Patients' Review of Communications

It is often beneficial to review with the patient (or give the patient the option to review) the contents of letters or copies of materials from the record before they are mailed. Because these materials may affect the patient in unanticipated ways in the future, the patient should be fully informed both about the content of the disclosure and the potential uses to which the materials may be put.

Review of reports is especially important in interactions with third-party payers. The general principle to follow in sharing information with payers is to send them the least amount of information needed to obtain reimbursement. Information sent to payers may also be entered by them into national data banks that store all health care data and that are accessible to all subscribing insurance companies. Patients may be shocked to learn later that an application for mortgage insurance or a new life insurance policy, for example, has been declined based in part on these records of mental health treatment. Understandably, then, accurate and limited information must be submitted, and patients should be informed of the "not-so-private life" of their health insurance data. Some third-party payers are reportedly lax about confidentiality in their offices, as well, and patients have learned about their diagnoses from neighbors and others who were employed by insurance companies. Some patients will prefer to forego third-party reimbursement rather than risk the potential harm caused by disclosure of the data.

When communications surrounding reimbursement are made by telephone (with the patient's permission), the nature of the contact and the identity and position of the person to whom information was shared should be documented in the record in the event that there is a future disagreement about reimbursement.

Nonconsensual Release of Information

As previously noted, in some situations psychologists may or must release information about patients without their consent and even over their objections. According to the APA *Ethics Code*,

> Psychologists disclose confidential information without the consent of the individual only as mandated by law, or where permitted by law for a valid purpose, such as (1) to provide needed professional services to the patient or the individual or organizational client, (2) to obtain appropriate professional consultations, (3) to protect the patient or client or others from harm, or (4) to obtain payment for services, in which instance disclosure is limited to the minimum that is necessary to achieve the purpose. (APA, 1992, section 5.05)

The most common situations that mandate disclosure, even over the objections of the patient, are when the therapist suspects child abuse and when the therapist is treating a potentially dangerous patient.

Child Abuse Reporting

Psychologists are required in every state to report suspected child abuse. Although the definition of child abuse varies from state to state, it can include one or more of four categories: nonaccidental physical injury, neglect, sexual abuse, and emotional abuse. The definition of abuse in every state includes, at the least, nonaccidental physical injury and neglect.

In order for acts to constitute child abuse, the child must be under the age of 18 and the acts must be done by a care giver, parent, or guardian or the paramour of the parent or guardian. Similar acts to persons over the age of 18 are not child abuse, but could constitute the basis for a criminal charge. Harmful acts done by adults other than parents or other care givers may also be handled by the criminal justice codes, but such acts would not be considered child abuse.

Child abuse reporting laws require psychologists, along with other mandated reporters, to report when they believe or suspect that abuse has occurred. Absolute proof of abuse is not needed. In fact, psychologists and other mandatory reporters are not expected to conduct investigations into their suspicions about abuse. Rather, they are required to report whenever they are suspicious. The laws are written so that, if errors are to be made, therapists should err on the side of reporting when none exists, rather than not reporting when abuse in fact has occurred. The agency to whom such reports are to be made varies by jurisdiction. The patient's record should contain clear documentation of the decision to report.

States vary on the reporting requirement when the perpetrator of abuse alone seeks treatment. Some states require reporting when a perpetrator comes into treatment alone. In other states the reporting requirement applies only when the abused child comes into treatment. In the latter instance the report of abuse would not need to be made if the abuser admits to the behavior while in therapy, ostensibly to encourage abusers to obtain psychological help.

In circumstances in which psychotherapists are not required by their state law to report abuse, they may be permitted or required to do so by other regulations or ethics codes. For example, as noted in the next section, psychotherapists may break confidentiality when it is necessary to protect the life or safety of an identifiable third party. Consequently, a psychotherapist may have an obligation to report a perpetrator if the therapist believes that a child is in imminent danger of harm.

Mandatory reporting laws try to encourage reporting by providing incentives as well as penalties for failing to report. The laws provide immunity from lawsuits for those making reports in good faith as well as criminal penalties for those failing to report as required.

The Duty To Protect

The "duty to protect" refers to the 1976 California Supreme Court decision (*Tarasoff v. the University of California et al.*) that established standards of conduct for psychotherapists who are dealing with patients who present an imminent danger of substantial harm to an identifiable person or an identifiable class of persons. According to *Tarasoff*, psychotherapists should use reasonable care in assessing dangerousness of their patients and, if they believe that the patient poses immediate danger to identifiable others, then the psychotherapist should act to protect the potential victim(s).

Although the original *Tarasoff* decision applied only to California, no state court has ever overturned it. Furthermore, it is consistent with the APA *Ethics Code* (section 5.05) and has been incorporated into the statutes of several states.

The steps that the psychotherapist should take to fulfill this obligation vary depending upon the circumstances and state laws. The acceptable actions may include, but are not limited to, warning the intended victim(s) or someone who is likely to warn the potential victim, notifying the police, initiating a voluntary or involuntary commitment, increasing the frequency of psychotherapy, involving the targeted victim in therapy (especially if the victim is a family member), referring the patient for medication, or referring the patient to a more structured therapy program such as a partial hospitalization program (Monahan, 1993; VandeCreek & Knapp, 1993).

Record keeping becomes important in these situations because litigation is likely to occur when patients harm themselves or others. Regrettably, no box score or formula can be given to positively identify a "dangerousness quotient." However, dangerousness can be predicted with a modest degree of certainty by considering such items as past acts of violence, accessibility of weapons, abuse of alcohol or other drugs, or membership in a social support system that condones or encourages violence (Monahan & Steadman, 1994). In these circumstances, psychotherapists should document their assessments and interventions carefully. Consultations with colleagues and experts are especially encouraged, with documentation of the consultation placed in the patient's record. Even if the psychologist makes a mistake in the prediction of dangerousness, the record can be used to document that the psychologist used reasonable judgment in making treatment decisions (VandeCreek & Knapp, 1993).

Other Nonconsensual Release Situations

According to the APA *Ethics Code*, psychologists may share patient information for consultations without the prior consent of the patient (section 5.05). When consulting, psychologists avoid sharing information that could lead to the identification of a patient. We believe, however, that in many instances patients will be reassured by their therapists' desire to consult about their cases, and we prefer to make this issue part of the therapeutic process. For example, a therapist might say to a patient who is worried about obsessions of hurting a spouse,

> Your strong fears of acting on your obsessions about hurting your spouse are very troubling to you and I know that you want to be reassured that you can resist acting on these obsessions. With your permission, I'd like to consult with an expert on such obsessions to reassure both of us that we are "on track" with our treatment plan.

These consultations should be documented in the patient's record.

Privileged Communications

As noted earlier, privileged communications is a legal concept barring patient communications, under certain circumstances, from being introduced by therapists in court. Privileged communication laws were written to encourage and protect certain professional activities. For example, it is believed that the benefits of the stronger therapeutic alliance resulting from the psychologist/patient privilege outweighs the harm caused by withholding some information from being introduced into courtroom proceedings.

All privileged communication laws have exceptions, however. That is, there will be occasions when privileged information will be introduced in court, even over the objection of the patient, primarily when another law supercedes the privilege law or the court determines that the privileged information is indispensable to the case (Knapp & VandeCreek, 1987).

On the other hand, patients may waive their privilege whenever it suits them. In addition, patients automatically waive the privilege when they enter their mental health into issue, such as through a psychological malpractice claim, a personal injury lawsuit with a claim of emotional damage, or an insanity defense. The privilege also does not apply to the results of court-ordered psychological examinations or other evaluations in which the patient has been advised that the results will be disclosed to the other party, regardless of the results of the examination. Psychologists are obligated to inform or remind such patients that these reports will be shared with other legitimate parties.

When patients indicate their intentions to initiate legal actions that may bring into issue the status of their mental health, their psychotherapists should inform them of the potential pitfalls of waiving their privilege and of having their records reviewed by the court.

LENGTH OF TIME TO KEEP RECORDS

It is helpful for providers to receive the records of previous treatment providers. That material may help them understand the dynamics and history of the patient. However, treatment records lose their value as time goes by, and in some cases old records may be harmful if released.

The determination of the minimal length of time to keep records is typically controlled by each agency's regulations and/or by other accrediting or credentialing bodies such as state licensing boards. When record retention is not governed by agency or licensing board regulations, guidelines from professional associations may be followed. According to the APA *Ethics Code* (1992), "[p]sychologists maintain and dispose of records in accordance with law and in a manner that permits compliance with the requirements of this Ethics Code" (section 5.04). The *Record Keeping Guidelines* (APA, 1993) specifies that in the absence of guidance from laws and regulations, complete records are maintained for at least 3 years after the last contact with the patient. Records or a summary are then maintained for an additional 12 years before disposal. If the client is a minor, the record retention period is extended until 3 years after the age of majority.

When records are discarded, they should be shredded, burned, or otherwise destroyed beyond recognition. Regrettably, incidents have occurred in which records thrown into the garbage have been retrieved by members of the public.

At times, however, providers may want to keep records longer than the minimal period required. One of the most significant reasons to retain records for longer periods of time is the potential for lawsuits by ex-patients. Typically the statute of limitations for adults to bring suit against health care providers is 2 or 3 years after the injury occurred or after a reasonable person should have known that the behavior in question constituted malpractice. It is not difficult to understand that a seriously disturbed patient might not be able to recognize the harm of a treatment for many years, perhaps until another provider is able to effect improvement. Courts have become especially forgiving of the statute of limitations in cases of sexual exploitation.

The statute of limitations for children typically begins when they reach the age of majority. Thus, their records must be retained longer than those of adult former patients.

DEATH OR RETIREMENT OF THE PSYCHOLOGIST

According to the APA Ethics Code (1992), "[a] psychologist makes plans in advance so that confidentiality of records and data is protected in the event of the psychologist's death, incapacity, or withdrawal from the position or practice" (section 5.09). Psychologists can provide in their wills for the transfer of records to another practitioner in the event of death. The practitioner who receives these records should notify all patients that the records are now in his or her possession. Patients may then request the transfer of their records to the practitioners of their choice or may leave them at the location of the new practitioner.

The retirement of a psychologist creates fewer problems because the psychologist should be able to anticipate the transition with patients. Psychologists may destroy out-of-date records. The psychologist will also have the opportunity to notify current and past patients of the anticipated retirement and make provisions for the distribution of these records.

SUMMARY

Records provide a paper trail of care of the patient. Practitioners need to be knowledgeable of their state laws, agency requirements, ethics codes, and other professional documents regarding record-keeping requirements. Patients have a right to be maximally informed about their records and generally have a right to review their contents. Records also may protect practitioners against allegations of negligence in the care of their patients.

REFERENCES

Abille v. United States, 482 F. Supp. 703 (N.D. Cal. 1980).

American Psychological Association (1992). *Ethical principles of psychologists and code of conduct.* Washington, DC: Author.

American Psychological Association (1993). *Record keeping guidelines.* Washington, DC: Author.

Handelsman, M., Kemper, M., Kerson-Craig, P., McCain, J., & Johnsrud, C. (1986). Use, content and readability of written informed consent forms. *Professional Psychology: Research and Practice, 17,* 514–518.

Knapp, S., & VandeCreek, L. (1987). *Privileged communications in the mental health professions.* New York: Van Nostrand/Reinhold.

Knapp, S., & VandeCreek, L. (1993). Legal and ethical issues in billing patients and collecting fees. *Psychotherapy, 30,* 25–31.

Levenstein, J. (1994). Treatment documentation in private practice II: PIRC progress notes. *The Independent Practitioner, 14*(5), 233–237.

Monahan, J. (1993). Limiting therapist exposure to *Tarasoff* liability. *American Psychologist, 48,* 242–250.

Monahan, J., & Steadman, H. J. (1994). *Violence and mental disorder: Developments in risk assessment.* Chicago: University of Chicago Press.

Pope, K., Tabachnick, B., & Keith-Spiegel, P. (1987). Ethics of practice: The beliefs and behaviors of psychologists as therapists. *American Psychologist, 42,* 993–1006.

Soisson, E., VandeCreek, L., & Knapp, S. (1987). Thorough record keeping: A good defense in a litigious era. *Professional Psychology: Research and Practice, 18,* 498–502.

Sturm, I. E. (1987). The psychologist in the Problem- Oriented Record (POR). *Professional Psychology: Research and Practice, 18,* 155–158.

Tarasoff v. The University of California et al. (1976), 551 P.2d 334.

VandeCreek, L., & Knapp, S. (1993). *Tarasoff and beyond: Legal and clinical issues in treating life endangering patients* (rev.). Sarasota, Fl: Professional Resource Press.

Woody, R. H. (1988). *Protecting your mental health practice: How to minimize legal and financial risk.* San Francisco: Jossey-Bass.

▶ 9

Special Issues Involving Children

PEGGY GRECO   DONALD K. ROUTH

▶ CASE EXAMPLE

Robert

Robert looks intently at the lid of a jar as he carefully puts it on a smooth surface and with a deft turn of his hand sets it into motion. He watches the lights and shadows as they spin across the walls and looks closer in fascination as the lid's rotation slows down and it clatters to a stop. Robert's reverie is interrupted by his mother, Miriam Q., who has been calling Robert's name to no avail. Miriam grabs the lid. "I told you—no more of that!" Robert throws himself to the floor, wailing and biting his arm in frustration.

Miriam Q. is a single mother with two children, 3-year-old Robert and 18-month-old Alicia. She realizes that Robert acts "strange," prefers to be alone, and is very quiet, but she is only recently beginning to recognize the serious nature of his difficulties. Alicia is starting to mimic her brother, at times throwing tantrums and screaming. Miriam Q. decides to seek help. This scenario is one of many that may cause a parent or other adult to seek services for their child for an emotional or behavioral problem.

This chapter covers special issues in clinical psychology pertaining to children and adolescents. The intent of the chapter is not to provide a comprehensive review of child and adolescent assessment or treatment, but rather to focus on special issues that are unique to the treatment of children. Differences between children and adults relevant to psychological intervention include children's ongoing maturation and their dependence upon others to care for them. These differences have several implications for delivery of clinical services to children: (1) A child's developmental status may affect the choice of treatment approaches, (2) persons other than the child are likely to be included in the treatment, and (3) particular difficulties such as abuse and neglect may arise in the context of children's dependence on adults. This chapter focuses on some of the specific clinical issues related to the unique developmental status of children. Topics covered include the significance of the child's developmental level in assessment and treatment, the role of family and nonfamily members in treatment, and the assessment of several problem areas specific to children such as child abuse and neglect.

Childhood is typically defined as lasting from birth until about age 12, with adolescence spanning the age range from about 13 to 18. For the purposes of this chapter, the term "children" is used to include both children and adolescents. Children are raised by a variety of care givers including biological parents, step-parents, adoptive parents, relatives, or nonrelated adults. To avoid confusion, the label "parent" is used to describe the adult who has legal custody of the child and who has primary responsibility for the child's upbringing.

Children who are identified as having difficulties may be evaluated by a variety of professionals in a number of different contexts. Professionals who assess and treat children and their families may include physicians, teachers, psychologists, social workers, physical therapists, and speech therapists, among others. Although parents and teachers are usually the first to identify child behaviors that are developmentally inappropriate, any of these professionals, or any other adult who has regular contact with a child, may initiate a referral to a child specialist. This chapter focuses primarily on psychologists and students receiving training in the field of clinical psychology as primary providers of assessment and treatment services for children. Psychologists may treat children in a variety of contexts including university-affiliated clinics, outpatient private practice settings, schools, publicly funded outpatient or inpatient institutions, medical clinics, and hospitals. Although it is not intended to examine fully every possible context for child assessment and treatment, this chapter presents examples of clinical intervention in some of the most common settings.

DEVELOPMENTAL FACTORS IN THE ASSESSMENT AND TREATMENT OF CHILDREN

The professional must consider a child's developmental stage throughout the treatment process, from problem identification to problem resolution.

Therefore, any clinical professional working with children should have a thorough foundation in normal child development. The accurate identification of unusual behaviors that may indicate developmental delay or psychopathology is not possible without this foundation. For example, seemingly slow development of speech at age 2 might not be cause for alarm given the normal variability in the emergence of language ability. However, the presentation of this same problem at age 3 might indicate a significant delay in language development and thus would be considered a more serious indicator of possible difficulties.

The term "development" as it applies to childhood and adolescence refers to age-related changes. Some of these changes may be relatively specific, for example, when an infant takes a first unassisted step. Others may be relatively general, for instance when a school-age child becomes increasingly able to cooperate with peers in work projects or play. On the whole, developmental changes tend to unfold gradually. Children develop in several spheres simultaneously but not always at a consistent rate. This can complicate the picture for a psychologist who must take a child's developmental status into account.

The three main spheres of development are usually considered to be cognitive, physical, and psychosocial. Cognitive development is related to how children gain and store knowledge of their environment and how they conceptualize the world; language acquisition, reasoning, and school learning are examples of skills that emerge as a part of cognitive development. Physical development involves biological maturation and includes changes in the body and in the way a child uses his or her body. Examples of physical development include the refinement of walking, playing sports, and the manipulation of objects. Psychosocial development refers to changes in feelings or emotions and in how children relate to other people. Psychosocial development includes more complex and sophisticated relationships with family, peers, and teachers, as well as a more fully developed personal identity or sense of self. When considering the impact of a child's developmental status on psychological treatment, it is important to consider the child's progression within the cognitive, physical, and psychosocial realms. The following case example demonstrates the relevance of normal developmental processes in these three spheres to the identification of problem areas.

▶ CASE EXAMPLE

Baby Kane

James, a graduate student in clinical psychology, is receiving training at a university clinic that has recently established a "Community Help Hour." The purpose of this service is to provide phone consultations for parents

(Cont.)

▶ CASE EXAMPLE *(Continued)*

with questions about common child development and behavioral problems. While working on the help line one evening, James received a call from Mrs. Kane, a young mother who was concerned about the behavior of her 8-month-old baby. Mrs. Kane described how when she departed from the room or left the child with a baby-sitter, her child showed little concern. Typically, the child would turn away from her mother and crawl happily on the floor. Mrs. Kane concluded by stating that she was worried that her child might be exhibiting signs of withdrawal.

James first responded by asking about the baby's cognitive, physical, and psychosocial development. The information provided by Mrs. Kane indicated that her baby had met normal developmental milestones. Over all, the baby was well adjusted; she had normal feeding patterns and a regular sleep schedule. Mrs. Kane's descriptions of the baby's interactions with others also indicated normal social development. James then inquired why the mother had become concerned about the child's behavior at this particular time. Mrs. Kane explained that she had just returned from a visit with her sister, who had a child of approximately the same age. Her sister's infant would protest loudly upon separation from her mother. Mrs. Kane's sister would exclaim proudly, "You see—my little angel really loves me!"

James was struck by the behavioral differences between two babies who were about the same age. However, because of his knowledge of normal development, he realized that factors such as differences in temperament and the emergence of separation fears could account for the discrepant presentations of these two children. James explained to Mrs. Kane that it was likely that her sister's baby was experiencing separation anxiety. "Separation anxiety" refers to an infant's being upset when separated from the care giver. At approximately 8 to 9 months of age, infants often begin showing separation anxiety and cry in distress when their mothers depart. James reassured Mrs. Kane that because of the variability in the time course and intensity of developmental behaviors such as separation anxiety it would not be unusual for her baby to behave differently than her sister's baby. James asked Mrs. Kane to phone again if she noted any other signs of withdrawal or if she noted that the baby's sleeping and/or eating patterns began to be affected.

Knowledge of normal developmental processes not only facilitates accurate problem identification, as illustrated by James's experience with the Kane baby, but may also help to determine the appropriateness of particular treatment modalities. Since children and adolescents are in the midst of rapid growth and developmental changes, unique techniques need to be employed to address their clinical problems; it is usually inappropriate, and possibly even harmful, to apply principles of adult treatment to children. For example, children who do not have the capacity for abstract thought would do poorly with insight-based therapies given their inherent limitation in understanding these concepts.

PARENTS AS PARTICIPANTS IN CHILD ASSESSMENT AND TREATMENT

After a problem has been identified using a developmental perspective, treatment is often begun by referral to an appropriate professional or agency.

▶ CASE EXAMPLE *(Continued)*

Robert

Miriam Q., whose son Robert's unusual behaviors and tantrums were described earlier, mentioned her concerns to her pediatrician, Dr. Wong. Dr. Wong noted that Robert had met developmental milestones pertaining to language more slowly than expected. Robert's motor abilities, however, were average for his age. Although Dr. Wong had not observed Robert interacting with other children, she was worried about the pattern of withdrawal from social contact and aggressive behavior described his his mother. Dr. Wong knew that children who are preverbal may get frustrated more easily when their demands are not met; however, she realized that the self-directed aggression displayed by Robert, such as biting his arm and occasionally hitting his head on the floor, was clearly unusual. Dr. Wong realized that Robert's development in the cognitive and psychosocial spheres might be impaired. She gave Mrs. Q. the telephone number of a child guidance clinic run by a local university. When Mrs. Q. called the clinic to make an appointment, she was asked to bring both of her children and a relative or friend who could watch the children while the therapist obtained a detailed history from Mrs. Q.

Unlike adults, who usually initiate treatment for themselves, children often have treatment sought out and arranged for them by others. Although the child is identified as the patient, referrals to clinical psychologists are typically initiated by the child's parents, and in all but a few instances a parent or legal guardian's consent must be obtained before treatment can begin. Parents often take primary responsibility for many aspects of treatment including making treatment appointments, monitoring compliance with recommendations, and implementing interventions in the home environment.

Especially when working with infants and younger children, therapists regard parents' involvement as central to assessment and treatment. Thus, psychologists who specialize in treating children often spend a significant proportion of their time working with adults.

Although parents are the most likely individuals within the child's environment to be involved in treatment, the therapist will at times involve a child's entire family when therapeutically indicated. The first step in deciding whether to involve a child's parents or other family members in the therapeutic process is to define "parent" and "family" for that particular child. The primary care giver may not always be a biological parent; children may be raised by step-parents, adoptive parents, relatives, neighbors, or even siblings. Our idea of the "typical" family has evolved away from the prototype of a father who works outside the home and a mother who works inside the home caring full time for the family. The divorce rate is high. Many divorced parents remarry, so that a significant proportion of children live in step-families, which may include step- or half-siblings. The therapist should identify the principal care givers and other family members important to the child, whether they are members of a "traditional" nuclear family or not, and then determine the appropriate level of family involvement in the assessment and treatment process.

In general, the extent of parental or family involvement in treatment can range from minimal (e.g., simply providing consent for treatment) to complete involvement in the therapy process. The degree of involvement will depend upon a number of factors including the child's age, developmental status, cognitive ability, the referral issue, and the treatment approach chosen. Greater parental involvement generally is necessary with young children, when the child has below average cognitive ability, or for referral problems directly related to the functioning of the family. Several examples of situations in which the therapist may decide to involve parents or additional family members are described here.

The following clinical example illustrates the integral role a parent may play in the assessment and treatment of childhood problems. In this case the child's young age and the interactional nature of his feeding difficulties required close involvement of his parents in the therapy.

▶ CASE EXAMPLE

Jamilah R.

Jamilah R. is an 8-month-old infant who was referred to a psychologist for failure to gain weight in the absence of organic disease and had been diagnosed with "non-organic failure to thrive" (NOFT). During the initial evalu-

(Cont.)

▶ CASE EXAMPLE   *(Continued)*

ation, observations were made of the parents and infant together in feeding situations. The psychologist noted Jamilah's response to food, evidence of distress, and parent–child interaction during feeding. Behavioral, emotional, and environmental concomitants of NOFT were recorded and addressed with the parents in subsequent treatment sessions. Jamilah's parents were given the responsibility for instituting treatment recommendations to promote weight gain. During later sessions the therapist observed implementation of these changes in the office and also monitored the parents' compliance with recommendations in other settings.

This example illustrates how parents may be the primary recipients of the therapist's guidance. In this case the parents were very active participants in the therapy process. They were responsible for following the treatment recommendations and reporting back to the psychologist. The next case illustrates how other family members in addition to parents can play an integral role in the therapy process:

▶ CASE EXAMPLE

Anne L.

Anne L. is an 11-year-old girl who was referred for extreme weight loss within the past 3 months. She recently received a comprehensive physical examination from her pediatrician and a gastroenterologist, both of whom found no physical etiology for her weight loss and pronounced Anne in good health. Anne says she is trying to lose weight on purpose and would like to weight 75 pounds, a figure that is significantly below her ideal body weight. Her parents are very upset by her weight loss and, upon the recommendation of Anne's pediatrician, have brought her to a clinical psychologist for treatment. During the initial interview, which included all of the family members, it became clear that family dynamics played an influential role in maintaining Anne's restricted eating habits. In the initial session the therapist learned about the family system by eliciting and observing patterns of family interactions. From the interaction patterns exhibited during the sessions it appeared that the Lees had a conflictual marriage, which Mrs. Lee attempted to cope with by distancing herself from her husband and becoming overly involved with her daughter. In subsequent sessions the therapist attempted

(Cont.)

▶ CASE EXAMPLE *(Continued)*

to identify and restructure maladaptive family interactions, with all family members playing an active role in this process.

In this case example of the disorder known as anorexia nervosa, the therapist decided it would be beneficial to involve all family members in treatment. We can hypothesize that the therapist's goal is to improve family functioning, which will eventually reflect itself in amelioration of Anne's eating problem.

The next case example illustrates the treatment of an adolescent in which parents had minimal therapy involvement. This case also describes a method for keeping parents informed as to the goals and progress of the prescribed intervention.

▶ CASE EXAMPLE

Betty

Betty is a 17-year-old young woman who was referred for significant anxiety related to test taking. Betty was a conscientious student who received primarily As and Bs. However, after beginning her senior year, she began to worry about admission to college, and her grades dropped. She became increasingly distressed about her test performance. Her anxiety level on test days increased to the point where Betty felt physically ill and expressed a desire to stay home from school. Lynne, a therapist in private practice who was asked to see Betty, decided that systematic desensitization would be an appropriate and effective choice of treatment. Betty's parents were seen during the initial session, and the rationale and process of treatment were explained to them. Betty was seen individually for weekly therapy. During her sessions she was trained in deep muscle relaxation. Once she became proficient at inducing a deep level of relaxation on her own, she was guided through a succession of distressing imaginary situations related to test taking. By applying relaxation to imagined anxiety-provoking images, Betty was able to reduce her anxiety in real-life testing situations. The therapist met once a month with Betty's mother during the final 15 minutes of a session. With the help of the therapist, Betty would summarize her therapy activities and progress to date.

In the three case examples just described, family members were involved to varying degrees in the assessment and treatment of their child. The decision to involve family members is a multifactorial process in which the therapist must consider the individual characteristics of the case as well as the impact on the therapeutic process. One issue that arises in any situation involving treatment of the child—independent of degree of family involvement—is how to provide information about the therapy process to family members or professionals such as teachers and pediatricians. The following additional material related to a case example already presented examines the topic of confidentiality in child assessment and treatment.

▶ CASE EXAMPLE *(Continued)*

Robert

Miriam Q. shook the hand of James, who introduced himself as a graduate student in clinical child psychology who would be working with the family. James began by explaining some of the clinic procedures. After discussion of the intake process, appointment making, and billing, James introduced the topic of confidentiality. He explained that although most therapy relationships were founded on the principle of confidentiality of information revealed during the therapy session, there were several exceptions that he wanted to discuss in greater detail. "Since I am currently a graduate student, all of my clinical work is supervised by a licensed clinical psychologist. My supervisor and I discuss families that I work with in order to make sure that they are receiving the best possible care—you are benefiting from our combined skills. I also need to let you know that I am legally and ethically required to inform the appropriate professionals or agencies if during our work together it is revealed that: (1) you intend to harm yourself or harm someone else, or (2) there is reasonable suspicion that your children or other children are being sexually abused, physically abused, or neglected." After answering Miriam's questions about the limits of confidentiality, James provided her with a brochure that explained in writing the clinic's policy on confidentiality and which listed his supervisor's name and phone number.

The Ethical Principles of Psychologists and Code of Conduct of the American Psychological Association (1992) and many state statutes provide for confidentiality of information disclosed during therapy sessions. Confidentiality is a central component of the ethical code of psychologists as well as of mental health professionals other than psychologists. Confidentiality protects the patient's right to privacy, helps maintain the patient's trust in the therapist (which promotes meaningful disclosure), and increases the public trust in mental health professionals in general. The APA's guidelines, however, do not specifically address special issues regarding therapy with children and adolescents.

Legally, minors are not guaranteed a right to the same degree of confidentiality as are adults. In most cases the parent or legal guardian has the right to be informed of treatment proceedings. However, as with adults, most children—especially adolescents—are more likely to participate actively in therapy with the assurance of confidentiality. Thus, the therapist should work with the family to reach an agreement on confidentiality that is consistent with ethical and legal principles and also takes the individual needs of the case into account.

The following general guidelines may be helpful when formulating an agreement on confidentiality:

1. Discuss the issue of confidentiality with parent and child at the beginning of the therapeutic relationship or as soon as possible thereafter. As recommended by the APA's ethics code, discussions of confidentiality should occur at the outset of professional (or scientific) relationships. Regardless of the policy adopted in a particular case, the therapeutic relationship is likely to benefit from clear explanation of this policy during the first session and periodically thereafter during the course of treatment.

2. When speaking to children about confidentiality, use developmentally appropriate terms. While an adolescent may understand the concept of confidentiality, this term may be better explained to a young child by using a simple, age-appropriate explanation such as "I won't tell anyone what you tell me unless we talk about it first."

3. At a minimum, provide regular summaries of treatment progress to the child's legal guardian. Before the initiation of an evaluation or treatment, parents should be given a clear rationale for the services and the likely effect of treatment on the child's presenting complaints. After the start of treatment, parents should be provided with regular updates on progress toward treatment goals. Although minimal parental involvement may be consistent with some treatment approaches, the therapist should consider possible negative consequences of parental exclusion from the therapeutic process. For example, if parents are not aware of the rationale for treatment or their child's progress toward therapy goals, they may either knowingly or unknowingly derail treatment.

4. Whenever possible and clinically appropriate, involve the child in regular meetings with the legal guardian. Depending upon the age of the child and the presenting problems, the child may be included in discussions with parents when the child's progress is reviewed. Having the child present during such feedback sessions provides an opportunity for the child to communicate his or her own concerns about therapy, facilitates communication between parent and child, and provides the parent with feedback on the child's progress while maintaining the confidentiality of specific information shared between the child and therapist.

5. Carefully explain the limits of confidentiality to both parent and child. The therapist may wish to disclose information for which the primary purpose is to facilitate treatment of the child by other health professionals, teachers, family members, or when sharing information with a supervisor when the clinician is a trainee. In cases in which information is to be shared with persons outside of the family, written consent from the child's legal guardian should be obtained. Children should be notified of such a disclosure even though they may not be asked to sign the official release-of-information form. As discussed in earlier chapters, there are specific instances in which the therapist is required by law to disclose information that may not require prior consent from the parent. In general, these situations are subsumed under the psychologist's duties to warn, protect, and report. If a psychologist becomes aware of a threat to a person's well-being, he or she must take the appropriate steps to warn or to protect the person who is at risk. In all fifty states, statutes require professionals to report evidence of immediate and probable harm to the child or others or when there is evidence of physical abuse, sexual abuse, or neglect. Taylor and Adelman (1989) suggest the following dialogue as a model for discussing the limits of confidentiality with children and adolescents:

> Although most of what we talk about is private, there are three kinds of problems you might tell me about that we would have to talk about with other people. If I find out that someone has been seriously hurting or abusing you, I would have to tell the police about it. If you tell me you have made a plan to seriously hurt yourself, I would have to let your parents know. If you tell me you have made a plan to seriously hurt someone else, I would have to warn that person. I would not be able to keep these problems just between you and me because the law says I can't. (p. 80)

6. Children and their parents may benefit from a written explanation of confidentiality. While verbal discussion of confidentiality allows for clarification of any misunderstandings, provision of written materials ensures comprehensive coverage of relevant points and provides a record to which the patient and the family can refer when necessary.

The APA ethical code emphasizes the importance of informed consent to participation in research as well as consent to treatment. There are generally considered to be three important components to informed consent for research

(Haas & Malouf, 1989). First, subjects should be provided enough information to be able to weigh the costs and benefits and make a decision about
participating in treatment or research; they should be *informed*. Second, subjects should be *competent* to make such a determination. Third, the consent
provided should be *voluntary*. When obtaining children's agreement to participate in treatment or research, special consideration must be given to the
child's capability to provide informed and voluntary consent.

As long as a parent remains the legal guardian, parental permission must
be obtained for a child to participate in treatment or in a research study. At
age 18, children are considered legally able to provide informed consent as
long as there are no limitations on their functioning that would affect their
ability to provide consent. Between the ages of approximately 7 to 18, a child's
"assent to participate" should be obtained, even though the child cannot legally provide informed consent. This process entails, for example, explaining a research study to the child in developmentally appropriate terms and
clearly explaining the child's role in the study. The child may be asked to
sign the consent form along with the legal guardian as an indication that he
or she understands the study and agrees to participate. Most clinics, hospitals, and universities have committees that review research projects to ensure that procedures for informed consent are followed (among other criteria). Studies in almost any institution must receive approval from the research committee (typically referred to as Institutional Review Board or IRB)
before commencing. Such boards act to protect the welfare of humans and
animals under their jurisdiction. As such, most research and/or clinical
projects require IRB approval regardless of scale. As a student, it is important to remain aware of this requirement; class projects such as interviewing
a college student or administering questionnaires to an undergraduate class
may need prior IRB approval.

THE ROLE OF TEACHERS

In addition to parents, clinical psychologists must often call upon other adults
in the community who have contact with the child to aid in assessment and
treatment. Teachers most often fill this role for a variety of reasons: They can
be invaluable sources of information in the course of assessing a child; they
are likely to have observed the child's performance in structured and unstructured academic situations as well as social situations; and they are often
the first to notice difficulties such as distractibility and learning disabilities,
which may be apparent only within academic situations. Teachers also hold
an advantage over parents in that they are able to compare the behavior of

each child to an informal norm derived from observing other children in the classroom. Thus, while parents may sometimes have difficulty judging whether their child's behavior is cause for concern, teachers have a ready-made comparison group with which to evaluate behavior. The following case example illustrates the importance of obtaining teacher ratings and of evaluating behaviors within the classroom setting.

▶ CASE EXAMPLE

Andy

Andy, a 5-year-old who had just begun kindergarten 3 months earlier, was referred for hyperactive and aggressive behaviors on the recommendation of his teacher. Andy lived at home in a rural area with his biological parents and was an only child. He enjoyed being outdoors and reported his favorite activities were target practice with his BB gun and basketball. Andy's mother agreed to the referral with some reluctance, as she had not observed any of the problematic behaviors noted by Andy's teacher. Given this discrepancy, the psychologist asked both the teacher and parents to complete a standard behavior checklist (a brief measure of child functioning in a variety of areas) in order to obtain an estimate of Andy's functioning within both the home and school settings. Additionally, the psychologist arranged an informal classroom observation period. Comparisons of the checklists completed by parent and teacher revealed a significant elevation on the Attention Problems scale of the teacher's checklist, while all of the scales on the parent's checklist were within the normal range.

During the informal observation period in the classroom, Andy was monitored in three different situations to obtain as broad a sampling of his behavior as possible: (1) during a highly structured academic task, (2) during a loosely structured group academic activity ("circle time"), and (3) during an unstructured play period. In each of these situations, Andy was observed for a 10-minute block of time and a simple count was made of behaviors that might indicate a significant problem. These behaviors were categorized as on-task (working quietly and productively) or off-task (fidgeting, tapping a pencil, aggression, talking, distracting others, staring, and withdrawal). For comparison purposes, a male classmate was chosen at random during each of the three observation periods and was rated on these same behaviors. Observation sessions were conducted between 9:00 and 10:30 in the morning. There were eighteen children, one teacher, and one teacher's assistant present in the classroom. The observations yielded the following results:

(Cont.)

▶ CASE EXAMPLE *(Continued)*

1. Highly structured academic task: Andy's behavior was first coded for 10 minutes during a structured academic task: (a math worksheet). Andy was rated as being on-task 20% of the time and off-task 80% of the time. His off-task behaviors were characterized by fidgeting, talking, and staring into space. During the same 10-minute observation period a male classmate of Andy's was rated as being on-task for 100% of the time during this same activity.

2. Loosely structured academic activity: Andy was rated as being on-task 60% of the time and off-task 40% of the time during a group activity that involved academic tasks such as naming colors, identifying the days of the week, and following teacher directions in a more relaxed situation with children sitting on the carpet in a circle. His off-task behaviors were primarily talking and giggling. Andy's activity level was noticeably higher than that of his classmates during structured play activities, although he complied with teacher directions throughout the activity. During the "hokey-pokey," while his classmates turned slowly in a circle, Andy turned in a circle while jumping up and down, waving his arms in the air, and sticking out his tongue. A male classmate of Andy's was on-task for 90% of the time and off-task for 10% of the time during this same activity.

3. Unstructured play period: During a period of unstructured play in a corner of the room set up to resemble a kitchen area, Andy was able to play appropriately for 75% of the time; he was off-task for approximately 25% of the activity. Andy would occasionally speak out loud to himself and would call out to other children who were in different areas of the room. These behaviors were noted to increase in frequency toward the end of the unstructured play period. A peer observed during the same period of time was on-task for 90% of the time and off-task for 10% of the time. Over all, during these three brief observation periods it was noted that Andy was somewhat active and distractible. The pattern of Andy's behaviors in the classroom indicated that his behavior worsened with greater academic demands. Thus, the parent–teacher discrepancy in behavioral ratings appeared to be a reflection of situational influences on Andy's behavior. In school, greater cognitive demands appeared to increase distractibility and hyperactivity, while at home, where Andy primarily spent his time playing, little variation was noted in levels of hyperactivity and distractibility. Given the increase in behavioral difficulties when asked to concentrate and perform academically, a full evaluation was recommended, to investigate the possibility of a cognitive deficit or learning disability, as well as to evaluate the diagnosis of attention-deficit hyperactivity disorder.

Teachers and parents sometimes disagree about the degree to which a child shows attention problems. Often the teacher will report such problems but not the parent, probably because the school makes far greater demands than do parents on a child's ability to concentrate and pay attention.

In addition to being instrumental in the assessment of children, teachers often are able to implement recommended classroom intervention strategies, as long as they are brief and nondisruptive to the remainder of the students. In the next case example, returning to the previous case of Robert, who was diagnosed with autistic disorder, the role of teachers in an intervention procedure is described.

▶ CASE EXAMPLE *(Continued)*

Robert

After receiving the diagnosis of autistic disorder as a result of a multidisciplinary evaluation initiated by James at the University Clinic, Robert was placed in a special education preschool classroom for five mornings a week and appropriate outpatient therapies were arranged to address his communication and social deficits. James kept in regular contact with Robert's classroom teacher to ensure that the same behavioral programs to extinguish inappropriate behaviors and to shape desired behaviors were in place both at home and at school. For example, James was working on appropriate eye contact during treatment sessions. Whenever Robert made appropriate eye contact with James, he was praised. Robert's classroom teacher used the same procedure, slightly modified to fit the constraints of the school day. Rather than rewarding Robert throughout the day, his teacher picked two discrete activities that involved socialization (circle time and play centers) and verbally praised Robert when eye contact occurred.

As in the case of Robert, involving the teacher in treatment is likely to improve the success of the interventions. Generalizability, or the likelihood that newly learned behaviors will be applied to novel situations, may also be increased. Teacher involvement is also important in cases in which the problem occurs predominantly (or solely) in the classroom or when the behavior has negative implications for school performance.

THE ROLE OF SIBLINGS AND PEERS

▶ CASE EXAMPLE *(Continued)*

Robert

James had been working with Robert Q. and his family for approximately 1 month to address behavioral management issues related to his autism. Several weeks after beginning treatment, he began to notice aggressive behaviors exhibited by Robert's 19-month-old sister, Alicia. Alicia has been mimicking Robert's tantrums. Recently, she began displaying aggressive behavior toward Robert, usually by hitting his head or biting him. In response, Robert's behavior problems have intensified, often leading to self-directed aggression. To address these issues, James instructed Mrs. Q. on providing clear and consistent consequences for aggressive behavior. He discussed the use of a brief time-out (removing the child from the situation for a short period of time) when Alicia became aggressive toward Robert. In addition, James and Mrs. Q. made a list of joint activities for Robert and Alicia, which would promote positive sibling interactions.

This case example illustrates how a child other than the identified patient may become a focus of treatment. It is important to consider the contribution of sibling and peer relationships to the difficulties of the child who is referred for treatment. Social interactions tend to be underemphasized in child assessment and treatment despite the clear negative implications of deficient social relationships.

Sibling and peer relationships are both relationships between children rather than between a child and an adult. However, peer and sibling relationships differ in several ways. First, interactions with siblings occur more frequently than peer interactions. Sibling interactions are also more enduring than those with peers. Last, sibling relationships involve more shared history than most peer relationships. During middle childhood, conflict is more common in sibling relationships than in peer relationships, and given the close proximity in which siblings exist, this conflict is harder to escape from. Because conflict does not cause the sibling relationship to dissolve, children must learn how to resolve or live with sibling strife. Thus, it is important for the clinician to assess the nature of sibling relationships and to intervene when appropriate.

A child's friends or peers are also important to consider in the assessment and treatment of children. Peer acceptance is important for normal childhood development, and peers play an especially influential role at certain times, for example during adolescence. A number of studies have found that children with poor peer relationships are at greater risk for later psychological maladjustment. For example, socially rejected children report higher levels of unhappiness and loneliness (Asher & Wheeler, 1985). These children tend to be actively disliked by their peers and are excluded from activities. Because these children are excluded from peer groups, they rarely have a chance to practice social interactions. This exclusion can affect the child's long-term adjustment. In the classic study by Cowen and his colleagues (1973), children who were rated as playing negative roles in the third grade were more likely to have mental health problems in early adulthood.

Given the significant short-term and long-term consequences of peer difficulties, the rationale for focusing on social relationship problems in children is apparent. Interventions pertaining to social interactions may address specific problematic behaviors or attempt to enhance positive social skills. Although the clinician may implement peer-focused interventions, peers themselves may play an active role in the treatment process as well. The potentially positive role of peers in the treatment of children has only recently been recognized. Therapeutically, peers can be used in contexts as diverse as social skills training for children with learning disabilities or autism to impulse control training with aggressive and hyperactive children. The following case example illustrates the use of peers in intervention with children and adolescents.

▶ CASE EXAMPLE

Joshua

Joshua is a 15-year-old male with mild autism. He lives with his parents and a younger sister, attends high school, and is receiving vocational training through a community-based sheltered workshop. Joshua is able to use verbal means of communication but is quite awkward when trying to speak in social situations; he tends to have difficulty with the more subtle aspects of communication such as turn taking and utilizing interpersonal cues. He has a few repetitive mannerisms such as flapping his hands by his face, but he has learned to control these movements when out in public. Joshua's hobbies include collecting numerical information about people, such as their birthdate or number of siblings, and collecting information about the city bus system and riding on city buses. When someone expresses an interest in his hobby, Joshua will launch enthusiastically into a detailed discussion of the latest city bus models and specifications.

Joshua joined a social skills group that was created to give adolescents with impairments a social forum within which to practice subtle aspects of

(Cont.)

▶ CASE EXAMPLE *(Continued)*

communication and social interaction. His group consisted of four adolescents with autism, four nondisabled high school students in the same age range from a service club, and a program director. The group met on a weekly basis and followed a program of structured teaching, which involved reviewing a particular skill and then putting the skills into practice during group activities and outings. During one meeting the adolescents broke up into pairs and practiced a short conversation in which the skills of greeting appropriately, turn taking in conversation, and good eye contact were practiced. For the last half-hour of the session, drinks and snacks were brought out, and during this "mixer" the adolescents were assigned to "meet" three people and engage them in conversation, using the skills practiced earlier in the session.

SPECIAL CLINICAL ISSUES OF CHILDREN: ABUSE AND NEGLECT

Psychologists and psychology trainees who work with children are likely to encounter the issue of child abuse or neglect. Clinicians may be asked to evaluate whether a child has been abused or neglected. In addition, in the process of treatment for an unrelated issue the possibility of abuse or neglect may arise. When there are indications of abuse or neglect, clinicians are required in all fifty states to report known or suspected child maltreatment. (See also Chapter 1.)

Although there is a clear requirement to report child abuse or neglect, the process of doing so varies from state to state and can be cumbersome and complex. The following guidelines attempt to clarify the reporting process and provide a framework for reporting suspected child abuse or neglect.

1. Become familiar with the regulations in your state for reporting neglect and abuse of children. Although reporting of suspected child abuse or neglect is mandated in all states, specific rules for making a report and the definition of abuse itself may vary across states. For example, the state of Missouri defines abuse to include physical injury, sexual abuse, or emotional abuse inflicted on a child other than by accidental means. The Missouri definition does not include spanking if administered in a reasonable way. Nebraska adopts a broader definition of abuse to include the knowing, intentional, or negligent placing of a child in a situation that endangers his or her life or physical or mental health.

2. Include a discussion of mandated reporting when reviewing the limits of confidentiality during the first session. Describe to parents the meaning of "mandated reporting" and explain the circumstances under which you would be required to report suspicions of child abuse or neglect. Reviewing the topic occasionally throughout the course of therapy facilitates greater understanding and cooperation if a need arises to make a report during the course of therapy.

3. When reasonable suspicion has been determined to exist, and an evaluation of other possible causes does not reveal an alternative explanation, immediately consult with a supervisor in regard to the ethical and treatment-related concerns about reporting the suspected abuse. Keeping in mind that the ultimate goal is protection of the child, the therapist will find it helpful to discuss with a supervisor the best method for proceeding with a report of suspected child abuse or neglect so that the risk to the child is minimized.

In regard to treatment-related concerns, many therapists believe that reporting suspected child abuse or neglect has a negative effect on the therapeutic relationship (Kalichman, 1993). However, empirical investigations of this issue have indicated minimal adverse effects of reporting suspected abuse on the therapeutic process. Nevertheless, it may be helpful to anticipate a family's likely response to reporting in order to minimize any possible negative effects on treatment.

4. Unless the safety of the child, a family member, or the therapist would be compromised, inform the appropriate members of the family of the need to report. If possible, have a family member participate in filing the report. When discussing the need to report with a family, it may be helpful to emphasize the following points: (a) There is a legal obligation to report and the therapist (or reporter) has no choice in the matter; (b) if an investigation reveals that there is no basis for concern, the case will be closed; (c) if there is reason for concern, the state protection agency will provide appropriate assistance and act to protect the child from further harm; and (d) the family's involvement in therapy will be regarded positively.

5. Be prepared for situations in which it is unsafe to allow the child to leave the clinic or treatment setting. At times, concern for the child's welfare may require an *immediate* report to the state protection agency and/or require police intervention. In these cases the therapist should immediately contact the supervisor and proceed according to a predetermined protocol for such situations. Such a protocol should include: (a) immediate communication with the therapist's supervisor and state protection agency if it has been determined that it is unsafe for a child to leave the treatment setting, and (b) contact with the police authorities and/or institution security force if there is a lack of cooperation from the adult accompaning the child and/or if the child or therapist is in immediate danger.

6. Be prepared to make a detailed and accurate report. Before filing a report of suspected child abuse or neglect, contact the appropriate agency to determine the exact information that will be required. Have all of these required materials organized and accessible when filing the report.

7. Keep careful and detailed documentation for all issues related to suspected child abuse or neglect (see Chapter 8). Document information collected during the course of your evaluation of suspected abuse, and keep careful records of all actions taken in reference to a case. Examples of items that should be carefully documented are discussions with a colleague in regard to the case and calls to child protection agencies to determine available services.

PEDIATRIC PSYCHOLOGY

Pediatric chronic illness can have a profound effect on the psychosocial status of children and adolescents. Children and adolescents with chronic illness often experience significant physical, emotional, and social stress. For example, children and adolescents with asthma may evidence an increase in general psychopathology (Kashani et al., 1988) and emotional difficulties such as depression and low self-concept (Mrazek, 1985). In particular, adolescents may have a difficult time because they are in the midst of continuous developmental changes. Adolescents who have a chronic illness must not only cope with normative developmental tasks but must do so while experiencing the demands and stressors particular to their illness.

Chronic illnesses often impose major limitations on habits and lifestyle that can increase stress on the family and child, interfere with opportunities for social interactions with peers, and lead to problems with disease management. Because of these stressors, children may require additional assistance in the form of psychotherapeutic intervention. Pediatric psychology, a special branch of clinical child psychology, attempts to improve functioning as it relates to a child's health and illness. This relatively new field is continuing to investigate the efficacy of illness-related psychological services.

Therapists who work with children with a chronic or acute illness must recognize and accommodate the unique aspects of working with children already described in this chapter and also acquaint themselves with the principles of pediatric psychology. The following case describes the treatment of a child with insulin-dependent diabetes. It illustrates how psychological functioning and disease status are often closely intertwined.

▶ CASE EXAMPLE

Ashley

Ashley R., a 13-year-old girl, has had insulin-dependent diabetes for approximately 4 years. At her most recent outpatient visit her endocrinologist, Dr. Rizzoli, noted that her disease management had deteriorated. When Dr. Rizzoli inquired about how closely Ashley was following her prescribed regimen, Ashley's mother complained about how irresponsible Ashley had become, to which Ashley hurled denials and insults in reply. Dr. Rizzoli asked the psychologist on the Endicrinology team to consult with Ashley and her mother to determine if psychological intervention was needed. The psychologist determined that over the past year, conflicts between Ashley and her mother related to Ashley's diabetes management had increased. Mrs. R. found herself nagging Ashley more and more about testing her blood sugar and making sure she was taking her insulin shots on time. Ashley's compliance with her regimen had decreased over the same period of time and she was experiencing greater physical difficulties as a result. This made Mrs. R. even more concerned, and, as a result, she had increased the intensity and frequency of her reminders to Ashley. After a brief assessment for the purpose of problem definition, the psychologist recommended follow-up services to help Mrs. R. and Ashley learn more effective methods of problem solving and to apply these methods to their conflicts about diabetes management. The psychologist scheduled a follow-up appointment to coincide with Ashley's next check-up at the Endocrinology clinic.

As illustrated in this case example, the pediatric psychologist usually works with children with acute or chronic illness in a medical setting. Because of the integrated nature of a child's physical and psychological status, there is often close collaboration between medical and psychological professionals. In addition to the goal of improved psychological functioning, psychological intervention may result in improved physical status as well.

SUMMARY

The work that clinical psychologists do with children and families is both rewarding and filled with challenges. In this chapter we have tried to present case examples representing a broad array of the problems such psychologists confront, including autism, normal developmental variations in behavior, failure to thrive, anorexia nervosa, test anxiety, attention-deficit hyperactivity disorder, child abuse and neglect, and the psychological aspects of physical illness. Because of the limited scope of the chapter, it has not been possible to convey how greatly our approach to each one of these problems has benefited from scientific research, as psychology has developed both as an academic discipline and as a profession (Routh, 1994). Perhaps the reader will be sufficiently interested in the material presented here to pursue it in more depth.

REFERENCES

American Psychological Association (1992). Ethical principles of psychologists and code of conduct. *American Psychologist, 47,* 1597–1611.

Asher, S. R., & Wheeler, V. A. (1985). Children's loneliness: A comparison of rejected and neglected peer status. *Journal of Consulting and Clinical Psychology, 53,* 500–505.

Cowen, E. L., Pederson, A., Babigian, H., Izzo, L. D., & Trost, M. A. (1973). Long-term follow-up of early detected vulnerable children. *Journal of Consulting and Clinical Psychology, 41,* 438–446.

Haas, L. J., & Malouf, J. L. (1989). *Keeping up the good work: A practitioner's guide to mental health ethics.* Sarasota, FL: Professional Resource Exchange.

Kalichman, S. C. (1993). *Mandated reporting of suspected child abuse: Ethics, law, and policy.* Washington, DC: American Psychological Association.

Kashani, J. H., Konig, P., Sheppard, J. A., Wilfley, D., & Morris, D. A. (1988). Psychopathology and self-concept in asthmatic children. *Journal of Pediatric Psychology, 13,* 509–520.

Mrazek, D. A. (1985). Childhood asthma. *Advances in Psychosomatic Medicine, 14,* 16–32.

Routh, D. K. (1994). *Clinical psychology since 1917.* New York: Plenum.

Taylor, L., & Adelman, H. (1989). Reframing the confidentiality dilemma to work in children's best interests. *Professional Psychology: Research and Practice, 20,* 79–83.

10

An Introduction to Psychotropic Medication

RANDY A. SANSONE   **BLAINE SHAFFER**

Psychotropic medications provide clinicians with potent therapeutic interventions in the management of patients with emotional problems. Our intent in this chapter is to provide an overview of the indications, benefits, and limitations of these drugs and to discuss the complex interface in drug management between the physician, the nonphysician clinician, and the patient. Throughout the chapter we have elected to use the trade names, rather than generic names, of the various drugs to facilitate the reader's recognition.

PSYCHOPHARMACOLOGY ESSENTIALS

To prepare the reader for this chapter, several pharmacology terms warrant definition.

Half-Life (t½): The half-life of a drug is the time required for 50% of the drug to be cleared from the body.

Steady State: Steady state is the stable level of a drug which will eventually occur in the body if the drug is administered at a constant rate. Steady state is typically achieved within a time period that equals 5 half-lives of the specific drug (i.e., a drug with a half-life of 1 day reaches steady state in 5 days).

Metabolism of Drugs: The metabolism of a drug is the process of bio-transformation that typically occurs in the liver for psychotropic drugs (the kidney for lithium), resulting in either the generation of active metabolites and/or inactive compounds. Impaired liver function (e.g., due to age or liver disease) prolongs the half-lives of drugs that are metabolized by the liver.

THE ANTIDEPRESSANTS

Predominant Clinical Indications

Antidepressant medication is most often prescribed for the treatment of depression. Acute discrete depressive episodes characterized by changes in body rhythms (i.e., neurovegetative symptoms such as changes in appetite, weight, or sleep patterns) appear to respond extremely well to antidepressants, regardless of the presence or absence of identifiable stressors or precipitants (e.g., individuals suffering from intense grief reactions respond to intervention with antidepressants).

Depressions that are longstanding (i.e., of several years duration, such as dysthymia) and/or which coexist with an underlying personality disorder have less robust responses to treatment with antidepressants. Although individuals with these types of depressions may experience some relief with antidepressant treatment, it is usually limited to a modest reduction in symptoms. This does not preclude treatment with antidepressants; however, the expectations of both the mental health professional and the patient need to be tempered.

Antidepressants are also prescribed for the treatment of mixed anxiety/depression syndromes, broad-spectrum anxiety disorders both acute and chronic, and panic disorder. Antidepressants with significant serotonergic activity have been particularly useful in the treatment of obsessive-compulsive disorder (OCD).

Although predominantly prescribed for depression and the conditions just listed, antidepressants have been useful in a variety of other clinical situations including attention deficit disorder, enuresis in children, chronic pain syndromes, and headaches.

Purported Mode of Action

The overwhelming majority of antidepressants appear to have some measurable impact in the central nervous system on the neurotransmitters norepinephrine and serotonin. For many antidepressants this impact occurs through *reuptake inhibition* (i.e., the prevention of the reuptake of the neurotransmitter into the pre-synaptic neuron that results in its degradation). Reuptake inhibition usually occurs within hours of initiating treatment with antidepressants, but the actual therapeutic benefit from an antidepressant does not occur until about 3 to 4 weeks into the treatment. Therefore, reuptake inhibition does not fully explain these drugs' mode of action.

In addition to reuptake inhibition, the antidepressants appear to alter or modify receptor sites on both pre-synaptic and post-synaptic neurons. The alteration of these receptors (e.g., beta adrenergic receptors) takes place over several weeks, which coincides with the onset of antidepressant activity in responders.

Although norepinephrine and serotonin appear to be the predominant neurotransmitters directly affected by the antidepressants (e.g., occasionally dopamine is also implicated), some investigators feel that these neurotransmitters really function as modulators, indirectly affecting or exerting an influence over a broad range of other neurotransmitters within the central nervous system.

In defining the mode of action of these drugs to patients, perhaps the easiest explanation is that these drugs "reverse" or "normalize" the underlying neurochemical changes that are believed to cause mood disorders.

Organizational Schema

These diverse drugs can be arranged into an organizational schema that enables easy recall (see Figure 10-1). Antidepressants can initially be divided into two groups: (1) monoamine oxidase inhibitors (MAOIs) and (2) non-MAOIs.

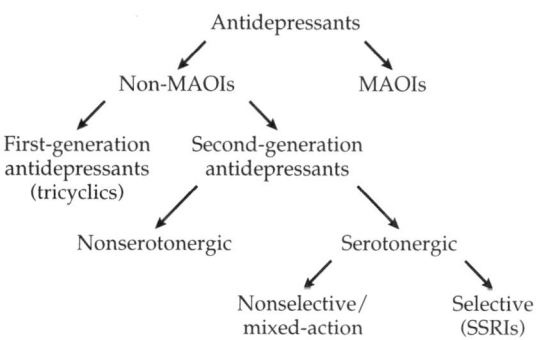

FIGURE 10-1 Antidepressant Organizational Schema

MAOIs

The MAOIs (e.g., Nardil, Parnate) are an interesting and unusual group of drugs. They are fairly efficacious in the treatment of atypical depressions (i.e., depressions characterized by mood lability, obsessive-compulsive features, hypochondriasis, somatic preoccupation, histrionic features, phobias, and anxiety) (Zisook, 1985) as well as panic disorder. Typical side effects may include orthostatic hypotension (i.e., light-headedness precipitated by a change in body position), weight gain, stimulation or sedation, and anticholinergic side effects (described under "TCAs").

MAOIs have unusual constraints, however. Individuals taking MAOIs need to strictly avoid: (1) foods that contain tyramine (high tyramine levels are often found in aged or fermented foods) and (2) certain types of medications (stimulant-type drugs called sympathomimetics) which include over-the-counter as well as prescription drugs (see Table 10-1). A food–drug interaction involving a MAOI may cause an elevation in blood pressure resulting in a headache (Tollefson, 1983) and possibly a stroke. These reactions (hypertensive crises) need to be promptly treated in an emergency room with medication (e.g., phenotolamine).

Non-MAOIs

The non-MAOIs can be divided into two groups: (1) first-generation antidepressants and (2) second-generation antidepressants. The first generation antidepressants represent an older group of drugs that all have tricyclic chemical structures (i.e., the tricyclic antidepressants or TCAs). The core molecular structure of these drugs contains three connecting chemical rings. The second-generation antidepressants are newer drugs. Most are chemically unique when compared to each other and they are not related to the tricyclics in any way except for: (1) Anafranil (a true tricyclic antidepressant) and (2) Asendin and Ludiomil, which have tricyclic-like chemical structures.

First Generation Antidepressants.   The first generation antidepressants can be organized according to their potential for sedation. This ordering is shown in Figure 10-2. Elavil is the most sedating TCA. Both Sinequan and Tofranil

TABLE 10-1   **Examples of Foods and Drugs Contraindicated with MAOIs**

Tyramine-Containing Foods	*Medications*
Aged, matured cheeses	Ephedrine
Smoked or pickled meats/fish	Phenylephrine
Aged meats/fish	Phenylpropanolamine
Yeast or meat extracts (bouillon)	Amphetamines
Red wines	Cocaine
Fava beans	TCAs

Increasing
Sedation

↑ Elavil	very sedating
Sinequan	moderately sedating
Torfanil	moderately sedating
Norpramin	mildly sedating
Aventyl/Pamelor	mildly sedating
Vivactil	nonsedating/stimulating

**FIGURE 10-2   First-Generation Antidepressants
Organized by Sedation**

are moderately sedating. Norpramin and Aventyl or Pamelor (referred to from this point forward as Aventyl/Pamelor) are both mildly sedating. Vivactil, reminiscent of the word "vivacious," is somewhat stimulating. The sedation hierarchy of the TCAs can be recalled by ordering their initial letters into the acronym, E-S-T-N-A-V ("Electroshock therapy needs amps and volts").

This ordering sequence (according to sedation) facilitates the recall of several other clinically pertinent relationships among these drugs (see Table 10-2). First, the standard psychiatric dose per day of the top four drugs is 150 mg. The standard psychiatric dose per day of Aventyl/Pamelor is 50–100 mg and of Vivactil's is 30–40 mg. Thus, the potency of these drugs increases as one goes down the list (i.e., the amount of required drug is less and therefore the drug is more potent).

Second, the three TCAs with the most clinically meaningful or reliable serum levels are clustered together—Tofranil, Norpramin, and Aventyl/Pamelor(APA Task Force; Yesavage, 1986). The suggested serum level for Tofranil, which is determined by adding together the imipramine level and the level of desipramine (the active metabolite of imipramine), is approxi-

TABLE 10-2   Clinical Relationships among the TCAs

	Standard Psychiatric Dose (mg/day)	Clinically Reliable Serum Levels (ng/cc)	Anticholinergic Activity
Elavil	150	—	****
Sinequan	150	—	***
Torfanil	150	225	***
Norpramin	150	125	*
Aventyl/Pamelor	50–100	50–150	**
↓ Vivactil	30–40	—	****

Increasing
Potency

mately 225 ng/cc. The suggested serum level for Norpramin is approximately 125 ng/cc. The suggested serum level for Aventyl/Pamelor is actually a range from 50 to 150 ng/cc, which is referred to as the "therapeutic window."

The third clinically pertinent relationship in this schema is the comparative anticholinergic activities of the TCAs. Anticholinergic activity, due to the blockade of cholinergic receptors, results in a collection of symptoms that may include dry mouth, blurred vision, rapid heart beat, constipation, urinary retention, impairment in the recall of newly acquired information, and confusional states. Higher levels of anticholinergic activity potentially result in more of these symptoms. The TCAs at the ends of the ordering (Elavil and Vivactil) are the most anticholinergic. Norpramin is the least anticholinergic, followed by Aventyl/Pamelor.

Many of the TCA's have unique individual properties. For example, Elavil has significant serotonergic activity which may account for its usefulness in primary care settings for treating headaches and chronic pain, two phenomena that appear to be related to serotonergic receptors. Elavil has an active metabolite, nortriptyline (Aventyl/Pamelor).

Sinequan blocks H_2 receptors at doses of 75 mg or more per day, which results in a significant reduction in gastric acid secretion (Mangla & Pereira, 1982). This effect is comparable to that achieved with Tagamet, an anti-ulcer drug that also blocks H_2 receptors. Both drugs facilitate the healing of ulcers.

Tofranil, the first TCA to be commercially marketed in the United States, has an active metabolite, desipramine (Norpramin). Norpramin is most notable for being the TCA with the lowest anticholinergic activity. Aventyl/Pamelor is most notable for being the TCA that is least likely to cause orthostatic hypotension, a common side effect of the TCAs. Vivactil is noteworthy because of its long half-life of 70–80 hours; the other TCAs have half-lives of approximately 24 hours.

In overdose, all of the tricyclics can cause cardiac arrhythmias that may result in death (Glassman & Preud'homme, 1993); approximately ten to twenty times the standard psychiatric dose per day of a tricyclic is lethal. Because of Vivactil's prolonged half-life, the typical cardiac monitoring period following a tricyclic overdose is extended to several days.

The TCAs, listed by both trade and generic names, are shown in Table 10-3. The available formulations, half-lives, and presence of active metabolites are also noted in the table.

While the TCAs are effective antidepressants, their side effect profiles (e.g., anticholinergic activity, sedation, orthostatic hypotension) and the risk of death with overdose have precipitated the development of other antidepressants, the second generation antidepressants.

Second-Generation Antidepressants.   In general, the second-generation antidepressants are significantly less anticholinergic and cardiotoxic than the TCAs. Unlike the tricyclics which all have a three-ring chemical structure,

TABLE 10-3   Tricyclic Antidepressants

Trade Name(s)	Generic Name	Formulations* (mg)	t ½ (hours)	Active Metabolites
Elavil Endep Amitril	amitriptyline	T: 10, 25, 50, 75, 100, 150 Cp: 10, 25, 50, 75, 100, 150 Injection	16	nortriptyline
Sinequan Adapin	doxepin	Cp: 10, 25, 50, 75, 100, 150 Oral concentrate	17	nordoxepin
Tofranil Janimine SK-pramine	imipramine	T: 10, 25, 50 Injection	18	despiramine
Tofranil-PM	imipramine pamoate	Cp: 75, 100, 125, 150 Injection		
Norpramin Pertofrane	desipramine	T: 10, 25, 50, 75, 100, 150 Cp: 25, 50	31	—
Aventyl/ Pamelor	nortriptyline	Cp: 10, 25, 75 Oral concentrate	31	—
Vivactil	protriptyline	T: 5, 10	78	—

*T = tablets; Cp = capsules

second-generation antidepressants generally are unique chemical formulations when compared to each other with the exception of the chemical cousins Desyrel (trazodone) and Serzone (nefazodone). A summary of the trade and generic names, formulations, half-lives, active metabolites, and usual dosage is shown in Table 10-4.

The second-generation antidepressants have been organized according to relevant neurotransmitter activity (see Figure 10-1). They can be divided into two groups: (1) nonserotonergic and (2) serotonergic. The serotonergic drugs can be further divided into: (1) mixed action or nonselective (i.e., drugs that either demonstrate mixed effects at various serotonin receptor sites or affect other receptors in addition to serotonin receptors) and (2) selective (i.e., drugs that selectively affect serotonin receptor sites similarly and not other receptors).

Second-Generation Antidepressants—Nonserotonergic.   These include Asendin, Ludiomil, and Wellbutrin. Asendin has a tricyclic-type chemical structure (Cohen et al., 1988). It is most noted for its metabolite, 7-OH

TABLE 10.4 Second-Generation Antidepressants

Trade Name	Generic Name	Formulations (mg)	t½† (hours)	Active Metabolites	Usuaul Dose (mg/day)
Asendin	amoxapine	T: 25, 50, 100, 150	8	7-OH amoxapine 8-OH amoxapine	200–300
Ludiomil	maprotiline	T: 25, 50, 75	51	?	75–150
Wellbutrin	bupropion	T: 75, 100	14	morpholinol threo-amino alcohol erythro-amino alcohol erythro-amino diol	300
Desyrel	trazodone	T: 50, 100, 150, 300	8	m-chlorophenyl-piperazine	150–300
Serzone	nefazodone	T: 100, 150, 200, 250	2–4	hydroxy-nefazodone m-chlorophenyl-piperazine	300–600
Effexor	venlafaxine	T: 25, 37.5, 50, 75, 100		o-desmethyl-venlafaxine	75–150
Anafranil	clomipramine	Cp: 25, 50, 75	30	desmethyl-clomipramine	150
Prozac	fluoxetine	Cp: 10, 20 Oral solution	24–72	norfluoxetine	20
Luvox	fluvoxamine	T: 50, 100	24	none	100–300
Zoloft	sertraline	T: 50, 100	24	desmethyl-sertraline	50–100
Paxil	paroxetine	T: 20	24	none	20

* T = tablets; Cp = capsules

† t½ of the parent compound

amoxapine, which blocks dopamine receptors like the typical antipsychotic drugs. Because of this, Asendin demonstrates bona fide antipsychotic activity and functions both as an antidepressant and an antipsychotic. These features establish a unique clinical role for Asendin in the management of psychotically depressed individuals. As with the typical antipsychotics, however, these dopamine effects can result in extrapyramidal symptoms (Goldstein, Dominguez, & Weiss, 1985—for example, dystonic reactions, akathisia, Parkinsonism, and tardive dyskinesia), which will be described in detail in the section, "Antipsychotics." Because of the potential for extrapyramidal symptoms, Asendin is routinely excluded as a drug choice for the treatment of nonpsychotic depression.

Ludiomil is the only antidepressant used in the United States that affects only norepinephrine receptors but not serotonergic or dopamine receptors. It is known to cause seizures. Unlike the other second generation antidepressants, Ludiomil (tetracyclic with a tricyclic-type chemical structure) is cardiotoxic in overdose.

Wellbutrin, the last drug in the nonserotonergic group, is thought to be a dopamine and norepinephrine reuptake inhibitor (not a dopamine blocker like the typical antipsychotics). Despite its half-life of 24 hours, which suggests once-per-day dosing, Wellbutrin is dosed two to three times per day because of the risk of seizures with large single doses. Wellbutrin is the only antidepressant with absolute clinical contraindications. These include: (1) the eating disorders anorexia and bulimia nervosa and (2) past/current seizure disorder. In one study the incidence of seizures was found to be unexpectedly high in bulimics (Horne et al., 1988). Relative contraindications (i.e., use caution) include all medical conditions that predispose to seizures (e.g., neurologic abnormalities, head trauma, withdrawal from depressants).

Second-Generation Antidepressants—Serotonergic, Mixed Action or Non-Selective. This group of drugs includes Desyrel, Serzone, Effexor, and Anafranil (a tricyclic). Desyrel demonstrates mixed serotonergic action (i.e., it is both an agonist and antagonist of serotonergic receptors). These effects may vary depending on the dose. Despite a short half-life of 8 hours, Desyrel appears to be efficacious with once-per-day dosing (Fabre, 1990). The predominant side effect is sedation (Fabre, 1990) which occurs about 30 minutes after ingestion; morning drowsiness can also occur. Because of the lack of addiction, many clinicians are prescribing Desyrel as a hypnotic (i.e., sleeping pill).

In some males, Desyrel has been known to precipitate priapism—painful prolonged erections (Warner et al., 1987). This is a fairly rare occurrence, but all male patients should be advised to promptly discontinue the drug with the development of any unusual penile discharges or abnormally timed or prolonged erections. This aspect of patient education should be documented in the patient's medical record. Priapism does not appear to be related to the dose or the duration of treatment with Desyrel. From a conservative viewpoint, some physicians avoid Desyrel as a first-choice antidepressant in male patients.

Serzone, a drug that is chemically similar to Desyrel (Sharpley, Walsh, & Cowen, 1992), also has mixed serotonergic action. It is a serotonin reuptake inhibitor as well as a serotonin agonist. Like Desyrel, Serzone is metabolized to m-chlorophenylpiperazine (mcPP). Compared to Desyrel, Serzone is less sedating.

Effexor predominantly affects serotonin receptors with secondary activity at norepinephrine receptors. This drug also inhibits the reuptake of dopamine (again, not dopamine blockade). Effexor may have particular efficacy for severe melancholic depression (Montgomery, 1993). Its side effect profile is similar in many ways to the selective serotonin reuptake inhibitors (SSRIs) and may include headaches, gastrointestinal disturbances (e.g., nausea), lightheadedness, and sexual dysfunction (Montgomery, 1993). In individuals with normal blood pressure, Effexor may cause an increase in the diastolic pressure. Therefore, physicians are advised to routinely check the blood pressures of patients on Effexor. The elevation appears to be dose-dependent and does not exclude patients with hypertension from treatment.

The last member in this group is Anafranil which is a bona fide tricyclic. It was placed in this group rather than with the TCAs because of the serotonergic activity of the parent compound, chlorimipramine or clomipramine. Anafranil is a mixed-action drug because its active metabolite (desmethylchlorimipramine/desmethylclomipramine) affects norepinephrine receptors. Like the SSRIs, Anafranil is highly efficacious in the treatment of OCD (Benkelfat et al., 1989). It has the typical tricyclic side effect profile including orthostatic hypotension, weight gain, anticholinergic activity, and cardiac conduction abnormalities/arrhythmias with overdose.

Second-Generation Drugs—Selective Serotonin Reuptake Inhibitors (SSRIs). The SSRIs are a unique group of antidepressants that selectively affect serotonin receptor sites. Because of their specificity, the side effect profile of these drugs is fairly narrow, similar, and mild. While they are all serotonin-specific, there is a strong suspicion that each may be acting at different subreceptor sites of serotonin (Saxena & Ferrari, 1992) and therefore a treatment failure with one SSRI does not predict treatment failure with another (Brown, 1992). A summary and comparison of the SSRIs is shown in Table 10-5.

The potential side effect profile of the SSRIs can be divided into four categories: (1) headaches; (2) gastrointestinal symptoms (e.g., nausea, bloating, abdominal discomfort, loose stools, diarrhea); (3) sexual dysfunction (e.g., inhibited sexual desire, delayed orgasm, sustained erections); and (4) psy-

TABLE 10-5   Summary and Comparison of the SSRIs

	Prozac	Luvox	Zoloft	Paxil
Serotonin receptor site affinity	low ———————————————————————→high			
Half-life, parent compound	1–3 days	1 day	1 day	1 day
Active metabolites	Yes	No	Yes	No
Activity of metabolite	Equipotent to parent compound	—	Weak	—
Half-life of metabolite	7–9 days*	—	2–3 days	—
Activating/ sedating	Activating	Mildly sedating	Neither	Mildly sedating
P-450 effects	Moderate	High	Low	Moderate
Weight effects	Initial decrease	?	None	Minimal increase

*Prozac inhibits its own metabolism in some individuals, such that at the end of 1 year, the half-life may extent to 19 days (Gelenberg, 1991a) and at the end of 2 to 3 years, 27 days.

chomotor effects from mild sedation to activation, including restlessness and difficulty sleeping.

From a cardiac standpoint, the SSRIs are fairly safe in overdose (i.e., lack of cardiac conduction abnormalities)(Dechant & Clissold, 1991; Leonard, 1992). When prescribed, they have few, if any, effects on blood pressure and heart rate, making them excellent choices for patients with cardiac problems.

The SSRIs may inhibit the metabolism of other drugs resulting in serum elevations of these drugs. This effect occurs through the inhibition of the metabolizing enzymes in the liver that are collectively referred to as the cyto-chrome P-450 system (Moltke et al., 1994). Individual SSRIs vary in their like-lihood to inhibit specific enzymes in the P-450 system (see Table 10-5), with Zoloft being the least likely and Luvox being the most likely to inhibit the system (Preskorn, 1992). This inhibitory effect appears to vary from indi-vidual to individual.

Abrupt discontinuation of some of the SSRIs—primarily Paxil and on occasion Zoloft—may precipitate a discontinuation syndrome that is charac terized by muscle cramps, nausea, mood lability, irritability and paresthesias. Discontinuation syndromes are uncomfortable but not life-threatening. Pa-tients who have taken these particular SSRIs for several months or more and wish to discontinue them should be advised to gradually taper the dosage downward over several weeks.

The SSRIs, as well as Anafranil, are highly effective drugs in the treatment of OCD (Griest, 1990; Fineberg et al., 1992). This may be related to their significant serotonergic activity. In the treatment of OCD these antidepressants may be prescribed at higher doses and for longer therapeutic trials (up to 10–12 weeks).

Duration of Antidepressant Treatment

All antidepressants require about 3 to 4 weeks to have an effect on depressive symptoms, although about 10% to 15% of individuals respond after 5 to 6 weeks of treatment (i.e., late responders). Therefore, if the patient can tolerate a particular drug and dosage, a full therapeutic trial of an antidepressant is 6 weeks. Responders must continue antidepressant treatment for 12 months or longer to prevent relapse. Individuals with chronic depression may continue antidepressant treatment for years.

THE ANXIOLYTICS

Predominant Clinical Indications

The anxiolytics are predominantly prescribed for the treatment of both acute and chronic anxiety. One subgroup of anxiolytics, the beta blockers (or ß-blockers), are particularly useful in the treatment of performance anxiety as well as akathisia (a type of extrapyramidal side effect that is discussed under "Antipsychotics"). High-potency benzodiazepines, such as Xanax and Klonopin (clonazepam), have been very effective in the treatment of panic disorder. Benzodiazepines have been extensively used for the treatment of withdrawal syndromes involving depressants such as alcohol and/or barbiturates. Finally, Klonopin, one of the high-potency benzodiazepines, has been useful in some individuals with mood instability.

Purported Mode of Action

The mode of action for the various anxiolytics is quite different depending on the type of anxiolytic. For example, the benzodiazepines act at benzodiazepine receptor sites and affect the neurotransmitter gamma-aminobutyric acid (GABA). Azaspirones act at the 5-HT_{1A} receptor site, a subreceptor site of serotonin. Beta blockers (ß-blockers from this point forward) are theorized to act through the peripheral blockade of ß-adrenergic receptors. Finally, the antihistamines, which affect H_1 receptor sites, appear to be non-specific sedatives unlike the other types of anxiolytics, which have anxiolytic-specific activity.

Organizational Schema

The anxiolytics can be divided into four groups: (1) benzodiazepines, (2) azaspirones, (3) ß-blockers, and (4) antihistamines. A useful acronym is B-A-B-A ("Bullies are born anxious").

Benzodiazepines

The benzodiazepines are a fairly similar, yet diverse, group of drugs. They are similar in regard to their mechanism of action, general side effect profile (e.g., mild sedation, cognitive impairment, uncoordination), potential hazards (e.g., cognitive impairment, addiction, withdrawal), and safety profile (exceptionally safe in solo overdoses but increasingly lethal with the addition of other drugs). In addition, they require a physician DEA number for prescription. Their diversity is primarily related to their individual half-lives, including the presence or absence of active metabolites, the high-potency features of the triazolo- (e.g., Halcion, Xanax) and nitro- (e.g., Klonopin) benzodiazepines, and individual unique features if present.

The commonly prescribed benzodiazepines are listed in Table 10-6 by the length of the half-life of the parent compound. They are divided into four groups: (1) short-acting (less than 20 hours), (2) intermediate acting (24 to 48 hours), (3) long-acting (60 or more hours), and (4) ultra long-acting (100 or more hours). (The reported half-lives of these compounds vary from reference to reference.) Formulations, dosage range, and the existence of any notable features for individual drugs are also noted in Table 10-6. The presence of any active metabolites, which extend the overall half-life of the parent drug, are noted in Figure 10-3. Note that: (1) several of the parent compounds are metabolized into a final common metabolic pathway, suggesting some similarities between these drugs; and (2) glucuronides are inactive compounds.

Although many patients who are prescribed benzodiazepines never increase doses and do not intentionally mix their medications with other drugs, this is a potential problem in patients with particular types of personality disorders (e.g., antisocial, borderline). As with all drugs, the risks (i.e., cognitive impairment, addiction, withdrawal) and benefits need to be carefully assessed for each patient.

Azaspirones

At the present time the azaspirone group has only one member, BuSpar (buspirone). Other azaspirones are in development (e.g., gepirone, ipsapirone, tandospirone), so that a group identity will be more meaningful in the future (Eison, 1989).

TABLE 10.6 Benzodiazepines

$t\frac{1}{2}$ Grouping	Trade Name	Generic Name	Formulations* (mg)	Dosage Range (mg/day)	Features
Short	Halcion	triazolam	T: 0.125, 0.25	0.125–.05	Hypnotic; amnesia risk
Short	Restoril	temazepam	Cp: 7.5, 15, 30	15–30	Hypnotic
Short	Serax	oxazepam	T: 15	45–120	—
Short	Ativan	lorazepam	Cp: 10, 15, 30	1–6	Reliable with intra-muscular injection
Short	Xanax	alprazolam	T: 0.25, 0.5, 1, 2	1–4	High-potency; greater addiction potential
Intermediate	Librium	chlordiazepoxide	Cp: 5, 10, 25	15–40	Unreliable with injection
Intermediate	Valium	diazepam	Injection T: 2, 5, 10 Cp: 15 Injection	5–40	Rapid absorption: "rush"; unreliable with intramuscular injection; greater addiction potential
Long	Tranxene Tranxene-SD	clorazepate	T: 3.75, 7.5, 15 T: 11.25, 22.5	15–60	Inactive parent drug
Long	Paxipam	halazepam	T: 20, 40	60–160	—
Long	Centrax	prazepam	Cp: 5, 10, 20	20–60	Inactive parent drug
Ultra-long	Dalmane	flurazepam	Cp: 15, 30	15–30	Hypnotic

* T = tablets; Cp = capsules

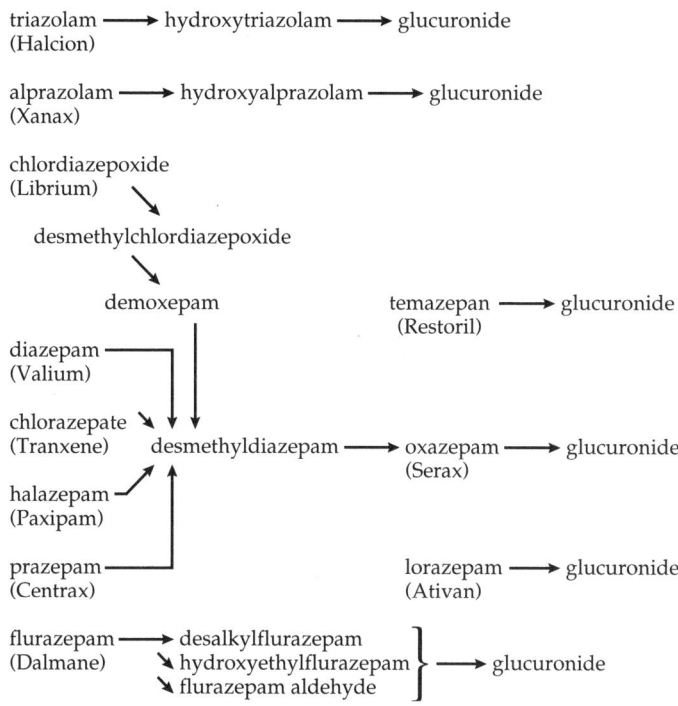

FIGURE 10-3 **Metabolic Degradation of Several Common Benzodiazepines**

BuSpar is an unusual drug compared to the other anxiolytics. It is not addicting (Lader, 1987), does not potentiate the effects of alcohol (Mattila, Arando, & Seppala, 1982), and does not cause any significant cognitive impairment. Unlike the immediate effects of the benzodiazepines, BuSpar's onset of action occurs in 7 to 10 days with full activity in 3 to 4 weeks. BuSpar is formulated as 5 mg and 10 mg scored tablets and the usual dosage is 30–40 mg/day. Common side effects may include nausea, light-headedness, and headache. The half-life of BuSpar is 6 hours and the drug must be dosed two to three times per day. BuSpar has only one active metabolite, 1-pyrimidinyl piperazine. The drug is extremely safe in solo overdoses. Anecdotally, patients with combined anxiety and ruminative/perfectionistic features appear to respond particularly well. Patients who have been on benzodiazepines in the past may have difficulty tolerating the lack of immediacy and the delayed onset of action with BuSpar.

ß-Blockers
ß-blockers appear to be particularly helpful in the treatment of the somatic manifestations of anxiety (e.g., tremulousness, rapid heart beat, shortness of

breath), but not with the psychological manifestations of anxiety (e.g., apprehension, fearfulness). For this reason, ß-blockers tend to be limited to patients whose anxiety syndromes are overshadowed by physical symptoms. In a psychiatric practice these patients are fairly uncommon.

ß-blockers have been very efficacious in the treatment of performance anxiety (e.g., stage fright, test anxiety) (Brantigan, Brantigan, & Joseph, 1982). Low-dose treatment (10–20 mg) with Inderal, the most commonly prescribed ß-blocker in psychiatry, 60 minutes before a performance reduces or eliminates the physiologic anxiety that accompanies performance expectations. As noted previously, ß-blockers have also been used in the treatment of akathisia.

ß-blockers are contraindicated in individuals who have bronchospastic problems (e.g., asthma), congestive heart failure, Raynaud's disease, and diabetes because of the deleterious effects of blocking ß-adrenergic receptors in these conditions. Therefore, all prospective candidates for ß-blocker therapy must be carefully screened for these conditions.

Side effects may include fatigue, irritability, dizziness, apathy, and possible depression. In psychiatry, ß-blockers are prescribed at fairly low doses; the rebound phenomenon seen at the discontinuation of high-dose ß-blockers is rare.

Antihistamines

Antihistamines, which may not have any anxiolytic activity beyond general sedation, include Vistaril (hydroxyzine) and Atarax (hydroxyzine). The advantage of prescribing antihistamines is that they are nonaddicting and have a high margin of safety in overdose. Therefore, they may be useful for the treatment of anxiety syndromes in personality-disordered and/or substance-abusing patients. Potential disadvantages include their side effect profile (e.g., anticholinergic side effects, confusion, sedation) and the possibility of their ineffectiveness over longer periods of usage (i.e., patients may develop tolerance).

Comparison of the Anxiolytics

A comparison of the features of the various anxiolytic groups is shown in Table 10-7. Because of these differing features, some may be more advantageous in particular clinical situations than others.

ANTIPSYCHOTICS

Predominant Clinical Indications

Antipsychotics are predominantly prescribed for the treatment of sustained hallucinations and/or delusions (e.g., schizophrenia, bipolar disorder, psychotic depression, organic mental disorders, and paranoid states).

TABLE 10-7 Comparison of Anxiolytic Groups

	Benzodia- diazepines	Azapirones	ß-blockers	Antihistamines
Controlled substances	yes	no	no	no
Onset of action	minutes/ hours	days (7–10)	minutes/ hours	minutes/hours
Sedation	possible	no	possible	yes
Addiction	possible	no	no	no
Withdrawal	possible	no	no	no
Safety in overdose	good	good	good	good
Medical contrain- dications	none	none	yes*	none

*For example, asthma, bronchospasm, Raynaud's disease, congestive heart failure

Antipsychotics may also be prescribed for the treatment of severe disso-ciation, impulse-control problems, violent or aggressive behavior, overwhelm-ing anxiety states, and treatment-resistant OCD.

Purported Mode of Action

The antipsychotics that are available in the United States all have activity at dopamine receptor sites. The traditional, classic, or "typical" antipsychotics all predominantly affect a subgroup of dopamine receptors called the D_2 re-ceptors. The newer antipsychotics, which also affect serotonergic receptor sites and may be more specific to dopamine receptors in the mesolimbic ar-eas of the brain, are referred to as the "atypical" antipsychotics. These in-clude the drugs Clozaril (clozapine), which affects serotonin and both D_1 and D_2 dopamine receptor sites, and Risperdal (risperidone), which affects serotonin and dopamine receptor sites.

Organizational Schema

Typical Antipsychotics
The typical antipsychotics can be organized according to anticholinergic activity (e.g., dry mouth, blurred vision, constipation, urinary retention);

sedation; and the potential for weight gain, endocrinologic changes, orthostatic hypotension, potency and extrapyramidal symptoms (EPS)(see Table 10-8). The organizing properties for this antipsychotic organizational schema are more relational because of the similar neurochemical spectrum of these drugs; they can be recalled using the acronym, T-M-T-S-N-P-H ("To maintain total sanity, never prescribe hallucinogens").

Some of these drugs have specific or notable features. For example, Thorazine was the first available antipsychotic in the United States (early 1950s). With chronic use, Thorazine may cause a slate-gray discoloration of the skin. Because Thorazine may cause corneal and lenticular opacities, some physicians recommend a yearly examination by an opthalmologist to check for these potential changes in patients' eyes. Thorazine may also cause abcesses when administered as an intramuscular injection.

Mellaril is the typical antipsychotic which some investigators feel may have the lowest incidence of EPS (described later in this section). Mellaril is the only antipsychotic listed in the organizational schema that does not come as an injectable. It is also the only antipsychotic that has a legally relevant absolute dose limit, which is 800 mg per day. Dosages above this limit may result in retinitis pigmentosa, a condition that initially manifests as difficulty with night vision and can progress to a gradual deterioration of vision. At doses of 200 mg per day or more, Mellaril may cause non-pathologic changes in electrocardiograms (EKGs or ECGs), which may complicate the interpretation of these recordings. Mellaril may have some mood-lifting features, although it is not primarily prescribed as an antidepressant. Finally, Mellaril may cause erectile and ejaculatory disturbances in males.

TABLE 10-8   Organizational
Schema for the Typical Antipsychotics

↑ Anticholinergic activity
↑ Sedation
↑ Weight gain
↑ Endocrinological changes (e.g., galactorrhea)
Orthostatic hypotension

Thorazine
Mellaril
Trilafon (Loxitane, Moban)
Stelazine
Navane
Prolixin
Haldol

Increasing potency
Increasing potential for EPS

Trilafon and Stelazine, which are fairly popular because of their moderate side effect profiles, are midrange antipsychotic drugs without any particularly unique features. Like Mellaril, Navane may have some mood-lifting features. Navane comes in two different injectable doses (2 mg/cc, 5 mg/cc). Prolixin was the first antipsychotic in the United States to be available as a long-acting depot injectable (Prolixin decanoate) as well as a routine injectable. Prolixin decanoate gradually releases from the injection site over 2 to 4 weeks, and side effects tend to peak during the first 3 to 5 days. The advantage of a depot antipsychotic is that it may reduce patient noncompliance; however, patients must still be sufficiently motivated for treatment to attend appointments. The disadvantage of a depot injectable is that should significant side effects develop, there is no quick clearance of the drug from the body. Therefore, side effects need to be treated symptomatically until the drug is metabolized and excreted.

Haldol, the most potent typical antipsychotic, is noted for its minimal anticholinergic, cardiovascular (i.e., impact on heart rate and orthostatic hypotension), and sedative effects. This side effect profile may be particularly useful for organically compromised and/or elderly patients. However, the potential disadvantage is the increased likelihood of EPS (to be discussed below). Haldol formulations include an oral concentrate that is odorless, colorless and tasteless. Like Prolixin, Haldol is also available as a routine injectable and a long-acting depot injectable (Haldol decanoate). A comparison of the decanoates of Prolixin and Haldol are shown in Table 10-9.

Two other typical antipsychotic drugs, Loxitane and Moban, warrant mention. Both are mid-range drugs in the organizational schema, akin to Trilafon and Stelazine. Loxitane is metabolically interesting because the parent compound (loxapine) is metabolized to amoxapine (Asendin), which has antidepressant activity. Amoxapine, in turn, is metabolized to 7-0H amoxapine

TABLE 10-9 **Comparison of Decanoates**

	Prolixin decanoate	*Haldol decanoate*
t ½	7 days	21 days
Steady state	1 month	3 months
Injection frequency	every 2–4 weeks	every 3–4 weeks
Oral medication supplementation	may or may not be necessary	often necessary
Serum levels	greater fluctuation	less fluctuation

(recall the metabolic pathway for Asendin, an antidepressant), which also has antipsychotic activity. In summary, Loxitane has both antipsychotic and antidepressant activity and may be helpful for patients who have both psychosis and depression. Unlike the other antipsychotics, which tend to induce weight gain, Moban is noted for its lack of weight gain.

The typical antipsychotics including generic names, formulations, and usual dosage per day are listed in Table 10-10.

TABLE 10-10　Typical Antipsychotics

Trade Name	Generic Name	Formulations* (mg)	Usual Dosage (mg/day)
Thorazine	chlorpromazine	T: 10, 25, 50, 100, 200 Capsules: 30, 75, 150, 200 Syrup Concentrate Parenteral	100–300
Mellaril	thioridazine	T: 10, 15, 25, 50, 100, 150, 200 Concentrate Suspension	50–300
Trilafon	perphenazine	T: 2, 4, 8, 16 Repetabs (8 mg) Concentrate Parenteral	8–16
Stelazine	trifluoperazine	T: 1, 2, 5, 10 Concentrate Parenteral	4–30
Navane	thiothixene	Cp: 1, 2, 5, 10, 20 Concentrate Parenteral	5–30
Prolixin	fluphenazine	T: 1, 2, 5, 10 Elixir Parenteral Decanoate (2.5 mg/cc)	1–15
Haldol	haloperidol	T: 1, 2, 5, 10 Concentrate Parenteral Decanoate (50 and 100 mg/cc)	1–15

*T = tablets; Cp = capsules

Atypical Antipsychotics

The atypical antipsychotics include Clozaril and Risperdal. In addition to the positive symptoms of schizophrenia (e.g., hallucinations, delusions), atypical antipsychotics appear to be particularly efficacious in treating the negative symptoms (e.g., apathy, emotional unresponsiveness, poor motivation) (Marder, 1992), as well.

Clozaril was the first atypical antipsychotic available in the United States. Clozaril affects serotonergic as well as D_1 and D_2 (dopamine) receptors. In contrast to the typical antipsychotics, there appears to be an exceedingly low prevalence of tardive dyskinesia with the use of Clozaril (Tully, 1988). Common side effects of Clozaril include sedation, rapid heart beat, and weight gain. The drug may also cause seizures (higher risk with higher doses) as well as severely depress bone marrow and the production of blood cells (i.e., agranulocytosis) (Lieberman, Kane, & Johns, 1989). For these reasons, Clozaril treatment requires baseline laboratory studies and weekly blood tests to assess the blood cell count. Presently this drug is primarily prescribed by psychiatrists, and laboratory studies are monitored by the pharmaceutical company as well as the physician.

Risperdal is the most recently available atypical antipsychotic. It is chemically different from Clozaril and affects serotonergic and dopamine receptor sites (Heylen & Gelders, 1992). Side effects may include fatigue, weakness, insomnia, and infrequent EPS (Borison et al., 1992). Risperdal does not require routine laboratory monitoring, nor does it seem to have any of the potential hematologic or neurologic risks associated with Clozaril (e.g., suppression of bone marrow, seizures).

Extrapyramidal Side Effects (EPS)

Extrapyramidal side effects are abnormal muscular movements caused by antipsychotics. They can be divided into four categories and are presented in order of their potential appearance following the onset of antipsychotic treatment. They include dystonic reactions, akathisia, Parkinsonism, and tardive dyskinesia. The acronym is D-A-P-T ("Draw A Person Test").

Dystonic reactions are dramatic, abrupt spasms of voluntary muscles that wax and wane over time. They typically appear within the first few doeses or days of antipsychotic treatment. They tend to occur more often in young males on high-potency antipsychotics (e.g., Prolixin, Haldol). Dystonic reactions can be painful and frightening for patients and often worsen with anxiety. Descriptions of classic dystonic reactions are noted in Table 10-11 These reactions dramatically resolve with either the administration of Cogentin or some other anticholinergic agent (e.g., Benadryl, Artane). Unlike the other dystonic reactions, laryngospasm, which results in the occlusion of the airway, is a medical emergency. It should be promptly treated

TABLE 10-11   Examples of Dystonic Reactions

Reaction	Description
Torticollis	Deviation of the head to the side
Retrocollis	Deviation of the head backward
Oculogyric crisis	Deviation of the eyes upward
Trismus	Gritting of the teeth
Laryngospasm	Intermittant occlusion of the airway due to spasm of the larynx
Opisthotonos	Arching of the body

with an intravenous injection of Cogentin, Benadryl, or a similar drug to hasten the response.

Akathisia is an uncomfortable restlessness that may appear after several days to weeks of antipsychotic drug exposure. Patients may appear to be in constant motion, unable to sit down for any length of time, and/or agitated. They may report a very uncomfortable sense of inner restlessness. Akathisia is less likely to respond to treatment with anticholinergic drugs such as Cogentin or Benadryl (only about one-third of patients respond), but ß-blockers (Inderal) appear to be helpful.

Antipsychotic-induced Parkinsonism, which develops over several days to weeks, resembles bona fide Parkinson's disease. Symptoms include a pill-rolling tremor, stiffness of the body, shuffling gait, an expressionless face ("masked facies"), drooling, difficulty with initiating and stopping movement during ambulation, and "en bloc" turns (i.e., gradual approximation of a turn, with the body remaining for the most part in one plane) rather than pivotal turns, which involve a smooth rotation of the body. Like dystonic reactions, this syndrome responds well to treatment with anticholinergic drugs and completely resolves with the discontinuation of the antipsychotic.

The final extrapyramidal reaction is tardive dyskinesia, which typically develops over months to years of treatment with antipsychotics. Tardive dyskinesia appears as involuntary, repetitive movements that usually begin around the mouth and face but can progress to affect the entire body. The principal concern with tardive dyskinesia is its limited reversibility in many patients despite the discontinuation of the antipsychotic medication. Therefore, patients beginning treatment with antipsychotics may be asked by the physician to sign a consent form that acknowledges the potential risk of tardive dyskinesia. Patients on antipsychotic drugs are closely followed during treatment for the development of this reaction. Some clinicians use a checklist, the Abnormal Involuntary Movement Scale, or AIMS, at routine intervals to help detect the appearance of and measure changes in abnormal movements.

Various treatments have been explored to reduce or eliminate the abnormal movements of tardive dyskinesia. However, treatment responses have been inconsistent (i.e., some individuals improve, some don't). Because of the potential risk of tardive dyskinesia and its erratic responses to treatment, physicians should carefully document their rationale for the use of drugs that might cause the impairment.

Neuroleptic Malignant Syndrome

Neuroleptic malignant syndrome (NMS) is an idiosyncratic antipsychotic-induced syndrome that is abrupt in onset and is characterized by: (1) central nervous system dysfunction (e.g., altered sensorium, tremors, dyskinesias, akinesia), (2) hyperthermia, (3) autonomic dysfunction (e.g., increased heart rate, sweating, pallor), and (4) muscular rigidity. This syndrome is infrequent, is often associated with high-potency neuroleptics, and occurs more frequently in males. The course intensifies over a 24- to 72-hour period, and the mortality rate is 20% (due to cardiac, respiratory, and/or renal failure). Treatment includes: (1) discontinuation of the antipsychotic drug, (2) supportive treatment (e.g., adequate hydration, antipyretics, cooling blanket), and (3) medication (e.g., bromocriptine, dantrolene, amantadine) (Sakkas et al., 1991).

ANTI-CYCLING/ANTI-MANIC DRUGS

Predominant Clinical Indications

Anti-cycling or anti-manic drugs are primarily prescribed for the treatment of acute mania or depression in bipolar patients as well as for the prophylaxis of both manic and depressive episodes. These drugs may also be used in patients with dramatic cyclothymia (i.e., severe moodiness) as well as the severe mood instability seen in some borderline patients.

Anti-cycling/anti-manic drugs may also be used for the treatment of aggression, impulse-control difficulties, and rage reactions. They may be prescribed as adjuncts to treatment in nonbipolar depressed patients who are not responding to antidepressants alone.

Lithium

Lithium was the first drug that is not an antipsychotic to be successfully used in the treatment of bipolar disorder. Lithium is available as a liquid (lithium citrate), routine-release 300-mg capsules/tablets (lithium carbonate), and sustained-release tablets of 300 mg (lithium carbonate, marketed as Lithobid) and 450 mg (lithium carbonate, marketed as Eskalith CR-450). The half-life of lithium is 24 hours and serum levels are routinely drawn every 5 days (i.e., at steady state) following a change in the dosage. When the desired level is achieved, lithium levels are drawn every 2 to 4 months depending on the stability and reliability of the patient. In the treatment of acute mania or depression the desired serum level is between 0.8 and 1.2 mEq/l (usually 1200 to 1800 mg of lithium per day). For maintenance and other psychiatric indications the serum level is typically adjusted between 0.6 and 1.0 mEq/l (usually 900 to 1200 mg of lithium per day).

Lithium, like Clozaril and the anticonvulsants, is one of the few psychotropic drugs that requires laboratory evaluation prior to prescription. The laboratory studies include electrolytes (low sodium can result in lithium retention), blood urea nitrogen (BUN) and creatinine to assess kidney function (the drug is excreted by the kidneys), thyroid function tests (lithium can cause hypothyroidism, so a baseline measure is important), and a white blood cell count with a differential (lithium can cause leukocytosis, a dramatic though benign increase in the white blood cell count). Some physicians will also include an EKG in the laboratory work-up of patients over 40 years of age or of younger patients with heart problems because lithium may cause minor changes in the EKG. These laboratory studies are repeated on an annual basis.

Lithium may cause a variety of side effects including sedation, hand tremor, frequent thirst, frequent urination, nausea, diarrhea, hair loss, metallic taste, and weight gain. At toxic levels, lithium may cause gastrointestinal disturbances (e.g., nausea, vomiting, diarrhea) as well as neurologic side effects (e.g., lethargy, uncoordination, unsteady gait, blurred vision) (Annitto, 1979). Lithium can be lethal in overdose. Because it is excreted by the kidneys, patients who have severely elevated lithium levels can undergo renal dialysis for the removal of the drug.

Potential treatment complications with lithium can include (1) hypothyroidism, which may be heralded by dramatic weight gain and require subsequent treatment with thyroid hormone; (2) leukocytosis, which causes no medical difficulties; and (3) diabetes insipidus. The latter condition is rare, manifests as copious urination (i.e., up to several liters of urine per day—well beyond mere frequent urination), and usually requires the discontinuation of lithium.

For years, investigators have wondered about the potential long-term effects of lithium treatment on the kidney. Although there may be some changes, the overwhelming majority of patients on long-term lithium treatment never experience changes in kidney function that require medical intervention (Jefferson, 1990).

Anticonvulsants

Over the past few years the anticonvulsants have been prescribed for lithium nonresponders or partial responders as an adjunct to lithium treatment (Zajecka (carbamazepine), 1993). The two most commonly prescribed anticonvulsants are Tegretol and Depakene (valproic acid) or Depakote (a combination of valproic acid and sodium valproate—divalproex sodium—that is less irritating to the stomach). A comparison of these drugs can be seen in Table 10-12.

Tegretol, Depakene, and Depakote can be challenging to work with because of potential drug interactions, potential medical complications, and the need for frequent laboratory assessment during the first few months of treatment. In addition, Tegretol induces its own metabolism for several months, which complicates the stabilization of a serum level. These drugs should be avoided during pregnancy.

PSYCHODYNAMIC ISSUES RELATED TO PSYCHOTROPIC MEDICATION

Unrealistic Expectations

The potential benefits of psychotropic medication in the treatment of patients are fairly clear. However, clinicians may encounter unrealistic expectations from patients and families about drug treatment. They may perceive the medication as a treatment that will eradicate their emotional problems, like an antibiotic in the treatment of an infection. This perception may compromise patients' participation in a psychotherapy treatment and/or adjunctive psychosocial interventions.

TABLE 10-12   Comparison of Tegretol, Depakene, and Depakote

	Tegretol	*Depakene*	*Depakote*
Formulations (mg)	T: 100, 200 Suspension	Cp: 250 Syrup	T: 125, 250, 500 Sprinkle capsules (125)
t ½ (hours)	15	10–15	10–15
Dosage range	800–1200 mg/day	up to 60 mg/kg/day	up to 60 mg/kg/day
Serum levels (ng/cc)	4–12	50–120	50–120
Side effects	lethargy, sedation, nausea, tremor, rash	nausea, tremor, lethargy, weight increase, transient hair loss	nausea, tremor, lethargy, weight increase, transient hair loss
Lab studies	required	required	required

Resistance to Medication

Patients may perceive the recommendation of medication as an indication that their clinical situation is particularly severe (e.g., "I'm not going crazy, am I?"). They may resist drug treatment, feeling that they must do everything within their capability to help themselves before it's "too late" (the "pull-yourself-up-by-the-bootstraps" philosophy). Unfortunately, this attitude may also be shared by family members, who may misinterpret the patient's clinical situation as end-stage.

Intervention with medication may also challenge the patient's or family's belief structure about psychiatric or psychological treatment (e.g.,"One must deal with what one is dealt in life"). The latter may include spiritual, religious, or cultural values and beliefs.

Treatment with medication is often more visible to the outside world than a psychotherapy treatment, both through the taking of medication and in the appearance of side effects. Patients and families may be realistically concerned about how others will interpret the medication, despite being at ease with it themselves. This is of particular concern for patients who are seeking employment situations or negotiating new relationships.

Finally, patients and families may be realistically concerned about the potential complications of medication (e.g., food–drug interactions with monoamine oxidase inhibitors, tardive dyskinesia with antipsychotics, addiction with benzodiazepines).

Before prescribing medications, one should actively discuss the patient's thoughts and feelings about taking a drug for an emotional problem. It may also be useful to ask about the possible reactions of family members, many of whom may be very supportive of medication intervention. Finally, patients should be asked if they anticipate any special difficulties or problems in being prescribed a psychotropic drug. Active discussion prior to and during the treatment may alleviate both unwarranted as well as realistic concerns.

Psychotropic Medication and the Borderline Patient

In patients with personality disorders, particularly borderline personality, intervention with medication can be fairly complicated. In general, these patients have a less robust response to medication (Zanarini, Frankenburg, & Gunderson, 1988), and the potential risks are higher.

The risks are many. Borderline patients may experience unusual sensitivity to drugs including idiosyncratic reactions as well as bona fide allergic reactions. From a psychodynamic standpoint, borderline patients engage in ongoing self-destructive behavior and the medication may be misused (e.g., purposefully combined with illicit drugs), underused, or overused including overdose. Borderline patients may also use medication-related issues to resist psychological exploration and/or foster tension between the psychotherapist and the physician. Over all, in work with borderline patients, the risk–benefit ratio must be carefully evaluated for each patient.

Psychotropic Medication and the Psychotherapist–Physician Relationship

In most cases, patient management is enhanced by a strong, mutually supportive relationship between the psychotherapist and the prescribing physician. Regular contact between the two may be particularly helpful when dealing with difficult patients (e.g., characterological patients, treatment nonresponders).

Splitting

One significant threat to the psychotherapist–physician relationship is splitting, in which distortion of information results in unhealthy alliances. Splitting may occur between the patient and the professional as well as between professionals. A deterrent to splitting is for professionals to: (1) anticipate splitting, (2) discuss their treatment philosophies and orientations with each other, and (3) contact each other at the first sign of apparent miscommunication. When confusion occurs, a useful guideline is to strongly consider the possibility of splitting until proven otherwise—through discussion with your fellow clinician.

Boundaries

Another dilemma may occur if either professional extends beyond the identified professional role with the patient. For example, the physician needs to limit the initial consultation and subsequent medication follow-up appointments to issues that relate to medication. The provision of psychotherapy during medication appointments is usually inappropriate, and physicians need to be alert to avoid this. Patients who initiate psychotherapy issues with the physician consultant need to be redirected to their psychotherapist unless there is a significant therapeutic impasse.

Likewise, nonphysician professionals need to be thoughtful around discussing medication issues with patients. It is helpful to avoid suggesting a particular medication when making a referral for medication evaluation. Specific drug suggestions tend to overly focus the patient on a drug that may not be the best choice in a given case. When prescribed, specific questions about the medication need to be redirected to the physician. It is appropriate to explore patients' side effects, tolerance to the medication, and the general response to psychotropic drug treatment. However, the nonphysician professional should not recommend to patients complex drug regimens, dosage changes, changes in the timing of medication, or stopping medication (unless there is an acute complication). When necessary, the therapist's concerns about medication should be directly addressed with the physician.

Philosophical Differences

If there is significant disagreement around the treatment philosophy and/or orientation, professionals need to discuss their differences. Both need to determine whether or not these differences will deter their professional working relationship in the management of the patient.

CONCLUSION

This chapter has endeavored to provide the reader with (1) an overview of four types of psychotropic medication and (2) an introduction to some of the psychodynamic issues related to medications and patients, their families, nonphysician clinicians, and physicians. However, the field of psychopharmacology is rapidly advancing. Updated information on psychotropic medications can be obtained from most medical libraries through literature searches. In addition, there are several excellent synopses of psychopharmacology (Gelenberg, 1991a; Kaplan & Sadock, 1993; Salzman, 1991; Schatzberg & Cole, 1991), and surely more will be published. It is hoped that the information in this chapter will function as a framework in which to encode further information as new psychotropic medications become available.

REFERENCES

APA Task Force (1985). Tricyclic antidepressants—blood level measurements and clinical outcome: AnAPA task force report. *American Journal of Psychiatry, 142,* 155–162.

Annitto, W. J. (1979). Recognizing lithium-associated neurotoxocity. *Drug Therapy, 9,* 45–51.

Benkelfat, C., Murphy, D. L., Zohar, J., Hill, J. L., Grover, G., & Insel, T. R. (1989). Clomipramine in obsessive-compulsive disorder. *Archives of General Psychiatry, 46,* 23–28.

Borison, R. L., Pathiraja, A. P., Diamond, B. I., & Meibach, R. C. (1992). Risperidone: Clinical safety and efficacy in schizophrenia. *Psychopharmacology Bulletin, 28,* 213–218.

Brantigan, C. O., Brantigan, T. A., & Joseph, N. (1982). Effect of beta blockade and beta stimulation on stage fright. *American Journal of Medicine, 72,* 88–94.

Brown, W. A. (1992). Are patients who are intolerant to one SSRI, intolerant to another? *Presented at the American Psychiatric Association Meeting, Washington, DC,* May 3–6.

Cohen, B. M., Harris, P. Q., Altesman, R. I., & Cole, J. O. (1982). Amoxapine: Neuroleptic as well as antidepressant? *American Journal of Psychiatry, 139,* 1165–1167.

Dechant, K. L., & Clissold, S. P. (1991). Paroxetine: A review of its pharmacodynamic and pharmacokinetic properties, and therapeutic potential in depressive illness. *Drug Evaluation, 41,* 225–253.

Eison, M. S. (1989). The new generation of serotonergic anxiolytics: Possible clinical roles. *Psychopathology, 22,* 13–20.

Fabre, L. F. (1990). Trazodone dosing regimen: Experience with single daily administration. *Journal of Clinical Psychiatry, 51,* 23–26.

Fineberg, N. A., Bullock, T., Montgomery, D. B., & Montgomery, S. A. (1992). Serotonin reuptake inhibitors are the treatment of choice in obsessive compulsive disorder. *International Clinical Psychopharmacology, 7,* 43–47.

Gelenberg, A. (1991a). Fluoxetine levels and interactions. *Biological Therapies in Psychiatry Newsletter, 14,* 1–2.

Gelenberg, A. (1991b). *Practitioner's guide to psychoactive drugs* (3d ed.). New York: Plenum.

Glassman, A. H., & Preud'homme, X. A. (1993). Review of the cardiovascular effects of heterocyclic antidepressants. *Journal of Clinical Psychiatry, 54,* 16–22.

Goldstein, B. J., Dominguez, R. A., & Weiss, B. L. (1985). Amoxapine in psychotic depression. *Journal of Clinical Psychiatry Monograph, 3,* 14–16.

Greist, J. H. (1990). Medication management of obsessive-compulsive disorder. *Today's Therapeutic Trends, 7,* 29–36.

Heylen, S. L., & Gelders, Y. G. (1992). Risperidone, a new antipsychotic with serotonin 5-HT2 and dopamine D2 antagonistic properties. *Clinical Neuropharmacology, 15,* 180A–181A.

Horne, R. L., Ferguson, J. M., Pope, H. G., Hudson, J. I., Lineberry, C. G., Ascher, J., & Cato, A. (1988). Treatment of bulimia with bupropion: A multicenter controlled trial. *Journal of Clinical Psychiatry, 49,* 262–266.

Jefferson, J. W. (1990). Lithium: The present and the future. *Journal of Clinical Psychiatry, 51,* 4–8.

Kaplan, H., & Saddock, B. (1993). *Pocket handbook of psychiatric drug treatment.* Baltimore, MD: Williams & Wilkins.

Lader, M. (1987). Assessing the potential for buspirone dependence or abuse and effects of its withdrawal. *American Journal of Medicine, 82,* 20–26.

Leonard, B. E. (1992). Pharmacological differences of serotonin reuptake inhibitors and possible clinical relevance. *Drugs, 43,* 3–10.

Lieberman, J. A., Kane, J. M., & Johns, C. A. (1989). Clozapine: Guidelines for clinical management. *Journal of Clinical Psychiatry, 50,* 329–338.

Mangla, J. C., & Pereira, M. (1982). Tricyclic antidepressants in the treatment of peptic ulcer disease. *Archives of Internal Medicine, 142,* 273–275.

Marder, S. R. (1992). Risperidone: Clinical development: North American results. *Clinical Neuropharmacology, 15,* 92A–93A.

Mattila, M. J., Aranko, K., & Seppala, T. (1982). Acute effects of buspirone and alcohol on psychomotor skills. *Journal of Clinical Psychiatry, 43,* 56–60.

Moltke, L. L., Greenblatt, D. J., Harmatz, J. S., & Shader, R. I. (editorial) (1994). Cytochromes in psychopharmacology. *Journal of Clinical Psychopharmacology, 14,* 1–2.

Montgomery, S. A. (1993). Venlafaxine: A new dimension in antidepressant pharmacotherapy. *Journal of Clinical Psychiatry, 54,* 119–126.

Moran, M. G., Thompson, T. L., & Nies, A. S. (1988). Sleep disorders in the elderly. *American Journal of Psychiatry, 145,* 1369–1378.

Preskorn, S. H. (1992). Selected topics on the pharmacokinetics and drug interactions of serotonin-selective reuptake inhibitors: An interview with Sheldon H. Preskorn, M.D. *Currents in Psychopharmacology, 11,* 5–6.

Sakkas, P., Davis, J. M., Hua, J., & Wang, Z. (1991). Pharmacotherapy of neuroleptic malignant syndrome. *Psychiatric Annals, 21,* 157–164.

Salzman, B. (1991). *Handbook of psychiatric drugs.* New York: Holt.

Saxena, P. R., & Ferrari, M. D. (1992). From serotonin receptor classification to the antimigraine drug sumatriptan. *Cephalgia, 12,* 187–196.

Schatzberg, A. F., & Cole, J. O. (1991). *Manual of clinical psychopharmacology* (2d ed.). Washington, DC: American Psychiatric Press.

Sharpley, A. L., Walsh, A. E. S., & Cowen, P. J. (1992). Nefazodone—a novel antidepressant—may increase REM sleep. *Biological Psychiatry, 31,* 1070–1073.

Tollefson, G. D. (1983). Monoamine oxidase inhibitors: A review. *Journal of Clinical Psychiatry, 44,* 280–288.

Tully, E. M. (1988). Clozapine: A review. *American Journal of Preventative Psychiatry & Neurology, 1,* 19–23.

Warner, M. D., Peabody, C. A., Whiteford, H. A., & Hollister, L. E. (1987). Trazodone and priapism. *Journal of Clinical Psychiatry,* 244–245.

Yesavage, J. A. (1986). Psychotropic blood levels: A guide to clinical responses. *Journal of Clinical Psychiatry, 47,* 16–19.

Zajecka, J. (1993). Pharmacology, pharmacokinetics, and safety issues of mood-stabilizing agents. *Psychiatric Annals, 23,* 79–85.

Zanarini, M. C., Frankenburg, F. R., & Gunderson, J. G. (1988). Pharmacotherapy of borderline outpatients. *Comprehensive Psychiatry, 29,* 372–378.

Zisook, S. (1985). A clinical overview of monoamine oxidase inhibitors. *Psychosomatics, 26,* 240–251.

11

Introduction to Assessment of Organic Disorders

ANTONIO E. PUENTE

THE QUESTION OF ORGANICITY

One of the classical questions in clinical psychology involves whether the patient has a functional or an organic problem. That is, does the patient have a problem that is tied to psychological factors (e.g., depression) or does it have a physiological basis (e.g., Alzheimer's). As a consequence, one of the basic questions in evaluating a patient is whether the patient has a psychologically based difficulty or could the problem be directly traceable to an organic substrate. Such questions are typical, for example, when evaluating elderly patients. Memory disorders are common in this population, and the referral question might be something like "Is the patient depressed or demented?"

Presently these kinds of questions seem to be less likely to be asked and probably have less validity as well (Puente, 1992). The focus has shifted away from simplified differential diagnoses to more functional issues. Hence, the question shifts from "Does the patient have a physiological substrate to his/her behavioral aberration?" to "Describe the problems present in the patient." In other words, instead of ruling out (or in) an organic problem, the task has shifted to describing and quantifying behavioral patterns.

The case of an elderly patient provides an illustration. If the patient is demented (of the Alzheimer's type), then one should expect difficulties with certain types of verbal learning that should deteriorate at a particular rate and pattern. Further, such patients do not typically respond to antidepressant medication intervention as would depressed patients.

Thus, the question of organicity becomes less relevant in current approaches to evaluating these patients. Further, some neuropsychologists (including this author) believe that all patients are "organic," at least to some degree. That is, all forms of psychopathology have physiological and nervous system substrates. Anxiety and depression have been found not only to have a neurochemical basis but neuropsychological complications as well (see Puente & McCaffrey, 1992, for further information). It becomes difficult, and generally irrelevant, to focus on whether there is organicity. Instead, the primary focus becomes analysis of the problem in question. While it would be impossible to provide an exhaustive analysis of brain disorders and clinical neuropsychology, this chapter provides a general overview of some of the most salient issues in clinical neuropsychology. Other scholarly efforts (e.g., Anderson, 1994) provide a more comprehensive and detailed analysis of the many issues covered in this chapter.

HISTORY AND APPROACHES OF NEUROPSYCHOLOGY

Historians of psychology have repeatedly referred to Ebbinghaus, who once said, "Psychology has a long past but a short history." The same sentiment applies to neuropsychology. Analysis of the Greeks would quickly reveal an interest in brain function as it relates to abnormal behavior. This concern continues with Descartes and other philosophers during the nineteenth century with the controversial phrenologists and culminates with the pioneering work of Broca and others. During the twentieth century particular focus on brain disorders occurred after World War II when veterans were returning home with missile wounds. Goldstein and Franz at St. Elizabeth's Hospital in Washington, DC evaluated these patients with a focus on understanding their unusual behavioral patterns (e.g., perseveration). Simultaneously, Karl Lashley at Harvard was stimulating interest in experimental and theoretical questions about brain function. His ideas of equipotentiality (all portions of the brain are roughly equally involved with the production of behavior) were tested with rats and monkeys in simple and complex learning experiments. The culmination of experimental research in the 1900s was the pioneering work of Sperry (Sperry, 1982) with split-brain patients. Sperry, Bogen, and several colleagues over more than 25 years carefully studied the effects of splitting the brain in half (commisurotomy). Their carefully designed studies helped reveal the unique functions of the left and right sides of the cerebral cortex.

During the last quarter of this century, neuropsychology has grown quickly and in a variety of ways. The experimental work has helped spawn the promising field of neuroscience, although within neuropsychology a strong experimental focus still exists in some circles (e.g., International Neuropsychological Society; Journal of the International Neuropsychological Society). In contrast, a more applied or clinical segment has also grown exponentially. The early work of Reitan (Reitan & Wolfson, 1984) and Golden (1981) in using psychometric tests to carefully quantify brain dysfunction gave rise to a group of neuropsychologists with interest and expertise in the assessment of "organic" disorders (National Academy of Neuropsychology; *Archives of Clinical Neuropsychology*). More recently, however, alternative methods of evaluation (more ecological and cognitive) have been proposed, and the rehabilitation of patients with brain injuries has also become a primary concern for clinical neuropsychologists. Puente (1990) provides a more thorough analysis of the major historical issues that contributed to the development of clinical neuropsychology as a professional specialty.

Components of Clinical Neuropsychology

Like other specialties in psychology, clinical neuropsychology has evolved from different areas within and outside of psychology. North American neuropsychology has drawn its foundations from psychopathology, psychometrics, and physiological psychology. Clinical neuropsychology focuses typically on the abnormal—what is wrong or different with the patient. Hence, the study of abnormal behavior has been a natural starting point for the assessment of "organic" conditions. With its rich history in intellectual assessment, psychometrics helps focus the quantitative analyses of abnormal brain function. This concept was eventually developed by Reitan into the first (and still widely used) neuropsychological battery, the Halstead-Reitan Neuropsychological Battery (Reitan & Wolfson, 1984). Finally, a thorough understanding of the physiological substrates of behavior, primarily neuroanatomical and neurophysiological, has become a critical cornerstone to clinical neuropsychology.

However, neuropsychology also can trace its roots to other related disciplines. The most closely aligned is neurology, especially its modern-day behavioral neurology orientation. Understanding of neurological principles is a given in the assessment of organic patients. In addition, basic principles of neuroscience and psychopharmacology play a key role in providing a backdrop for the emerging specialty of neuropsychology.

In summary, neuropsychology is a combination of a variety of specialties within and outside of psychology. Indeed, the currently accepted definitions of a clinical neuropsychologist as developed by both the National Academy of Neuropsychology and the Division of Clinical Neuropsychology

(Division 40) of the American Psychological Association embody this multi-disciplinary approach to understanding brain dysfunction.

Biopsychosocial Approach

As outlined previously, neuropsychologists have traditionally used a psychometric analysis of brain dysfunction. Underlying this approach is the assumption that an understanding of both brain function and psychometrics is essential to careful measurement of brain activity. This approach is embodied in Lezak's benchmark book *Neuropsychological Assessment* (1994).

However, such an approach, as solid and sensible as it may appear, still leaves out an important aspect of the equation. Specifically, the patient is not factored into this critical analysis. People who present with brain damage have a rich personal history. The variables that could be involved would include but not be limited to, developmental stage, sex and gender, handedness and lateralization, socioeducational status, bilingualism, and motivational factors. In addition, all forms of psychopathology from anxiety to schizophrenia, have an underlying and concomitant set of neuropsychological substrates. For example, a patient with a head injury would often have some anxiety, even depression. Those disorders, in and of themselves, would cause neuropsychological changes that would complicate the clinical picture.

Thus, it is extremely important to place the patient within a complex biopsychosocial context (Puente & McCaffrey, 1992). A patient does not simply have a head injury for example, but a head injury with a prior history of substance abuse, marital problems, and now financial difficulties that may prevent the patient from seeking appropriate interventions. All of these factors may, on their own, actually outweigh the complications associated with the brain injury alone. Combining the brain injury with these additional problems thus results in an extremely fluid and difficult situation to assess and understand.

Confounding Factors

Much as the patient must be understood as part of a biopsychosocial context, other factors must be taken into account that often are ignored or misunderstood. Two major examples will be discussed in this section.

Brain injuries are rarely static (Long, 1992). For example, in a cerebrovascular accident or a head injury the recovery is fairly predictable. However, some basic behaviors will emerge first, such as the ability to walk, whereas more complicated behaviors, such as planning and organization, might emerge last, if at all. The recovery should be much faster at the beginning and often follows a quickly flattening curve—that is, more recovery early and slower and less recovery later. An evaluation completed several days post stroke or injury would be drastically different from one completed several months later and another several years later. It is imperative to understand the disease process as well as the current state and progress of the patient's symptomology.

Another factor of great importance is secondary gains. Patients may respond willfully or otherwise to either subtle or rather obvious secondary gains (Binder, 1992). Such gains would then influence the results of any evaluation and the recovery process. In litigation it has been suggested by some people, especially attorneys and insurance adjusters, that "compensation neurosis" often occurs. In these situations the patient presents as having more problems than actually is the case in the hope of receiving greater compensation (e.g., financial award) for the injuries. Recent evidence suggests that this situation may not occur as often as was previously thought. However, consider the case in which a neuropsychological evaluation determines whether a person convicted of first-degree murder would receive the death sentence. The motivating factors to appear more impaired are obvious. In some instances the opposite may be true, such as an elderly person being evaluated for Alzheimer's. In these situations the patient presents as having fewer problems than actually may be the case. Denial may be used by the patient as a means of covering up the presenting problems. However, in other situations the problem may be more neurologically mediated and the patient is neglectful or unaware of the problems in question. These cases are often simultaneously challenging and difficult to understand and rehabilitate.

ETIOLOGY OF ORGANIC DISORDERS

Even though it was previously suggested that all forms of abnormal behavior have a neuropsychological substrate, it would be beyond the scope of this chapter to ascertain the etiology or physiological concomitants for all major psychopathologies. For the purposes of this chapter, and for most neuropsychologists, organic disorders will be defined as those psychopathologies whose origin is clearly (and easily) defined as being associated with change in neurological function. The major causes for neuropsychological syndromes will be discussed next.

Head Trauma

Head trauma occurs most frequently in young people, presumably because of a higher incidence in risk-taking behaviors (Rimel, Jane, & Bond, 1990). The frequency of occurrence is 140 out of 100,000, and 2:1 in males relative to females. Trauma to the brain can occur with shifting forces within the cranium. Specifically, an external force is applied to the head causing the brain and the cranium to move at differential times. Due to the mechanics of the brain within the cranium vault, the cranium moves first, forcing the brain to move next. Then the cranium returns to its original location, to be followed once more by the brain. Each time this occurs, the brain collides with the cranium, causing injuries to the respective areas. In addition, some researchers have hypothesized that axons are sheared away from the soma, causing eventual neuronal death. Generally, there are two types of head injuries. If the skull is fractured and the brain is exposed (e.g., missile wound), it is considered an open skull injury. The risk for infection obviously increases in these cases. Closed head injuries are more complex psychologically in that the brain is not exposed but physical forces might affect several areas within the brain. It is important to note that modern neuroradiological techniques (e.g., MRI) will often not reveal the existence of these problems, causing false negative diagnoses on the part of medical professionals (especially emergency room personnel).

Dementia

Dementia is broadly defined as a progressive, often fixed and irreversible deterioration of complex mental functions, especially intellectual and memory ones. Different types of dementias exist, with some being more frequent than others. The one that has received by far the most attention and is considered most frequent is Alzheimer's (Cummings & Benson, 1983). This disorder occurs in less than 3% of people less than 75 years of age but increases to close to 50% in those over age 85. Although not well understood, recent investigations have reported deterioration of neurofibrils of the cerebral cortex. Other forms of dementias include Parkinson's, Huntington's, and AIDS. In each of these cases the initial symptomology is subtle and difficult to distinguish from some forms of psychopathology, especially depression.

Cerebrovascular Accidents

Cerebrovascular complications can occur in response to a variety of problems and occur in about 100 of every 100,000 people, again more frequently in men (Frye-Pierson & Toole, 1987). Some causes for strokes include congenital defects, hypertension, and hyperlipidemia (i., plaque build-up in the blood vessels). A thrombosis is defined as a clot in the blood vessel that is stationary and blocking circulation. If the clot moves from one point to another, then it is considered an embolism. Arteriosclerosis, or narrowing of the arteries, impedes circulation and subsequently results in alterations of neurocognitive functions. If a bleed occurs, then cerebral hemorrhaging will result in neuronal death in nearby regions. Sometimes a blood vessel will be on the verge of breaking, due to the ballooning of an artery.

Metabolic Disorders

Ingestion of a toxic substance, especially in excessive quantities, will increase the likelihood of damage to the nervous system (Hartman, 1995). Illicit substances such as most commonly used drugs (e.g., crack cocaine) will produce irreversible effects often mimicking those of cerebrovascular accidents. Even regular ingestion of large amounts of marijuana over a period of time has been shown to affect memory capacity. Long-term alcohol abuse is often associated with significant damage to temporal lobe structures, reflected by impairment in the acquisition and eventual storage of new information.

A new group of metabolic disorders has become more commonplace in modern industrial and chemical manufacturing (Hartman, 1995). It has been known for some time that exposure to lead could result in harm to central nervous system (CNS) functioning. However, recent evidence suggests that other related metals and toxins, such as formaldehyde, can also significantly and sometimes irreversibly alter CNS function.

Other Etiologies

It is impossible in a chapter of this length to address all the reasons for the development of CNS pathology. The list would be lengthy and nearly impossible to complete. Congenital problems are typically overlooked as reasons for CNS complications. However, mental retardation in a classical sense is organicity occurring before or during birth. Other problems have also become more commonplace and require attention by individuals interested in assessing for organicity. AIDS and other medical conditions (including but not limited to diabetes, chronic obstructive pulmonary disease, etc.) can have a critical and damaging effect on brain functioning. Another way to reformat this issue is to realize that any significant alteration of the environment causing physiological changes to the body (e.g., stress causing hypertension causing mini-strokes) can result in eventual and measurable neurocognitive deficits that should be considered in understanding the patient.

ORGANIC SYNDROMES

The variety of syndromes secondary to injury to the brain is almost limitless. The number of disorders affecting the brain and their unique interaction with the patient make each situation special. However, this section will address syndromes associated with some of the major disorders. Other syndromes that are evaluated by neuropsychologists but are not included in this section are Parkinson's disease, multiple sclerosis, Huntington's disease, progressive supra nuclear palsy, brain tumors, immunodeficiency virus (e.g., AIDS), and a variety of psychopathologies (e.g., schizophrenia).

Head Injury

Closed head injury can be categorized according to the original level of function after the experience of head injury (Long, 1992). One measure of initial functioning, the Glasgow Coma Scale, is used to determine whether the injury is severe (0–8), moderate (9–12), or mild (13–15). Of course, the more severe the head injury, the more severe the subsequent neuropsychological deficits. The following problems are often noted in these cases: orientation, attention, general intelligence and understanding, memory, motor, sensory functioning, and personality. In cases of mild head injury the patient often presents as having psychiatric problems. Since secondary psychological problems are not uncommon in these situations, care must be taken to separate the organic from the functional problems.

Stroke

It is difficult to present a standard syndrome for stroke patients in part because the type and location of the cerebrovascular problem determine the eventual effect. Two types of problems will be briefly discussed, as they tend to be most common in neuropsychological practice. Ischemic strokes often occur in the left frontal lobe adjacent to Broca's area. This stroke often results in an incapacity to communicate adequately verbally (i.e., aphasia). Vascular dementia or multi-infarct dementia is often confused with early Alzheimer's. One major difference is the variability of neurocognitive function in the vascular dementia. That is, while Alzheimer's presents as a relatively steady and downward regression of intellectual function, vascular dementias often "come and go" with neurocognitive complications presenting only intermittently.

Epilepsy

As with strokes, there are different types of epilepsies including tonic-clonic, absence, simple partial, and complex partial. Again, each case is unique, resulting in difficulties in obtaining a clear picture of epilepsy. However, the following problems have been discovered in some forms of epilepsy (Bennett, 1992): attention, memory, intellectual, sensory, motor, and executive functioning. As with other forms of brain complications, it is critical to note that in many cases of epilepsy, patients function extremely well and do not present with measurable neurocognitive deficits.

Alzheimer's

One of the most feared disorders of the elderly, Alzheimer's is a progressive and fairly predictable deterioration of neurocognitive functions (LaRue, 1992). With changes in mental status, attention, memory, intellect, language, visuospatial functioning, and executive functions, one of the most difficult issues is distinguishing Alzheimer's from depression. Problems with memory and visuo-motor-spatial function coupled with expressive speech difficulties are commonly seen in Alzheimer's patients but not in depressed patients without the orgnanic disorder.

Alcohol and Drugs

As with other brain syndromes, it is difficult to establish a specific alcohol or drug syndrome, as each case varies according to frequency, intensity, and type of drug used as well as constitutional or patient factors (Hartman, 1995). Alcohol, however, can cause significant changes in attention, memory, intelligence, communication, sensory and motor functioning, and executive functions. Illicit drug use, such as marijuana, will produce specific and often permanent effects in many of the neuropsychological variables noted in alcohol. Also of interest are nonillicit neuotoxins often found in the workplace. Carbon monoxide, copper, lead, mercury, solvents, and toluene can have serious and long-lasting neuropsychological sequalea. The long-term effects will vary according to the amount and length of exposure as well as subject characteristics. However, symptoms such as short-term memory complications, slowed speed of processing, and alterations in personality (e.g., irritability) are often seen in these patients.

SECONDARY EFFECTS OF ORGANIC DISORDERS

A focal theme in this chapter has been that patients must be understood in the context of their complex biopsychosocial existence. Brain damage does not occur in a vacuum, but affects individuals and their social networks. This section addresses those problems and how best to factor them in understanding the effects of brain damage on the overall functioning of the patient.

Affective Status

Probably the most common nonneurologically based problems associated with significant alterations of brain function are changes in patient's affective status (Newman & Sweet, 1992). Recent research has found that a large percentage of patients who have experienced brain injury also suffer from depression. Depression can be masked as neurological problems. For example, the following problems that are directly attributable to depression could appear to be related to the brain dysfunction; lack of motivation, decreased speed, decreased memory functioning, lack of long-term planning, and several physiological changes (e.g., sleep and appetite disturbances).

Although less common, other problems could surface as a function of the brain trauma. These problems include but are not limited to anxiety, somatization, mania, and schizophrenia. The long-term consequences of brain damage may in turn also produce permanent and negative characterological changes resulting in personality problems as well. An example of this might be an individual who uses the brain damage and the subsequent disability status as a coping mechanism for a previously unsatisfactory personal life. In these situations a permanent and negative alteration of personality functioning.

Familial Effects

Lezak, in her Presidential Address to the International Neuropsychological Society (1988), said that "brain damage is a family affair." When a person within a social network experiences brain damage, the delicate balance that holds together a social network or family unit is also affected. Take, for example, the case of a person who is the primary breadwinner of the family and no longer can provide the necessary income support for the rest of the family system. This reduction in income will result in numerous alterations of the family structure and function including additional stress for all involved, loss of self-esteem, rearrangement of hierarchical status, and increased responsibility of others (including children). It should come as no surprise that divorce is almost twice as prevalent in families of people with brain damage when compared to the general population.

Vocational Effects

It is not unusual for brain damage to affect vocational abilities and status. By definition, neuropsychological disorders are disorders of cognition. Such changes inevitably affect even the most basic of work abilities. Speed, processing, acquisition, retention, recall of new information, and other capabilities all affect even the simplest work behavior (e.g., manual labor). Thus, brain injury often affects a person's ability to perform in gainful employment. Interestingly, many neurocognitive symptoms do not arise or are not discovered until patients are shielded from complex neurocognitive demands. Initial support from co-workers usually quickly diminishes, resulting in unexpected mental demands on the patient. Initial patient responses might include irritability and depression followed by a variety of psychophysiological stress-related symptoms, such as headaches and increased perception of pain.

It is not unusual for brain injury to have legal implications since financial hardships are bound to occur. If the injury occurred at work, then the worker should be eligible for some type of worker's compensation. A rating is assigned to permanent and partial disability after maximum medical improvement has occurred. In cases in which workers cannot be gainfully employed at all, then they should be able to receive Social Security benefits. In both situations the ultimate goal is the establishment of functional abilities and limitations based on neuropsychological test results. In personal injury and criminal cases the financial and personal stakes are often higher, and, consequently, more comprehensive evaluations are typical. In all of these scenarios, however, malingering must be considered. That is, the evaluation must take into consideration potential secondary gains for the patient.

EVALUATION OF ORGANIC DISORDERS

Standard psychological evaluations take approximately 4 to 5 hours to complete. The focus is often quite specific (e.g., personality structure) and the recommendations and report are concomitantly brief. Neuropsychological evaluations are much more comprehensive and detailed. For example, most neuropsychological evaluations take about 10 hours to complete (Putnam & DeLuca, 1990). The following sections provide a brief introduction to the assessment of organic problems.

Records

Every neuropsychological evaluation begins with a review of prior records. Such a review sets the foundation for the eventual contact with the patient. Records that would be useful include but would be not limited to medical, educational, vocational, armed services, criminal, and even driving. Each record provides a brief glimpse into the patient's premorbid functioning coupled with an introduction of the current physiological and behavioral condition of the patient.

Medical records are often an initial starting point in this review. They provide information about the etiology of the disorder as well as subsequent treatments. Obviously, such records are often difficult to understand for the nonmedical professional, who must take care to become familiar with the more common terms and concepts. Educational records are also extremely important, especially in forensic cases, since they often provide the best illustration of premorbid intellectual functioning through grades, conduct marks, absences, and standardized test scores. Finally, if work return is an issue, job descriptions as well as prior yearly evaluations would be helpful in establishing vocational capacity.

Interview

The interview should typically include the basics of a standard psychological interview. In addition, information about a variety of neurocognitive functions should be considered. These might address sensory, motor, communication (e.g., language, writing, etc.), attention, learning, memory, problem-solving, personality, and affective status. Typical interviews might last up to 2 hours and might include brief contacts over a span of several days. Also, collateral interviews with significant others, such as family members, would be useful. The basic idea is to develop a hypothesis of what problems might exist by relating the interview data to the information obtained from the records review. This hypothesis would then help establish how best to proceed with the actual testing of the patient.

Screening Instruments

A comprehensive evaluation might take over 10 hours to complete, so it is often not efficacious to pursue a standard assessment. In such cases, briefer evaluations might be warranted. Berg, Franzen, and Wedding (1994) have published the best guide to performing such evaluations. Several issues are highlighted by these authors. All things being equal, it is important to realize that a screening evaluation is simply that, a screen. Thus, caution should be taken in subsequent decision making based on a limited database, which might include false positives or false negatives (i.e., inclusion of a non–brain-damaged patient in the category of brain-damaged or vice versa).

There are two general approaches to screening exams (see Berg, Franzen, & Wedding, 1995). One is to use standardized screening instruments geared specifically for that purpose. Examples that address a wide variety of functions include the Luria-Nebraska Screening Test and the Kaufman Screen. Other tests are specifically geared for specific populations. Two examples of these are the Dementia Rating Scale (for dementia patients, including Alzheimer's) and the Brief Test of Head Injury (especially useful for patients with closed head injuries). Regardless of the approach, it is important to once more emphasize that caution should be used in decisions based on limited data.

Complete Evaluations

In certain settings, such as private practice and neurology inpatient services, more comprehensive evaluations are needed to carefully address subtle problems. These evaluations require much more expertise, time, and resources because they involve a large variety of tests. Generally, there are two opposing approaches to these comprehensive evaluations. The standardized approach, thought to have originated in North America, applies the same tests regardless of the problem. The two most commonly used batteries today are the Halstead-Reitan Neuropsychological Battery and the Luria-Nebraska Neuropsychological Battery. They take, respectively, about 8 and 2 hours to administer. The alternative approach is often called the flexible approach, originating with European and Russian neuropsychologists and now associated with the Boston school (namely Kaplan). In this approach the evaluation is tapered according to the problem in question. While this latter approach has gained in popularity during recent years, a combination of the two is most often used in clinical practice.

Reports

An evaluation is only as good as its subsequent reports. Reports should mimic a case study, publishable in a scientific or professional journal. Neuropsychological reports tend to be exhaustive, comprehensive, and quite lengthy. They could be broken down into a variety of sections, and the following is but one method of doing so: identifying information, reasons for referral and evaluation procedure, premorbid history, prior medical history, history of current disorder, clinical interview, testing behavior, test results, and summary/conclusion/recommendations. The report should provide enough information for the evaluation to be replicable. Similarly, it should be sophisticated enough to stand up under peer scrutiny but not be so focused and jargon-laden that it is of little value to nonneuropsychologist professionals (e.g., physicians).

A CASE HISTORY

The following case example illustrates some of the complexities of neuropsychological clinical studies. Note that the patient presents with a history of serious emotional complications as well as complex environmental stressors. Also, as in this case, it is not unusual for neuropsychologists to come into a case relatively late in the treatment process.

▶ CASE EXAMPLE

John

John is a 35-year-old male from a large city in the Midwest who relocated to Wilmington, North Carolina. His premorbid history is interesting and complicated. Several members of his immigrant family suffer from serious

(continued)

▶ CASE EXAMPLE   *(Continued)*

affective disorders, including bipolar disorders and clinical depression. John has three master's degrees and had been a special education teacher. He also tutored and was active in civic activities. In addition to an active social and family life, he had been married 10 years to a highly successful business administrator whom he described as "very cold." After several years of psychiatric treatment with appropriate medications, he attempted suicide on three separate occasions. On the third attempt, he was close to being successful and was found after being inside his car for several hours passively inhaling carbon monoxide.

After being hospitalized for several days, John eventually regained consciousness. His sensorium was cloudy for another month or so. Upon discharge, he was transferred to a university-based psychiatric facility, where he underwent an initial neuropsychological evaluation and extensive multidisciplinary treatment. He regained much of his basic skills, including motor, sensory, and communication skills. However, numerous other problems were still evident, including even greater dissatisfaction with all aspects of his professional and personal life, especially his marriage. He moved to Wilmington, filed for divorce, and consulted the author of this chapter.

Extensive follow-up neuropsychological examination ensued. The evaluation involved review of prior psychiatric records, initial medical hospitalization, eventual psychiatric hospitalization, and discussions with several family members including his wife. Two interviews preceded a comprehensive neuropsychological evaluation, which included portions of the Luria-Nebraska and the Halstead-Reitan batteries combined with other tests focusing on frontal and temporal lobe functions. In addition, personality and affective issues were assessed with tests including the MMPI.

Results of the testing confirmed and extended the original findings, which suggested serious problems with planning, organization, judgment, attention, acquisition, storage, and recall of recently learned information. Serious emotional problems were also present. As a consequence, a treatment program was initiated using biofeedback (for relaxation), cognitive restructuring (to assist in remediating cognitive problems), psychotherapy (for emotional support and adjustment), and psychiatric consultation (for medication management). In addition, disability and retirement issues were addressed, as was an eventual divorce and readjustment to a new community.

This case, although somewhat unusual, reflects the importance of three major issues addressed in this chapter. First, patients must be understood within a complex biopsychosocial context: Patients with brain damage have a lengthy history. Secondly, neuropsychology is a hybrid specialty in which understanding of traditional subjects, such as psychopathology, must be combined with an understanding of the classically more difficult areas, including physiology. Finally, organic cases, as a rule, are more complex and challenging than regular clinical cases. However, they also reveal much more about maladaptive behavior and human nature.

FINAL WORDS

One of the most difficult situations found in early clinical exposure and training is that of the organic patient. Such patients present with very unusual and often difficult-to-understand behavior. Early training in psychology, both at the undergraduate and beginning graduate school levels, the focus is primarily (if not exclusively), on psychopathology as a psychosocial problem, with the origins of the maladaptive behavior being primarily environmental or behavior (e.g., inadequate learning). An alternative approach is to consider that all forms of psychopathology are organically based. Indeed, some neuropsychologists, neurologists, and even psychiatrists subscribe to this radical notion. An alternative is that at least some forms of maladaptive behavior can be directly traceable to a change in physical (e.g., brain) function. In these cases the behavioral presentation is different, as are the assessment, treatment, and prognosis. The clinical novice must use caution and knowledge to better understand these patients.

SUMMARY

This chapter has focused on both theoretical and applied information. That is, an understanding of the etiologies and syndromes is a prerequisite for understanding organic disorders. In addition, a background in psychopathology, psychometrics, and physiological psychology would be beneficial addressing neuropsychological issues. Often, the clinically oriented student is not prepared academically for dealing with more physiologically based problems. Thus, a more biologically based curriculum would enhance the basic foundations needed for these cases.

The applied focus is equally important in organic cases. Several issues have been emphasized here. First, patients present within a complex biopsychosocial context. Every effort must be made to understand that context. This would include, for example, a working knowledge of educational attainment. Secondly, evaluation for organic problems requires assessment of a wide variety of subtle cognitive functions, which requires a relatively long testing time coupled with a greater variety of tests. Finally, secondary issues (e.g., financial compensation) as well as affective problems (e.g., depression) often cloud the clinical picture. Hence, great care must be taken to control or tease out these factors.

Future Directions

It has been argued that while neuropsychology is experiencing a vibrant present, it has similarly enjoyed a long and moribund past. However, the future for a neuropsychologically based psychology is also possible. Indeed, some have argued that William James originally defined psychology as neuropsychology, and that current trends within the field of psychology presage an eventual return to the original concepts of James. It is important to note that the only psychologist to win a Nobel Prize was a neuropsychologist—Sperry. Maybe this distinction is but a benchmark of what aspects of psychology in general and clinical psychology in particular are viewed by society at large as being critical. Regardless, understanding of brain dysfunction hinges on a unique combination of clinical and academic expertise, a bridge hard to cross and often ignored in psychology.

REFERENCES

Anderson, R. M. (1994). *Practitioner's guide to clinical neuropsychology.* New York: Plenum.

Berg, R., Franzen, M., & Wedding, D. (1995). *Screening for brain impairment* (2d ed.). New York: Springer.

Bennett, T. (1992). *The neuropsychology of epilepsy.* New York: Plenum.

Binder, L. (1992). Malingering and deception. In A. E. Puente & R. J. McCaffrey (Eds.), *Handbook of neuropsychological assessment: A biopsychosocial approach.* New York: Plenum.

Cummings, J. L., & Benson, D. F. (1983). *Dementias: A clinical approach.* Boston: Buttersworth.

Frye-Pierson, J., & Toole, J. F. (1987). *Stroke: A guide for patient and family.* New York: Raven.

Golden, C. J. (1981). *Diagnosis and rehabilitation in clinical neuropsychology.* Springfield, IL: Thomas.

Golden, C. J., Hammeke, T. A., & Purisch, A. D. (1978). Diagnostic validity of a standardized neuropsychological battery derived from Luria's neuropsychological tests. *Journal of Consulting and Clinical Psychology, 46,* 1258–1265.

Hartman, D. (1995). *Neuropsychological toxicology* (2d ed.). New York: Plenum.

LaRue, A. (1992). *Aging and neuropsychological assessment.* New York: Plenum.

Lezak, M. (1988). Brain damage is a family affair. *Journal of Clinical and Experimental Neuropsychology, 10,* 111–123.

Lezak, M. (1994). *Neuropsychological assessment* (3d ed.). New York: Oxford University Press.

Long, C. (1992). *Handbook of head trauma.* New York: Plenum.

Newman, P., & Sweet, J. (1992). Depression. In A. E. Puente & R. J. McCaffrey (eds.), *Handbook of neuropsychological assessment: A biopsychosocial approach.* New York: Plenum.

Puente, A. E. (1990). Historical perspectives in the development of neuropsychology as a professional specialty. In C. R. Reynolds & E. Fletcher-Janzen (Eds.), *Handbook of child clinical neuropsychology.* New York: Plenum.

Puente, A. E. (1992). The status of clinicl neuropsychology. *Archives of Clinical Neuropsychology, 7,* 297–312.

Puente, A. E., & McCaffrey, R. J. (1992). *Handbook of neuropsychological assessment: A biopsychosocial perspective.* New York: Plenum.

Putnam, S., & DeLuca, J. W. (1990). The TCN Professional Practice Survey: Part I. General practice of neuropsychologists in primary employment of private practice settings. *The Clinical Neuropsychologist 2,* 199–243.

Reitan, R. M., & Wolfson, D. (1984). *The Halstead-Reitan neuropsychological battery.* Tucson, AZ: Neuropsychology Press.

Rimel, R. W., Jane, J. A., & Bond, M. R. (1990). Characteristics of the head injured patient. In M. Rosenthal, M. R. Bond, E. R. Griffith, & J. D. Miller (Eds.), *Rehabilitation of the adult and child with traumatic brain injury* (2d ed.) (pp. 8–16). Philadelphia: Davis.

Sperry, R. W. (1982). Some effects of disconnecting the cerebral hemispheres (Nobel Lecture). *Science, 217,* 1223–1226.

▶ 12

Training Issues in Clinical Psychology

DONALD K. FREEDHEIM

JAMES C. OVERHOLSER

The education of a clinical psychologist requires a long and rigorous program that includes academic work, scientific research, and clinical training. The student must be prepared for a minimum of 4 years, and more likely 5 or even 6 years, of graduate work, including a full-year internship in a clinical setting. The progress of the students' work on their doctoral dissertation often determines whether their training will extend beyond this time.

As in all scientific and health-related fields, the rapidly evolving knowledge base requires that the student be prepared to continue learning beyond the graduate years. Graduate education at its best should teach the student to study psychology and should provide a basis for further study as the field progresses. The process of study, habits of observation, and theoretical foundations learned in graduate school will stay with students throughout their professional careers. The success of any program can only be measured by the proficiency of its students. If students have learned to evolve as the field evolves, the graduate years will have provided the best launching pad for professional lifes that will be fulfilling and, optimally, contribute to the further development of the field.

Throughout this chapter the student's training activities and responsibilities will be discussed as they change through a variety of roles, including clinical trainee, supervisee, internship applicant, intern, post-doctoral fellow, and scientist-practitioner. We will begin with a look at training goals, and how models for teaching have developed to meet these goals. We will then discuss the training sequence, with examples of practicum experiences and initial therapy training. All these activities are precursors to the full-time internship. Last, we will look briefly at the role of the post-doctorate training program and re-training opportunities. We hope this overview of clinical training program will be helpful to students anticipating their graduate work in clinical psychology, as well as to those who may be contemplating the field as a possible career.

TRAINING GOALS

During the early stages of clinical training the student should expect to learn about a wide range of topics, including exposure to many different forms of psychopathology and a wide range of treatment options. Students often have specialized interests in particular areas, and many want to begin this specialization fairly early in their training. However, it is often helpful for students to postpone the in-depth specialization until later in their training (e.g., at the post-doctoral level). Early training should expose students to many topics that have direct or indirect relevance to their ultimate career goals. During graduate school, students must remember they are being trained to become psychologists, and therefore should become familiar with the entire field of psychology (Matarazzo, 1987). Later they can learn different applications within the general field of psychology. It is surprising how often students begin with apparently strong interests in a particular area (e.g., schizophrenia or child abuse), but when exposed to a broad range of topics, they find something that interests them much more (e.g., suicide or disorders of childhood). These shifts in interests and goals are easy to adapt to during the early stages of training but can be more disruptive if they occur later in training. Also, many students find ways in which training in one area (e.g., behavior therapy for weight management) can have clear implications in other areas (e.g., impulse control in borderline personality disorder). Thus, the breadth of training provided early to students can lay the foundation on which to build more specialized interests later.

In all aspects of training, students are expected to develop competence in a variety of clinical skills. Professional competence has been defined as including five overlapping domains: factual knowledge, generic clinical skills, orientation-specific technical skills, clinical judgment, and interpersonal attributes (Overholser & Fine, 1990). Factual knowledge is the easiest to develop, whereas clinical judgment can take a lifetime of learning.

Graduate work should prepare students to be competent and confident with the tools they will use in the field. But they also must learn a process of study, which will serve them throughout their careers. Throughout graduate training, students are given numerous opportunities to learn both the content and the process of clinical psychology. Also, students learn efficient ways of studying the field of psychology. These study habits are essential so students and practitioners can adapt to the ever changing field of psychology.

Perhaps the most important asset a faculty member or clinical supervisor can bring to clinical training is a genuine interest in the material and an enthusiasm for learning. Because much of a psychologist's knowledge base becomes obsolete within 10 to 12 years (Dubin, 1972), it is imperative that professionals retain an interest in learning that continues well beyond the end of their formal education. An important goal of professional training programs is to cultivate a lasting interest in the general process of learning and the use of the scientific method (Flexner, 1925). A sole focus on learning specific facts, studies, or techniques will ensure obsolescence or incompetence in future years.

MODELS OF TRAINING

There are a number of models for training in clinical psychology, and a graduate program may be identified closely with one or another of them. A training model includes two primary elements: first, the balance between an emphasis on the science and on the practice of clinical psychology and, second, the dominant theoretical orientation held by the faculty members.

The model endorsed by a clinical psychology training program serves several functions: It provides a general theoretical basis for the clinical work and research conducted by faculty and students, it serves as a guide for conceptualizing behavior and behavior deviance, and it endorses certain training sites where the students will have practicum experiences during their graduate years.

In terms of theoretical orientations held by faculty members, the dominant schools include psychodynamic, cognitive-behavioral, and humanistic. Although many programs encourage eclectic approaches that incorporate elements from a variety of perspectives, there has been a subtle move away from eclecticism toward integration (see Norcross & Goldfried, 1992, for a recent discussion of the uses of integration in psychotherapy).

Many psychology programs today attempt to follow the scientist-practitioner model. This model is also referred to as the Boulder Model because it was first advocated in 1949 at the training conference at the University of Colorado in Boulder, Colorado (Cohen, 1992). In the years following this important conference there have been a number of other conferences that have refined the criteria for training in clinical psychology and have taken into account factors such as the importance of including sensitivity to diversity in our culture and the emergence of freestanding schools of psychology

(Peterson, 1992). Prominent among the later conferences were the 1958 Miami Beach meeting, which clarified clinical training issues; the 1965 Chicago conference, which focused on diversification in clinical training; and the 1973 Vail meeting, which recognized professional training in graduate schools (for detailed discussion of these and the other training conferences, see Cohen, 1992). Essentially, the scientist-practitioner model encourages competence in both the science of psychology and its applications. The scientist-practitioner model attempts to develop professionals who fully integrate aspects of science and practice so that their research work has direct relevance to clinical applications and their clinical work is based on sound research (Perry, 1990). Some psychologists (e.g., Frank, 1984) feel the scientist-practitioner model does a disservice to many practitioner-oriented students, forcing them to learn material and techniques that are not compatible with their personality styles or their career goals. However, the scientist-practitioner model can be implemented adequately when faculty members provide students with opportunities to conduct research in applied settings, demonstrating the integration of science and practice (Goldfried, 1984). When the model is implemented properly,, even practitioner-oriented students will be exposed to the use of the scientific method and can learn an objectivity that is useful in all professional settings. Hence, it has been argued (McFall, 1991) that all forms of professional activity conducted by psychologists should have a firm grounding in science, and all clinical assessments and interventions should be scientifically valid.

In most training programs it becomes very difficult to maintain the balance across scientist and practitioner interests. Many different factors can pull clinical psychologists into one end or the other (see Table 12-1). The scientist focuses on work that is generalizable to other populations in other settings, attempting to gain a national reputation. The scientist's career is advanced by research publications and grant funding. In contrast, the practitioner works to apply the treatments to help specific individuals. The practitioner benefits from a local reputation that facilitates client referrals. Thus, it is often more accurate to describe psychologists or their training programs in terms of the degree to which they adhere to the scientist-practitioner model, with an emphasis on more of the scientist or more of the practitioner aspects of their work.

In terms of research, it is important that all students, regardless of program emphasis, are exposed to the scientific examination of clinically relevant issues. When students become involved with analog research (e.g., mild depression induced in normal college students) or irrelevant to the provision of clinical services, it is much more difficult to learn the scientist-practitioner model. However, when students are able to conduct research on applied topics and in applied settings, they are more likely to appreciate the blending of the science and practice of psychology (Goldfried, 1984). Such

TABLE 12-1   **Comparison of Forces Pulling Psychologists toward Scientist or Practitioner Goals**

Dimension	Scientist	Practitioner
Primary job function	conducting research	providing services
Primary focus	theory	application
Useful qualifications	specialist	generalist
View of psychopathology	nomothetic	idiographic
Type of intervention	structured across patients	individualized
Basis for treatment	published research	previous cases
Basic cognitive	critical thinking	empathic acceptance
strategy	logical	intuitive
Cognitive Style I	quantitative	qualitative
Cognitive Style II	research grants	clinical services
Financial incentives	national publications	local presentations
Activities	national leading to	local leading to referrals
Goal for reputation	promotion	referrals
Degree Sought	Ph.D.	Psy.D.

experience can help students develop an attitude of critical thinking, which is important in approaching both research and clinical issues in psychology. Students grounded in the basics of research will be better able to evaluate the information (viz., data) derived from clinical cases and it is hoped, will be better able to view their own approaches critically and objectively.

During the early stages of clinical training it is important for students to retain a strong basis in research. When first working with patients who have a particular psychological problem and attempting to devise a treatment plan, students should review the literature that pertains to the assessment and treatment of the disorder. This background work may uncover types of treatment that have been found to be especially helpful and some that have failed. In either case, students will be in a better position to provide treatment that has empirical evidence supporting its use.

Unfortunately, many practitioners do not rely on research when devising their treatment plan because they feel most research ignores the complexities of the clinical work (Morrow-Bradley & Elliott, 1986). Instead of arguing over who should be blamed, it is better for training programs to strive toward a synthesis of science and practice, making sure that professionals on both sides of this invisible line work to strengthen the communication and interrelationships between science and its applications (Phillips, 1989). Thus, it is important for students to learn the value of research in guiding therapeutic decisions. Students can gain a better understanding of the strengths and limitations of the published research as it relates to their own clinical work. Also, students can learn to use the scientific method to guide their work, developing hypotheses about clients' problems and critically evaluating the appropriateness and utility of these hypotheses.

THE TRAINING SEQUENCE

When first exposed to the provision of clinical services, students often begin with training in structured assessment techniques and basic interviewing skills. Training in assessment can include the use of projective techniques such as the Rorschach Inkblot Technique and the Thematic Apperception Test. The administration and scoring of these tests require a reasonably high degree of clinical skill and can give students many opportunities to begin learning how to work with clients while serving in the role of a professional.

Learning how to conduct psychological assessments can be relatively straightforward. Students are exposed to different methods of assessment, including structured ability tests (e.g., Wechsler Adult Intelligence Scale), psychometric personality inventories (e.g., Minnesota Multiphasic Personality Inventory), and projective methods (e.g., Incomplete Sentences Blank). After learning the theoretical and empirical basis for each instrument, students are usually given the opportunity to administer some of these tests in a supervised field setting. Here they can receive feedback on the proper techniques for the administration, scoring, and interpretation of most standardized tests.

Training in clinical interviewing skills emphasizes how to talk with and how to listen to clients. This training includes basic issues surrounding the use of questioning clients to gather information necessary for obtaining a detailed psychosocial history and for deriving a psychiatric diagnosis. Attention is also placed on the establishment of a proper therapeutic relationship based on empathy, warmth, and genuineness (Rogers, 1957).

Learning how to conduct psychotherapy is a complicated and lifelong process. During the early stages of their training, students may be allowed to observe psychotherapy sessions performed by a licensed psychologist. This observation requires the informed consent of the client. After the session, the student can ask questions about the content and process of the therapy session. Although a valuable opportunity, there are many complications involved when arranging for a student to observe psychotherapy sessions. The student must respect the nature of confidentiality that protects the material discussed during a therapy session. The client may feel threatened by the presence of an observer. Because of the potential damage to the therapeutic relationship, many therapists are reluctant to allow students to observe their therapy sessions face to face or even through a one-way mirror.

When direct observation is not possible, tape recordings of sessions can be used. Clients can be asked to give their written permission to allow the session to be audiotaped. Videotapes can be made so students can later watch segments of a previous therapy session. However, some clients become fearful that the videotape could haunt them years later, should it be used in a public demonstration. Clients seem more agreeable to the use of audiotape recordings because their identity can be more easily camouflaged. Nonetheless, audiotapes can allow students to listen to actual therapy sessions and get a feel for the often uneven flow of therapeutic discussions. There have been many published transcripts of good sessions conducted by the leading experts in the field. These published transcripts have "optimal moments" laced throughout every session. Tapes made in-house have the hidden benefit of allowing students the opportunity to listen to unedited transcripts of everyday sessions with good and bad parts included that can help students set realistic standards for evaluating their own work. Training tapes can be purchased from many vendors.

The American Psychological Association has recently developed a series of psychotherapy teaching videotapes with therapists demonstrating various approaches to therapy with actors in unrehearsed sessions (APA, 1994). A teaching guide accompanies the videos developed for courses and training sessions in psychotherapy. As with audiotapes, both "good" and "bad" moments in therapy can be observed and assessed by the viewer. Although each therapist develops his or her own style with experience, viewing therapy in action is a valuable teaching aid, which can add an important dimension to one's training.

Conducting role-played interactions of psychotherapy sessions during a class presentation can be helpful for students. The role plays may have students serving as either therapist or client. Role-played interactions can demonstrate the fluid nature of therapy and the numerous choices a therapist makes when deciding to emphasize or ignore different aspects of the discussion. Also, role-played interactions demonstrate the therapist's ability to process information throughout the interaction, gently guiding the flow of the session. As students improve their knowledge and confidence over time, they may be capable of playing a more active part in the role-played interactions.

When students begin therapy with their first client, the faculty supervisor should closely monitor the flow and content of the sessions. This process may involve direct observation by the supervisor in the room as co-therapist, or observing through a one-way mirror. More likely, because of the complications with direct observation methods, the supervisor will listen to audiotapes of the therapy sessions and later discuss the session with the student therapist. These supervisory meetings play a prominent role in the student's ability to learn the process of psychotherapy and can greatly enrich the quality of the clinical training.

STYLES OF SUPERVISION

Supervision of psychotherapy can be difficult for both therapist and supervisor. Student therapists must struggle with evaluation anxiety and insecurities about their abilities as a therapist. Supervisors must retain a focus on the growth of the student as a therapist and must encourage that growth. When both student and supervisor perform their roles adequately, clinical supervision can be a powerful stimulant to the academic growth process.

It is often helpful for supervisors to adapt their style to the needs of each particular supervisee. Students early in their training have different needs from students who are ready for internship. Thus, a developmental approach to supervision has been recommended (Stoltenberg & Delworth, 1987). Beginning students often want and need a fair degree of structure to guide their work with clients. If supervisors provide limited guidance, the level of anxiety may be substantially increased in the novice therapist. As the supervisee matures and gains added experience, the supervisor can allow greater freedom and autonomy in performing clinical work.

When students begin their clinical training and first serve in the role of supervisee, it can be threatening to have an experienced professional closely monitor their work and give them feedback on ways to improve. Optimally, the supervisor can keep a focus on positive growth and not dwell on minor mistakes made during the clinical work. However, many supervisors leave behind their clinical skills and focus on minor problems to the exclusion of positive growth. Also, some supervisors appear disinterested in the student's skill or progress and provide the minimal amount of actual supervision. This is unfortunate because the supervisor's attitude can determine whether supervision is experienced as a supportive opportunity for growth, a painful oral examination, or a perfunctory meeting to meet state regulations.

Students can maximize the use of supervision by using the experience as an opportunity to learn by trying out new therapy techniques and styles. Although students may make mistakes, these mistakes can provide excellent opportunities for new learning. If students feel anxious about the meetings with their supervisor, they should discuss with the supervisor their feelings and the reasons why they feel anxious. The best supervisees are those who can accept the role of trainee and come to supervision ready to learn. (For a more detailed discussion of issues pertaining to working with supervisors, see Chapter 3 of this volume.) From a supervisor's perspective, a good supervisee is not one who feels he or she already knows all the correct responses, but one who wants to learn new ways of dealing with clients.

Perhaps the most basic goal of supervision is to ensure that an adequate quality of care is provided to all clients. Thus, in certain difficult situations (e.g., a client expresses suicidal or homicidal thoughts) the supervisor may have to take a directive approach in supervision to ensure no harm is done.

However, when intake supervisors have adequate time to properly pre-screen potential clients, these crisis issues should be infrequent.

Another important goal of supervision is to allow students the opportunity to develop their own clinical skills and gain experience with a variety of clients, assessment techniques, and therapeutic strategies. Some supervisors strive to balance directing the flow of sessions with a more Socratic, reflective style (Overholser, 1991). As supervisors allow supervisees to develop their own style of therapy, students become more willing to experiment with new approaches.

Another important goal of supervision is to foster supervisees' abilities to evaluate their own work realistically and constructively. This self-evaluation skill is critical to the therapist's ability to performadequately when no longer being supervised. Some student therapists become overly critical of their work, tending to compare their performance in therapy with that of the experts they have observed in films or training videotapes. These students need to appreciate the strengths and abilities they have and focus on the gradual development of more refined therapy skills. Other student therapists lack a self-critical attitude and have difficulties differentiating therapeutic interactions from supportive social contacts with friends and family members. These students need to view a therapeutic relationship as special in many ways and need to avoid responding to clients in ways that are socially appropriate, but lack therapeutic purpose.

Supervision should help supervisees learn new and more complex ways of working with various clients. This works best when a teamwork approach develops between supervisor and supervisee, both working in the best interests of the client. The supervisor should emphasize process over content, so the student learns *how* to think about clinical issues, not simply *what* to think. The supervisor can help the student confront different treatment options and decide how best to proceed. When students are given a variety of opportunities to work with different clients in a variety of settings, they can develop the basic clinical skills needed to function as a clinical psychologist.

TRAINING OPPORTUNITIES

Pre-Internship Clerkships and Clinical Practica

An essential aspect of each student's education is the experience outside the department in a clinical setting. The timing of these clerkships varies widely among graduate programs. In some programs the experience might not be available until the student is ready for a full-time internship. In most schools, however, there is an attempt to have students gain experience in clinical settings well before they go on internship.

One of the best ways to introduce this experience is to integrate it with the assessment and intervention courses offered at the university. Although this approach takes much cooperation and coordination with community resources, the experiences can be valuable for the students. At Case Western Reserve University (CWRU), students taking the assessment course in the first year of their graduate program complete evaluations in clinical field settings. These evaluations are supervised by staff at the setting and provide the students with an initial experience in a mental health hospital or agency.

During the second year the students are assigned to a mental health setting for an 8-hour-per-week placement. The emphasis of the clinical work is in the area of assessment, with opportunities for students to thoroughly evaluate a client, present the data to staff, and participate in the interpretation of the assesssment data to the client. The field setting can be a community mental health center, outpatient clinic, residential center, or inpatient hospital. During the third and fourth years, students at CWRU participate in 16 hour per week clerkships, sometimes paid, in which they begin intervention techniques, case consultation, and at times community consultation, in addition to further assessment work. At the completion of the clerkships, the students are well prepared for full-time internships, which will round out their clinical training at the graduate level.

In addition to the experiences the students have with intervention in their field setting, the department at CWRU offers four year-long practica in basic therapeutic approaches. These practica are psychodynamic, cognitive-behavioral, client-centered, and child/family therapy. Each practicum includes a seminar and individually supervised cases. During the seminar, students are presented with the theoretical and empirical basis of that particular type of therapy as well as general issues relevant to all forms of psychotherapy. Students meet individually with a licensed psychologist for supervision on their cases. Also, students can bring their case material to the seminar for discussion. We require the students to take at least two practica during their third and fourth years of graduate work, but many students opt to take a third practicum to enhance their repertoire of techniques.

Pre-doctoral Internships

After graduate students have completed most of the requirements for the doctoral degree, they are ready to serve as interns at a clinical training site. Many internships have been formally approved by the American Psychological Association (APA). All approved internships are listed with accreditation status and address in the December issue of the *American Psychologist*. A complete listing of internship sites with a short description of each site is published in the *Internship and Postdoctoral Programs in Professional Psychology Directory* published by the Association of Psychology Postdoctoral and

Internship Centers (APPIC). This directory includes a summary of the number of intern slots, the current stipend, applicant requirements and restrictions, and the availability of various rotations and specialty tracks.

Preparing for internship and the application process should begin early. Megargee (1990) provides detailed explanations of the entire internship application process. From the beginning of their clinical training, students should keep records of clients they have seen and the types of assessment they have performed. In this way, students will have recorded much of the information that will be needed when they begin applying for internship (see below for details of information to be recorded).

There are numerous factors that influence the selection of an appropriate training site (Grace, 1985). These factors include APA approval, geographical location of the program, population served (e.g., adult versus child), type of training site (e.g. medical center, veterans hospital, outpatient counseling center, consortium), the predominant theoretical orientation held by faculty at the internship site, the quality and reputation of training, emphasis on different responsibilities (e.g., research, assessment, therapy), clinical and research specialization areas of the faculty, diversity of program, and (lastly), the stipend. Although difficult to estimate during the selection process, after completing their internship most interns rate the quality of supervision as the most valuable aspect of the experience (Weiss, 1975). Many applicants use some combination of these factors when deciding which internship site is best suited to their needs. Most importantly, applicants should select internship sites that correspond to their long-term career goals.

When interns apply, the training site will be evaluating them to estimate the "match." This term refers to the degree of correspondence between the responsibilities the site needs its interns to assume and the capabilities, qualifications, and interests of the intern. Training sites examine a number of factors, including whether the student has come from an APA-accredited program, whether the student is enrolled in a clinical (or counseling) specialization, the theoretical orientation of the student, the student's breadth and depth of clinical experience (across disorders, treatments, and modalities), research experience (publications and presentations), the student's specialized interests (e.g., childhood depression), and the quality of the student's academic training. Both academic preparation and clinical experience play important roles in the selection of interns (Stedman et al., 1981). Factors such as GRE scores and grade point average typically play little role in the selection process (Drummond, Rodolfa, & Smith, 1981). Also, decisions will be influenced by the applicant's personal qualifications as revealed through letters of recommendation, interviews with internship faculty and staff, and the applicant's personal statement (Petzel & Berndt, 1980). No single factor is likely to make much difference in the selection, but the combination of factors will help the selection committee determine who best satisfies the needs of their site.

Students should request by mail the application materials from several internship sites at least a year before they expect to begin the internship year. On the application form they will be asked to list the specific numbers of clients treated and tests administered. Early in their graduate training, students should begin keeping track of the number of clients seen with different disorders (e.g., anxiety, affective, schizophrenia); the number of clients across the age span (e.g., child, adolescent, adult, geriatric); and the number of tests administered, scored, and interpreted (e.g., IQ, Rorschach, TAT, MMPI, Bender).

Students should be prepared to deliver a curriculum vita that is well organized and thorough yet concise. The vita provides important documentation of the students' background and abilities. Not only does it record education and training experiences; it also demonstrates students' organizational and writing skills. Many students inquire about the ideal format for a curriculum vita. Although there is no standard form, conciseness is probably the best guideline. As an example of an informative, yet not overbearing vita, we have included a sample in the exhibit at the end of this chapter.

Students will also be asked to write a goals statement describing their interests and background and their compatibility with the training opportunities offered by a particular internship site. It is important that applicants be honest in describing their interests and goals; otherwise they may end up at an internship site not well suited to their long-term interests.

Finally, some internship sites ask applicants to include a sample psychological report they have prepared. When doing so, applicants should ensure that the patient's consent has been obtained and all information has been removed that could reveal the patient's identity (Megargee, 1990). All application materials should be mailed with a cover letter that includes a brief introduction and explanation of the application materials enclosed. Also, students should request three to five previous supervisors to write letters of recommendation. It will be the students' responsibility to make sure the letters are sent on time. It is usual practice for the chair of the clinical program to write a general letter to the internship site, outlining the areas of clinical training emphasized in the program, an overall evaluation of the student's functioning in the program, and verifying the student's status as eligible to begin the pre-doctoral internship.

After the written materials have been mailed, students should prepare for on-site and telephone interviewing. Most internship sites expect interested applicants to visit their training site during January or early February of the year preceding the start of the internship. At the interviews, students should expect to be asked specific questions about their experience with particular tests and disorders. Students may be asked to describe a success or failure experience they have had in therapy. Applicants may be asked to discuss their goals for the internship year, explain what led them to apply to that particular internship site, discuss their strengths and weaknesses as a psychologist, and describe their long-term career goals. During all interviews, students should be prepared with intelligent answers as well as their own questions to ask about the internship. When students have no questions about the internship site, it could be interpreted as a lack of interest (Monti, 1985) or inadequate preparation. Students should know their vita and be able to discuss their experiences in detail. After a day filled with interviews, applicants should record their observations and impressions. This summary can be important after applicants have interviewed at six or more different sites and it becomes difficult to remember their impressions of each of these sites.

The applicant's job is not done after interviews have been completed. Waiting until notification day does not mean simply waiting. The applicant can call the internship and send follow-up letters, thanking faculty and staff for their time and expressing interest in their program. This follow-up is important for expressing interest in their site and demonstrating a likelihood of accepting an offer should they make one.

Notification day is the second Monday in February. On notification day, internship sites call their top applicants to offer them a spot in their internship class. By the time of notification day, students should know which site is their top choice and should have been in touch with faculty there. When students receive an offer, they have until noon of the next day to give their decision. Although some applicants will receive offers from several internship sites, it is proper etiquette to keep one site on hold at a time (Belar & Orgel, 1980). Thus, if the applicant's interests in different sites have been ranked, the applicant can promptly turn down the lower-ranked site. This allows the site to make an offer to another applicant.

While on internship, students can expect to be kept very busy, serving as professionals in a service provider position. Often this activity involves participating as a multidisciplinary treatment team member. For many interns, this is their first intensive exposure to psychiatric inpatients in a hospital setting where biological factors are viewed as more important. Also, psychology interns will learn how to interact with professionals from other fields who may view mental illness from a more biological or social basis (Kingsbury, 1987). While on internship, students are supervised in individual and group psychotherapy formats. All work performed by the intern must be supervised and co-signed by a licensed psychologist. However, some of the actual case supervision is provided by other mental health professionals. Thus, the intern may work closely with the attending psychiatrist when providing services on an inpatient unit. Supervision is often provided on a regularly scheduled basis and on an "as needed" basis when emergencies or novel situations arise. Interns may be expected to carry a heavier caseload than they were accustomed to during previous training, now seeing inpatients, outpatients, and conducting assessments, and perhaps running a therapy group.

Post-doctoral Fellowships

Just as earlier stages of training are used to lay a solid foundation with a broad base of knowledge in psychology, post-doctoral fellowships can be used to provide greater depth and specificity of training. A post-doctoral program is an important opportunity to extend clinical experiences under intensive supervision. The post-doctoral training allows students to gain advanced experience working with certain specialized populations, assessment techniques, or approaches to intervention. During the post-doctoral year, students may be able to combine research and clinical work on interests that closely match their long-term career goals. Most states now require a year of post-graduate supervised training for licensure, and a full-time fellowship fulfills the requirement. Unfortunately, there are relatively few opportunities for paid fellowships and such funding is usually not as predictable as pre-doctoral funds. Information about post-doctoral fellowships can be obtained through the APPIC guide, the APA *Monitor,* and from established internship sites that may also offer clinical training fellowships.

The AAP is currently studying many issues surrounding specialization in psychology and the role of pre- and post-doctoral training in developing specialists. Proposals have been made for national residency programs and other means for institutionalizing specialty training. Students should keep abreast of developments in the field so that they may take advantage of opportunities for post-doctoral training as they evolve in the near future.

RETRAINING PROGRAMS

There is a continuing need to provide retraining programs for professionals who have completed doctoral degrees in other areas of psychology but who then wish to pursue clinical work. As with post-doctoral training programs, these programs are scattered throughout the country, and not all programs offer retraining every year. Also, there is usually no outside funding support for students wishing to enter such programs.

Although there is no set curriculum for retraining programs, they usually involve 2 years of clinical course work with part-time supervised clinical experience. The student is then ready to apply for an internship, competitive with all pre-doctoral students. Therefore, retraining usually takes 3 years before the student is qualified as a graduate in clinical psychology.

SUMMARY AND CONCLUSIONS

Preparation for a professional career in clinical psychology can be time-consuming and emotionally draining. However, it can also be interesting, exciting, and stimulating. Many aspects of clinical training are filled with opportunities for personal as well as professional growth. The student is able to learn about many forms of psychopathology and their treatment. The student can develop skills in specialized areas of interest and can appreciate how information from one area can generate useful ideas for approaching other problem areas.

Because we are in a young field that is constantly changing, training in clinical psychology is a lifelong process. There is no end goal; rather there should be ongoing appreciation of learning and excitement about the field.

EXHIBIT A

EXHIBIT: Sample Curriculum Vita

VITA
AMY FLOWER

Home: Office:
2610 Hammond Road   Department of Psychology
Cleveland Heights, OH 44106   Case Western Reserve University
(216) 555-8762   Cleveland, OH 44106
                                               (216) 555-3926

EDUCATIONAL BACKGROUND:

9/87-present   **Case Western Reserve University, Cleveland, OH**
                M.A., August, 1989; Ph.D. candidate in Clinical Psychology--APA
                approved.

1/85-5/87   **Clark University, Worcester, MA**
                B.A., 1987, *Summa Cum Laude;* Phi Beta Kappa; High Honors in
                Psychology.

8/83-12/84   **DePauw University, Greencastle, IN**
                Phi Eta Sigma and Alpha Lambda Delta honor societies.

CLINICAL EXPERIENCE:

9/90-6/91   **Clinical Practicum Placement, Department of Child Psychiatry,
                MetroHealth Medical Center, Cleveland, OH**
                Conducting child and family psychotherapy, parent guidance,
                and psychological assessments of children. (15–20) hours per
                week; supervised 2 hours per week.)
                Supervisors: Dennis Smith, Ph.D.; Sue Jones, Ph.D.

8/30-6/91   **Psychology Intake Worker: The Free Medical Clinic of Cleveland**
                Volunteer one evening per week conducting intake interviews with
                adults who enter the psychology clinic seeking help with
                problems including chronic mental illness, drugs/alcohol
                addiction, physical abuse, and sexual abuse. Referrals are made
                to psychotherapists, to a drug/alcohol group, to a batterers group,
                or to community services outside of the clinic. (3–5 hours per
                week; supervised on a per case basis.)
                Supervisor: Jane Black

8/89-8/90   **Clinical Practicum Placement, University Counseling Services, Case Western Reserve University**
Conducted long-term and short-term outpatient psychotherapy with graduate and undergraduate college students. Completed psychological assessment of a 22-year-old female undergraduate. Co-led support and psychoeducational groups, including "A transfer student forum," "International women students' support group," and "How to talk about sex." Member of the planning committee for a city-wide conference entitled "Women at work: Rivalry, competition, and sisterhood." (15–20 hours per week; supervised 2.5 hours per week.)
Supervisors: Jes White, Ph.D.; Bettina Lof, Ph.D.

9/88-5/89   **Clinical Practicum Placement, Beech Brook Residential Treatment Center, Pepper Pike, OH**
Conducted psychotherapy with individual children, ages 4–11, and with their families. Completed psychological assessments of children 4–12 years old. Treatment was conducted through a variety of Beech Brook affiliated programs, i.e., residential and day treatment, a community mental health center, and foster care. (15–20 hours per week; supervised 2.5 hours per week.)
Supervisor: Jeffrey Frank, Ph.D.

9/87-12/87   **Play Therapist, Rainbow Babies and Children's Hospital, Cleveland, OH**
Directed play activities with children on the Medical Behavioral Unit.

10/85-5/87   **Sexuality and Contraceptive Counselor, Clark University**
Worked in a student-run contraceptive and sexuality counseling center, providing education and referrals.

5/86-8/76   **Rehabilitation Staff, Worcester State Hospital, Worcester, MA**
Worked with adult inpatients on skill-building tasks.

8/84-12/84   **Peer Counselor, DePauw University**
Performed general counseling and made referrals to the campus counseling center for an all-female college residence. (supervised 3 hours per month.)

9/83-5/84   **Student-Friend Program, Greencastle, IN**
Spent 1–2 hours weekly as a companion to poor rural elementary school children with learning disabilities and/or family problems.

(Cont.)

EXHIBIT A *(Continued)*

THERAPY AND ASSESSMENT PRACTICA:

9/90-5/91 **Cognitive Behavioral Therapy Practicum, Case Western Reserve University**
Class consists of weekly lectures and case presentations. Conducting weekly individual cognitive behavioral therapy with a 29-year-old male with borderline personality features. (supervised 1 hour per week.)
Instructor and Supervisor: James Reed, Ph.D.

9/90-12/91 **Client Centered Therapy Practicum, Case Western Reserve University**
Unofficially auditing this course, which consists of weekly lecture and supervision of taped student role plays. (supervised 1 hour per week.)
Instructor and Supervisor: Fred Kilian, Ph.D.

6/90-7/90 **Psychology Intake Training, The Free Medical Clinic of Cleveland**
Participated in seven weeks of intensive training on crisis intervention, interviewing skills, sexual abuse and rape, sexually transmitted diseases, and substance abuse.
Instructors: Cynthia Thorp, Ph.D.; Jane Black

9/89-6/90 **Psychodynamic Psychotherapy Practicum, Case Western Reserve University**
Class consisted of weekly case presentations and discussion within a psychoanalytic framework, with particular emphasis on object relations theory. Conducted weekly psychodynamic psychotherapy with a 20-year-old female with dependent personality features. Therapy focused on identity issues and concerns around separating from parents. (supervised 1 hour per week.)
Instructor: Sandra Hope, Ph.D.; Supervisor: Donald Freed, Ph.D.

9/88-5/89 **Child and Family Therapy Practicum, Case Western Reserve University**
Class consisted of weekly discussion of treatment of children and families. Students presented cases from their outside clinical placements.
Instructor: Jane Black, Ph.D.

3/88-4/88   **Adult Assessment Practicum, Department of Neurology, University Hospitals of Cleveland**
Administered cognitive and personality tests and submitted test reports for two men in their early thirties who had each suffered head injuries in the past year.
Supervisor: James Reed, Ph.D.

11/87   **Child Assessment Practicum, Beech Brook Residential Treatment Center, Pepper Pike, OH**
Administered cognitive and personality tests and submitted a test report for a 13-year-old female resident being considered for transfer to a community public school.
Supervisor: Jeffrey Frank, Ph.D.

TEACHING AND RESEARCH EXPERIENCE:

1/91-5/91   **Teaching Assistant for Graduate Psychology Course "Methods of Assessment: Childhood," Case Western Reserve University**
Will assist in the teaching of child testing and child and family interviewing methods to first-year clinical graduate students.
Instructor: Daniel Weiss, Ph.D.

1/90-present   **Dissertation Research in Clinical Psychology, Case Western Reserve University**
Conducting research to determine factors contributing to resiliency in young adult children of alcoholics. Prospectus defense completed and passed on 10/19/90. Data collection begun.
Advisor: Lee Lomer, Ph.D.

1/90-5/90   **Instructor for Undergraduate Psychology Course Entitled "The Psychology of Prejudice," Case Western Reserve University**
Designed and taught this 1 credit hour course. The course covered psychological theories concerning prejudice, with discussions regarding racism, sexism, and religious prejudice.

9/88-7/89   **Master's Thesis in Clinical Psychology, Case Western Reserve University**
Thesis entitled: "The relationship between self-concept development and achievement motivation in fourth grade children."
Advisor: Lee Lomer, Ph.D.

1/88-8/88   **Research Assistant to Lee Lomer, Ph.D., Case Western Reserve University**
Tested over 60 twins, between the ages of 6 and 12 years, with the WISC-R, WRAT-R, and PPVT-R as part of research in Behavior-Genetics.

(Cont.)

EXHIBIT A   *(Continued)*

1/88-4/88	**DAS Standardization Tester, The Psychological Corporation, Cleveland, OH** Tested children as part of standardization for the development of an intelligence/achievement test.
9/87-5/88	**Research Assistant to J. Flam, Ph.D., Case Western Reserve University** Tested over 30 three-year-olds with the Stanford-Binet Intelligence Test and the PPVT-R.
1/86-5/87	**Honors Thesis in Psychology, Clark University** Thesis entitled "Some differences between transfer and non-transfer college students: Planning, coping with conflict, and adjustment."

RELATED GRADUATE COURSE WORK:

8/87-12/87	Methods of Assessment: Childhood.
1/88-5/88	Psychopathology of Childhood.
1/88-5/88	Methods of Assessment: Adulthood and Old Age.
8/88-12/88	Introduction to Intervention.
8/88-5/89	Intervention Practicum: Child and Family Therapy.
1/89-5/89	Measurement of Behavior.
1/89-5/89	History and Systems of Psychology.
8/89-5/90	Intervention Practicum: Psychodynamic Therapy.
1/90-5/90	Advanced Psychopathology (Adult).
8/90-5/91	Intervention Practicum: Cognitive Behavioral Therapy.
8/90-12/90	Intervention Practicum: Client Centered Therapy (Audit).

PRESENTATIONS AND PUBLICATIONS:

Flower, A. Self-concept and achievement versus affiliation motivation in fourth grade children. Submitted as a poster presentation to the Society for Research in Child Development, binennial conference, April 1991.

Flower, A. (in press). Diagnosing alcoholism: Toward a multisource approach. In Stout, Levitt & Ruben (Eds.), *Handbook for assessing and treating addictive disorders.* Westport, CT: Greenwood Press.

Flower, A., Hope, S., & Reed, J. (1987). Planning and coping with conflict: Transfer vs. non-transfer college students. Paper presented at Eastern Psychological Association 58th Annual Meeting, Arlington, VA.

REFERENCES:

By request.

REFERENCES

APA Psychotherapy Videotape Series (1994). Washington, DC: American Psychological Association.

Belar, C., & Orgel, S. (1980). Survival guide for intern applicants. *Professional Psychology, 11,* 672–675.

Cohen, L. D. (1992). The academic department. In D. K. Freedheim (Ed.), *History of psychotherapy: A century of change* (pp. 731–764). Washington, DC: American Psychological Association.

Dubin, S. (1972). Obsolescence or lifelong education: A choice for the professional. *American Psychologist, 27,* 486–498.

Drummond, F., Rodolfa, E., & Smith, D. (1981). A survey of APA- and non-APA–approved internship programs. *American Psychologist, 36,* 411–414.

Flexner, A. (1925). *Medical education: A comparative study.* New York: MacMillan.

Frank, G. (1984). The Boulder model: History, rationale, and critique. *Professional Psychology: Research and Practice, 15,* 417–435.

Goldfried, M. (1984). Training the clinician as scientist-professional. *Professional Psychology: Research and Practice, 15,* 477–481.

Grace, W. (1985). Evaluating a prospective clinical internship: Tips for the applicant. *Professional Psychology: Research and Practice, 16,* 475–480.

Kingsbury, S. (1987). Cognitive differences between clinical psychologists and psychiatrists. *American Psychologist, 42,* 152–156.

Matarazzo, J. (1987). There is only one psychology, no specialties, but many applications. *American Psychologist, 42,* 893–903.

McFall, R. (1991). Manifesto for a science of clinical psychology. *The Clinical Psychologist, 44,* 75–88.

Megargee, E. (1990). *A guide to obtaining a psychology internship.* Muncie, IN: Accelerated Development.

Monti, P. (1985). Interviewing for internships. *The Behavior Therapist, 8,* 205–206.

Morrow-Bradley, C., & Elliott, R. (1986). Utilization of psychotherapy research by practicing psychotherapists. *American Psychologist, 41,* 188–197.

Norcross, J. C., & Goldfried, M. R. (Eds.) (1992). *Handbook of psychotherapy integration.* New York: Basic Books.

Overholser, J. C. (1991). The Socratic method as a technique in psychotherapy supervision. *Professional Psychology: Research and Practice, 22,* 68–74.

Overholser, J.C., & Fine, M. (1990). Defining the boundaries of professional competence: Managing subtle cases of clinical incompetence. *Professional Psychology: Research and Practice, 21,* 462–469.

Perry, N. (1990). Scientist-practitioner training. *The Clinical Psychologist, 43,* 47–49.

Peterson, D. R. (1992). The doctor of psychology degree. In D. K. Freedheim (Ed.). *History of psychotherapy: A century of change* (pp. 829–849). Washington, DC: American Psychological Association.

Petzel, T., & Berndt, D. (1980). APA internship selection criteria: Relative importance of academic and clinical preparation. *Professional Psychology, 11,* 792–796.

Phillips, B. (1989). Role of the practitioner in applying science to practice. *Professional Psychology: Research and Practice, 20,* 3–8.

Rogers, C. (1957). The necessary and sufficient conditions of therapeutic personality change. *Journal of Consulting Psychology, 21,* 95–103.

Stedman, J., Costello, R., Gaines, T., Schoenfeld, L., Loucks, S., & Burstein, A. (1981). How clinical psychology interns are selected: A study of decision-making processes. *Professional Psychology, 12,* 415–419.

Stoltenberg, C., & Delworth, U. (1987). *Supervising counselors and therapists: A developmental approach.* San Francisco: Jossey-Bass.

Weiss, S. (1975). The clinical psychology intern evaluates the training experience. *Professional Psychology, 6,* 435–441.

▶ 13

Professional Issues in Psychology

GEORGE STRICKER   SHEILA COONERTY

JEROLD R. GOLD

The education and training leading to the doctoral degree in psychology provide the intellectual background and skills necessary to enter the profession of psychology. The profession itself allows the practitioner to use his or her training in many ways. In addition, there are further benchmarks of achievement as well as professional responsibilities that must be mastered. The purpose of this chapter is to define the roles and responsibilities of the clinical psychologist as well as to outline the professional issues relevant to that role. Specifically, these issues are professional licensure, continuing professional education, the National Register of Health Care Providers, the diplomate in psychology, and malpractice and malpractice insurance.

THE CLINICAL PSYCHOLOGIST

Resnick (1991) introduced a document defining the field of clinical psychology and the roles and responsibilities of its practitioners. We draw heavily on that document in this section. Clinical psychologists further the science of psychology, human welfare, and the profession of psychology through research, teaching, and services that address emotional, intellectual, biological, psychological, social, and behavioral maladjustment and psychopathology. In order to understand fully the role that clinical psychologists play, we must consider the areas of knowledge covered by their training, the skills essential to using that knowledge, and the psychologists' involvement in the integration of present knowledge with theory and further research.

Areas of Knowledge

Clinical psychologists are expected to have a broad knowledge of the social, cognitive/affective, and biological bases of behavior. In addition, an understanding of individual differences is an essential aspect of training. These areas of knowledge are not unique to clinical psychology, but they are certainly essential foundations upon which the specialty is built. Significant advanced training in the areas of personality and psychopathology is more likely to be unique to clinical psychologists. It is expected, therefore, that clinical psychologists are knowledgeable about normal and abnormal adjustment across the lifespan as well as being knowledgeable about appropriate assessment and intervention techniques.

Professional Skills

The major skill areas that are essential to the practice of clinical psychology are those of assessment, intervention, consultation and program development, and supervision of psychological services. Each of these will be described briefly here.

Assessment

In assessing adjustment, maladjustment, and psychopathology, clinical psychologists use a variety of tools. First, a knowledge of human behavior must be used to help the professional decide on *who* or *what* should be assessed. An adequate assessment of a client/patient may include the individual as well as the family system or relevant group of which the individual is a part. Clinical psychologists must make an informed decision as to the best tools for such an assessment, as well as the appropriate areas of functioning (cognitive, emotional, social, or behavioral) to be assessed. The major tools of assessment include behavioral observations (e.g., a psychologist observes a child in his nursery school class), clinical interviewing (e.g., a psychologist meets with the child in a play interview and the parents in an interview to ascertain the nature and history of the child's problem), and psychological tests (e.g., the psychologist administers intelligence tests as well as using an assessment of social maturity to gain a clearer sense of the child's functioning).

In addition to carrying out the assessment itself, clinical psychologists must be skilled in integrating the information they gather into a comprehensive description of the client's/patient's functioning. Finally, they must be capable of communicating those results in oral and written form to all concerned parties.

The capacity to make a comprehensive assessment of a client/patient is also an integral part of clinical psychologists' formulations of a plan for intervention or treatment, in that such plans must be based on a detailed and thorough knowledge of the problem and person to be treated.

Intervention

As noted, intervention begins with assessment and the formulation of an appropriate treatment plan. Clinical psychologists then must choose the correct intervention from the variety of techniques available. Appropriate interventions are directed at the prevention as well as the treatment of all types of psychopathology (i.e., emotional conflicts, personality disturbances, psychotic symptomatology, and skill deficits) that underlie a person's distress or maladjustment. In addition, interventions may be directed toward the promotion of good adjustment rather than simply the correction of maladjustment.

The most common intervention techniques are those of individual psychotherapy, marital and family therapy, group therapy, social learning or cognitive training, and environmental consultation and design. A broad range of theoretical approaches (e.g., psychoanalysis, psychodynamic theory, behavioral theory, cognitive theory, family systems theory) can be used in making such interventions. Psychologists' choice of theoretical approach depends on their training; some clinicians consistently carry out all interventions from one theoretical point of view, whereas others integrate approaches or let the needs of the person direct the choice of approach as well as technique.

Consultation and Program Development

In addition to using their skills in direct intervention, psychologists use their particular expertise to promote psychological understanding and possibly to coordinate intervention with others who may have a role in intervention. This may involve as simple a consultation as discussing a person's problem with a psychiatrist as an aid in choosing appropriate medication. Or it may involve acting as a consultant to an entire inpatient treatment staff in regard to an individual client/patient or to difficulties within the institution itself. Psychologists often are called upon to use their understanding of group processes and systems to help other mental health professionals create the best therapeutic environment for those under treatment.

Similarly, such knowledge of group processes and systems theory allows psychologists to assume a unique role in designing therapeutic programs and psychological services. The research background of clinical psychologists is often of help in evaluating the effectiveness of such programs and services.

Psychological Supervision

As clinical psychologists combine experience with expertise, they often function in the role of supervisor for other clinicians of all backgrounds, as well as for nonprofessionals. Because assessment and intervention in maladjustment and psychopathology are the specialties of clinical psychologists, and an understanding of groups and systems is also part of the training, clinical psychologists are often in a unique position to understand the needs and roles of mental health staff. Such supervision may be intensive supervision in regard to individual therapy sessions or a broader supervision of the workings of a system or group. Thus, clinical psychologists often are assigned the role of team leader on inpatient treatment teams or overall coordinator of outpatient services.

Research and Theory Development and Integration

A major aspect of clinical psychology training and a major role of professional psychologists is that of ongoing research and theory development. This involves not only research itself but the evaluation of present knowledge in the light of new research findings and theoretical paradigms. Professional psychologists see research and theoretical development as integral parts of their role, not as isolated academic pursuits. Thus, in all settings, from formal academic ones to hospital and clinic settings to private practice, research is carried out and presented to other professionals through conferences and scientific meetings. New theoretical paradigms then are tested further or enlarged upon. In addition to the presentation of such newly acquired knowledge to other professionals, some vehicle often is found to disseminate findings to the broader public.

PROFESSIONAL LICENSURE

The doctoral degree in psychology does not, in itself, allow for admission to the profession. Before psychologists can become practicing professionals, using the title of "psychologist," they must become licensed by the state in which they practice. This license is the government's way of guaranteeing the public that those professionals claiming to be psychologists have met at least the minimal qualifications necessary to practice the profession. Although some states provide a license in clinical psychology, most states offer a generic license in psychology , and individuals then are restricted to practicing within their areas of competence. Requirements for licensing vary from state to state; in most cases the requirements cover several general areas: education, experience, and an examination. Each of these areas will be reviewed generally here; however, it must be noted that actual requirements, particularly as to licensing exam scores, do vary from state to state. A student interested in the licensing laws for a state should contact that state's department of education, which oversees licensing of all professions.

Education

The typical educational requirement for licensure is the doctoral degree, either in psychology or, in some states, a substantial equivalent thereof. Some states allow licensing at a master's degree level. The degree must be granted from a program registered with the state department of education. If the psychologist's education was completed in another state than the one where the license is requested, he or she must apply to the department of education to have the degree-granting institution evaluated for equivalency with a registered program.

Experience

The experience requirement for licensure varies from state to state. However, most states require a fixed amount (e.g., 2 years) of supervised employment in appropriate psychological activities, with a specified amount to be completed post-doctorally. In most states, strict rules cover the duration of employment as well as the intensity of the supervision. In other words, a minimum of weekly hours in a psychology position may be required as well as a duration (e.g., 2 years) of experience. The experience itself must involve activities considered to be essential to the role of psychologist. Positions that involve mostly routine, nonprofessional work are not considered to be qualifying experiences.

In addition to the quantity and quality of the experience, an essential requirement is that it be supervised. Although states may vary in the amount of supervision required, in general, applicants must show that they have been supervised by a licensed psychologist on a regular basis (e.g., weekly).

Examination

The examination for licensure may include, but does not always include, some combination of a multiple-choice examination, a written essay exam, and an oral exam testing knowledge of state laws and clinical ability.

Examination for Professional Practice in Psychology (EPPP)

The EPPP is the multiple-choice examination constructed by the American Association for State Psychology Boards and used by almost every jurisdiction in the United States and Canada. The exam covers the broad range of subjects expected to be mastered by a psychologist. The applicant is allowed 4 hours to complete the exam.

The EPPP is intended to evaluate the knowledge that should have been acquired by any candidate who has a doctoral degree in psychology followed by 1 or 2 years of post-doctoral experience. Candidates are expected to have acquired a broad basic knowledge of psychology regardless of individual specialties. The exam attempts to assess competence in five dimensions:

1. Problem definition and diagnosis
2. Design, implementation, and assessment of intervention
3. Research and measurement
4. Professional/ethical/legal issues
5. Applications to social systems

The pass point for the exam is set by the state board for psychology in each state, and may vary considerably from state to state. In addition, each exam is assessed for comparative difficulty, leading to possible adjustments in the pass point from exam to exam. Most applicants with the required education and experience should be able to pass the test.

Oral and Essay Examinations

In general, oral exams and essay exams are meant to test applicants' ability to apply their knowledge to the practical world of professional psychology. Oral exams are conducted by one or several senior psychologists, whose questions center around a functional knowledge of the laws in the relevant state or around a case presentation. Essay exams ask applicants to apply their education and training to questions posed. In both cases the performance of the applicant is measured against the criteria for passing.

Not all states have oral or written exams. Many states simply require a passing grade on the EPPP.

Exemptions

Every state allows individuals in certain positions to be exempt from licensing laws. For instance, individuals working in federal, state, and municipal agencies, or in educational institutions, may be exempt from such licensing laws within those institutions. In addition, students designated as psychology trainees or psychology interns as part of their training are exempt from licensing laws. Persons who have received their doctoral degree and are acquiring the necessary experience may be exempt for a varying period of time, although the state may require that the title of psychologist not be used.

Finally, it should be noted that the title "psychologist" is the certifiable title. It is possible for someone to work as a therapist using the title "therapist" in states where that title is not certifiable. However, to do so while training to be a psychologist is considered unethical behavior in some states.

CONTINUING PROFESSIONAL EDUCATION

Most clinical psychologists believe emphatically that the education of the members of the profession cannot and does not end with the attainment of the doctoral degree. This belief is reflected in, and made statutory by, the licensing laws of most states. As already discussed, most states require psychologists to complete at least 1 year of supervised experience after completing the doctorate in order to qualify for initial licensing to practice psychology. Beyond that, many states require specified amounts of continuing education credits in order for the psychologist to renew the license.

Ongoing training and supervision are traditional and enduring parts of the employment of most newly graduated clinical psychologists. Although the specifics of this post-doctoral education may vary widely from job to job, most recent graduates receive 1 to several hours of ongoing individual or group supervision. In these relationships, novice clinical psychologists review their clinical work, assessment activities, research, or teaching with a more senior member of the psychology staff or faculty. This kind of supervision generally continues until the psychologist is judged by senior psychologists to be fully capable of independent work. However, many psychologists voluntarily seek out job related supervision on an ongoing or periodical basis for many years. Ongoing academic or clinical education frequently is available to the clinical psychologist in the form of case conferences, seminars, peer supervision, workshops, or lectures that are offered by the psychology department or by other units of a hospital, outpatient clinic, or university.

In addition to these on-the-job post-doctoral educational opportunities, there exist more intensive venues for post-doctoral education in general clinical psychology or in speciality areas. Of greatest interest and importance are the various postdoctoral clinical fellowships that combine employment and ongoing training, and the various post-doctoral institutes that offer long-term, intensive specialty training while the psychologist is otherwise employed.

Post-doctoral Fellowships in Clinical Psychology

Post-doctoral fellowships are paid educational experiences of intensive work and study for a period of 1 to 4 or 5 years following graduation. They may involve broad training in all scientific and applied aspects of clinical psychology or be situations in which the psychologist specializes in work with a particular approach, problem, or population. These fellowships are based in universities, medical centers, psychiatry departments, and outpatient clinics. The general clinical fellowships are the equivalent of the residencies that are required of physicians who wish to qualify as specialists. Currently clinical psychology does not have a specific requirement for post-doctoral specialty training, although there is an active debate in the profession concerning such a requirement. Some well-known clinical fellowships include those at the Menninger Foundation in Topeka, Kansas; the post-doctoral fellowship at the Austen Riggs Psychiatric Center in Stockbridge, Massachusetts; and the Yale University fellowships. Clinical psychology fellows in such settings do a variety of assessment, therapeutic, consultative, and research activities in an intellectually charged atmosphere. Many hours are devoted to clinical supervision, scholarly pursuits, and collegial interchange.

Other post-doctoral fellowships offer clinical psychologists the chance to learn specific advanced skills in assessment, intervention, and research in topics that their doctoral education may have touched on only briefly. For 1 or more years the psychologist becomes a junior staff member or investigator, working alongside, and under the supervision of, more senior experts in that particular specialty. In these experiences, psychologists may perfect skills in working with populations who have unique problems and needs and perhaps will emerge equipped with empirical and clinical knowledge and skills that are on the cutting edge in that speciality.

The availability of such fellowships seems to vary with the availability of funds, supervisors, and academic and clinical needs. Many are advertised in the employment section of the *Monitor,* the official newspaper of the APA. Others are represented in the listings of internships and fellowships published by the Association of Psychology and Postdoctoral Internship Centers.

It would be impossible to come close to listing completely the number of specialty areas in which post-doctoral fellowships are available. A random and highly arbitrary list includes Health Psychology, Behavioral Medicine, Clinical Neuropsychology, College Mental Health Services, Psycho-Oncology, Psychoimmunology, Substance Abuse, Child and Spousal Abuse, Family Systems and Therapy, Child Therapy, Cognitive Behavior Therapy, Short-Term Dynamic Psychotherapy, Cross-Cultural Psychotherapy, Treatment of Serious Mental Illness, Psychotherapy with Asian Americans, Psychotherapy with Hispanic American, and so on. It probably is not far from the truth to state that there exists a potential training site to match almost every interest.

Post-doctoral Institute Training

Institute training at the post-doctoral level involves 1 to several years of part time work in a variety of specialty areas. This training rarely is integrated completely into the psychologist's work life as is the post-doctoral fellow-ship; most people complete this aspect of their educational life while work-ing part time or full time (Gold, 1990). These experiences are hefty in their time demands and economic cost; most require 12 to 20 hours per week and an investment of $2,000 to $5,000 per year. However, most graduates regard these outlays as time and money that was well spent, for which psycholo-gists are recompensed personally, professionally, and financially. The insti-tute allows clinical psychologists to focus broadly and intensively upon the enhancement of their clinical and theoretical skills or to develop practical and academic expertise in areas of psychology with which they have had little prior experience. As such, the subject matter, goals, and results of the postdoctoral fellowship and institute training may overlap significantly. What differs is the practical setting.

There is a plethora of institutes and post-doctoral training programs avail-able to clinical psychologists. Traditionally, most have been freestanding edu-cational, professional, and clinical centers that evolved around a particular school of thought or clinical method. The prototypes of these programs are the autonomous psychoanalytic institutes that, since the 1940s, have accepted psychologists for training in the theory and practice of psychoanalysis. These include such well-known institutes as the William Alanson White Institute and the National Association for the Advancement of Psychoanalysis; both in New York City; the Topeka Institute of Psychoanalysis; and centers in many metropolitan areas across the country. In the last two decades a few post-doctoral institutes offering psychoanalytic training to psychologists have opened in universities. The first of these were the postdoctoral programs at the Department of Psychology of New York University and at the Derner Institute of Advanced Psychological Studies at Adelphi University. Training at these centers involves several years of supervised clinical work, a compa-rable time spent in theoretical and clinical course work, and a personal in-volvement in psychoanalysis.

Currently clinical psychologists may choose from an almost unlimited array of specialties that go well beyond psychoanalysis. There exist insti-tutes and post-doctoral programs that offer theoretical and conceptual train-ing in Gestalt Therapy, Individual (Adlerian) Psychology, Rational-Emotive Therapy, Cognitive Therapy, Behavior Therapy, Short-Term Dynamic Psy-chotherapy, Couples and Family Therapy, Jungian Therapy, Existential Psychotherapy, Child Psychotherapy, and many other interventions and theo-ries. Typically, these program require a part-time, multiyear involvement in classroom and supervised clinical activities. All of the institutes offer clinical psychologists some opportunities for ongoing involvement in a professional community that shares their clinical, scholarly, and theoretical orientation and interests. Many of these centers become the focus of the psychologists' professional network, and often there are activities and involvement available for the graduates of such programs. For example, many of these institutes publish professional and scientific journals. They also sponsor professional societies, conferences, workshops, and continuing education programs, often employing the graduates of the program as faculty in these activities, and eventually in the main training program as well.

Conferences, Workshops, and Seminars

Probably most post-graduate education in clinical psychology occurs in venues that are shorter and more modest in scope than the experiences just described. This does not make these training events any less valuable. Psychologists at every level of experience take part in conferences of the various professional and scientific societies to which they belong (e.g., the APA or the Society for Personality Assessment, to name just two). At these meetings, workshops, panels, and paper and poster sessions allow psychologists to keep up to date on new advances in the field, to learn new skills, and to update technical and theoretical knowledge. Many established scientific, academic, and professional groups sponsor similar meetings that last for periods that vary from an hour or two to a week or more that similarly give psychologists and other professionals the opportunity to keep up to date. Many of these organizations are accredited by the APA to offer continuing education credits to program participants. These credits are useful in documenting a professional's ongoing educational involvement and probably will be required more frequently in the future to keep the psychologist's state license active and to satisfy the reimbursement requirements of health insurance plans. For example, New York State now requires all licensed psychologists to submit proof of a completed course in the detection and reporting of child abuse in order to renew a psychology license.

Most psychologists receive a steady flow of advertisements and announcements of these events, often held in enticing domestic and foreign vacation spots. The most comprehensive single source of information about continuing education is the *Monitor,* which lists hundreds of certified sponsors and activities in each monthly issue.

Finally, home study, on formal and informal terms, may be the single greatest area of continuing professional education for clinical psychologists. An incredible number of journals, books, audiotapes, videotapes, software, and CD-ROM packages seems to be available. It is possible to earn continuing education credits through certified home study programs, but, more frequently, clinical psychologists simply try to keep up with this flood of information informally, to the best of their ability.

NATIONAL REGISTER OF HEALTH SERVICE PROVIDERS

The National Register of Health Service Providers, as its name implies, was established as a centralized listing of all psychologists who are appropriately trained and credentialed to offer health services. The purpose of the listing is to aid consumers in identifying professionals who are appropriately trained. To be listed in the Register, the potential registrant must have a doctoral degree from a regionally accredited institution, be licensed, and have 2 years of supervised experience, 1 year of which was in an internship and one of which was post-doctoral. For the most part, any licensed psychologist with training in a health care specialty, such as clinical psychology, can be listed in the Register if he or she makes application. The review of the application includes the evaluation and verification of credentials, but it does not require an examination. Being listed in the Register is not mandatory, and not all licensed psychologists are listed there.

THE DIPLOMATE IN PSYCHOLOGY

The diploma awarded by the American Board of Professional Psychology (ABPP), leading to the title "Diplomate," is considered certification at an advanced professional level in psychology. Prior to the establishment of licenses in each jurisdiction, the ABPP diploma was the only benchmark of status other than the doctoral degree. Since licensure has become a common practice, the diplomate is seen as assurance of an advanced level of competence.

Psychologists are eligible for candidacy if they meet the following requirements:

1. The completion of a doctoral degree meeting specific training standards
2. The completion of an internship
3. The completion of 4 years of acceptable qualifying experience, 3 of which must be post-doctoral. Experience must be the equivalent of full time (30 hours per week for 50 weeks)
4. Present engagement in professional work in the area of practice in which the individual wishes to be examined
5. Evidence of continuing education in the profession of psychology during the years of post-doctoral experience
6. Evidence of membership in a major psychological organization (e.g., APA)
7. Licensure in the state where the candidate actually practices

When a psychologist meets these basic requirements, he or she is eligible for candidacy. After all credentials have been verified, the candidate must submit two written work samples demonstrating (1) an assessment case and (2) an intervention case. If that work is acceptable, an individual exam is scheduled. The specific nature of the exam varies according to the specialty. In general, however, it covers 5 to 6 hours and has at least four Diplomate psychologists examining the candidate over previously specified areas and against previously specified criteria.

Diplomas currently are offered in the following specialties: Clinical, Counseling, School, Industrial/Organizational, Clinical Neuropsychology, Forensic, Family, Health, and Behavioral Psychology. In addition, several additional specialties, such as psychoanalysis, currently are seeking diplomate status.

MALPRACTICE AND MALPRACTICE INSURANCE

All professionals who serve the public must be aware of the great need to avoid causing harm to those they serve. Psychologists who work clinically with distressed persons or who do research in clinical areas certainly need to mind the motto "First, do no harm." However, no less than any other group, psychologists are imperfect beings. On many more occasions than we would like, our interactions, interventions, and behavior with clients/patients, research subjects, or students may affect those persons in ways that seem harmful to the individual.

Accidental or purposeful harm to any professional client/patient caused by a psychologist may fall in the category of professional malpractice. *Malpractice* itself is a legal term that is defined as practical negligence: The practitioner fails to live up to conventional standards of care and knowledge; departs from ethical and legal standards for practice; or intentionally acts in ways that violate the interests, rights, and well being of the client/patient (Cohen, 1990).

We live in a highly litigious society, and medical doctors and other health care providers increasingly have come under the scrutiny of an unhappy public. As a result, physicians have been sued for malpractice at extraordinary rates during the last two decades, and costs for medical malpractice insurance have moved into astronomical realms. There is some debate about the realities of this explosion as it applies to clinical psychology: Most recent data suggest that we as a profession are sued far less often, lose cases much less often, and are the subject of relatively small financial settlements when compared to physicians (Cohen, 1990). However, even if we are not in the center of the explosion of malpractice action, we still are implicated far more frequently than in decades past.

How might we concretely define negligent practice as a clinical psychologist? First, we must examine the parameters of "usual and customary" practice, a task that is far from easy. These parameters are set by a number of bodies of psychologists and legislators at several levels of civil and legal rigor. First, certain expectations for and sanctions about the practice of psychology are stated explicitly in the laws of the states and municipalities in which the psychologist practices. Failure to follow these laws can result in criminal prosecution for the psychologist, as well as in being found civilly negligent. An example of these types of legislative parameters is the laws recently passed in several states that require a psychologist to report any person who is suspected of child abuse to the appropriate authorities.

The licensing or certification laws under which the psychologist's credentials are granted usually define the range of activities in which the person may engage and rule out others: Licensure as a psychologist includes the practice of psychotherapy but does not permit other health services, such as prescription of medication, spinal manipulation, or extraction of teeth. Practice outside the scope of licensure also makes one vulnerable to criminal and civil actions by the government and by individuals.

Much of what we do as clinical psychologists also is guided by ethical and practical standards that have been developed by such professional groups as the APA, and various state, county, and other local psychological associations. These standards for professional behavior and practice are not legal or statutory; however, they frequently are consulted by judges and juries in determining the specifics of "usual and customary" practice. Thus, each member of the profession must be up to date and as fully aware as possible about these guidelines. These guidelines explicitly forbid certain types of activities by the psychologist. Most important in this regard is the prohibition of sexual contact between the psychologist and his or her clients/patients, research subjects, or students. They also rule in certain requirements for clinical, instructional, and research activities. For example, the psychologist is expected to protect each client's/patient's confidentiality, to obtain informed consent about agreement to be in treatment or to be a research subject, to evaluate the effects of all interventions on all subjects, and to avoid abandoning a client/patient before treatment is completed. Other issues covered in these guidelines include certain very specific prescriptions for practice that must be followed. We must, for example, refer any actively suicidal patient for psychiatric evaluation, or risk a violation of the guidelines for usual and customary practice.

Many of the other ethical and professional guidelines for practice in psychology are concerned with less focused but equally important issues related to the range of the individual psychologist's education, training, and competence. As we saw in the first section of the chapter, clinical psychology is a broadly defined profession, and there is no one member of the profession who can (or should) be competent in all aspects of it. The psychologist must take care to offer only those services in which he or she has been trained adequately and in which the psychologist is up to date about the latest methods, advantages, and risks. The psychologist who treats couples without having been trained to do so, who offers to mediate divorces after attending one lecture on the topic, or who assesses neuropsychological deficits with techniques learned on an internship 30 years past may well be guilty of negligent professional behavior.

Finally, much of the definition of "usual and customary" is derived from the clinical and scientific literature of our field and from related fields such as psychiatry, social work, and medicine. When the psychologist makes assessments or diagnoses, or offers treatments, these actions are more likely to be considered appropriate in the legal sense if there are substantial literature citations that back up those decisions. Selecting an intervention for which there is no prior support may move the field along; however, it also may be viewed dimly by judges and juries.

Some experts in the field have suggested that many clinical psychologists suffer from a phobia about being sued that actually is unwarranted (Brodsky & Schumacher, 1990). Some studies have suggested that the mean, median, and modal number of lawsuits each member of the profession will experience will be zero (Cohen, 1990). However, as the old saying goes, an ounce of prevention is worth a pound of cure. Careful study of and adherence to the statutory and professional guidelines that govern psychological practice will go a long way to lessen one's risk, as will adequate record keeping and consultation with attorneys and other informed persons in potentially litigious situations.

All psychologists should protect themselves further by ensuring that they are covered by adequate professional liability (malpractice) insurance. Graduate students, psychology interns, and most psychologists who work for institutions, agencies, or universities may be covered by insurance that is held by their employer or academic setting. Psychologists who are in independent practice must purchase this insurance privately. At the present time, professional liability insurance is offered in the United States through one private insurance company and through group plans that are sponsored by the American Psychological Association Insurance Trust (APAIT) and by the American Psychological Society. These plans cover the psychologist's legal fees if he or she is sued and will pay settlement costs of various amounts (limits range from $100,000 to $5,000,000 depending upon the policy selected) if the psychologist is found guilty of negligence. An exception to the usual limits of coverage may be made if the psychologist is found guilty of having been sexually involved with a client, in which case much lower limits of coverage usually are in force. The costs of this coverage vary according to the type of policy selected. *Claims-made* policies are cheaper but only offer coverage while the policy is active. *Occurrence-based* policies cost more but cover the psychologist even after he or she has retired or given up practicing. Certain types of interim policies ("tails") usually are available to cover those who have chosen claims-made coverage. Insurance costs also vary according to the psychologist's years of experience in the field, his or her geographic location, and his or her history of prior lawsuits. In general, 1994 costs roughly were in the range of $300 to $2,000 per year for an individual psychologist.

CONCLUSION

In these pages we have attempted to summarize the complex post-graduate challenges, responsibilities, and opportunities that await the newly minted professional clinical psychologist. In an ever developing field that exists in a highly complicated world the practice of psychology involves unique interaction with government, the legal system, and a host of professional requirements and organizations. We hope that this does not scare off the prospective student, but instead gives him or her a sense of the rich and multifaceted life of the practicing clinical psychologist outside of the office or laboratory.

REFERENCES

Brodsky, S. L., & Schumacher, J. E. (1990). The impact of litigation on psychotherapy practice. In E. Margenau (Ed.), *Comprehensive handbook of private practice* (pp. 664–676). New York: Gardner Press.

Cohen, R. J. (1990). The professional liability of behavioral scientists. In E. Margenau (Ed.), *Comprehensive handbook of private practice* (pp. 651–663). New York: Gardner Press.

Gold, J. (1990). The effects of private practice on the therapist's personal and family life. In E. Margenau (Ed.), *Comprehensive handbook of private practice* (pp. 503–513). New York: Gardner Press.

Resnick, J. H. (1991). Finally, a definition of clinical psychology: A message from the president, Division 12. *The Clinical Psychologist, 44,* 3–11.

► # 14

Evolution of Professional Issues in Psychology

Training Standards, Legislative Recognition, and Boundaries of Practice

ROBERT J. RESNICK   **PATRICK H. DeLEON**

GARY R. VANDENBOS

Professional psychology is an autonomous health profession providing clinical services within organized health care settings and private practice. Professional psychologists are highly trained professionals, possessing specialized clinical skills and expertise. Clinical psychologists serve as directors of state departments of mental health, as directors of psychiatric hospitals and community mental health centers, on the faculties of almost all medical schools as well as the faculties of psychology professional schools, and on the faculties of a range of other academic programs, and they are a strong and successful component in the private practice provision of health and mental health services.

Professional psychologists are trained at the doctoral level, with many clinicians having developed specialized post-doctoral skills and knowledge. Professional psychologists are licensed in all states in the United States, and there are a variety of specialized credentialing bodies, such as the American Board of Professional Psychology (ABPP), which recognize specialized post-doctoral training and proficiencies. "Freedom of choice" legislation in over 80% of states ensures patient access to needed psychological care, and psychologists are legislatively permitted hospital privileges in a growing number of states. The most recent emerging practice initiative involves expanding the boundaries of clinical practice in psychology to include psychopharmacological training and prescription privileges, which will be discussed in the second half of this chapter.

Professional psychology in the 1990s is a highly visible, prestigious, and critical health care profession. It has not always been that way. Professional psychology, as a health care profession has functionally emerged, developed, and matured in the last 50 years.

In 1945 there were 4,183 American Psychological Association (APA) members) (APA, 1945); this number has grown by 1995 to exceed 80,000. (See Chapter 15 for a detailed description of the APA.) The number of employed psychologists in both the civilian and military services in 1944 did not exceed 4,100 (Marquis, 1944), but by 1995 over 60,000 doctoral psychologists were qualified and licensed to provide psychological services to the U.S. public. In addition, by 1994, there were 289 APA-accredited doctoral programs in professional psychology in the United States and Canada (American Psychological Association, 1994). It is amazing that professional psychology has been able to grow and develop in the way that it has without psychologists possessing "homes of our own" (Rogers, 1980) where psychology had full autonomy and direct clinical responsibility for both inpatient and outpatient care.

The achievement of professional psychology's current status did not come without struggle and conflict. Such conflict has occurred both within the discipline of professional psychology and between psychology and related disciplines, most particularly psychiatry (for a history, see Cummings & VandenBos, 1983). Such conflict and discourse are a normal part of an evolving field and its changing place in a changing society, as professions evolve and develop, and societal values and goals, as reflected in legislation in public policy, evolve and change in response to societal forces.

The status and recognition psychology has achieved in the last 50 years are remarkable. On the one hand, this is a testimonial to a relatively small number of visionary leaders and advocates for the profession. However, in some circumstances governmental bodies, both legislatures and executive units, have challenged, and even forced, the profession of psychology to expand, develop, and refine itself. It is clear that, because of psychology's newly emerging maturity, professional psychology has only partially controlled and defined the professional issues agenda that has led to the present status and recognition of the field.

From our vantage point of having served in the governance and management of the APA and having worked on the state and national levels on behalf of professional psychology for more than two decades, it has become an all-too-familiar experience to see professional psychology forced by others to address specific professional issues, rather than professional psychology having a clear vision for its own autonomous clinical practice and relevant professional training. We believe professional psychology must begin to more comprehensively plan its own future—and then work to achieve it.

Our practitioners are extraordinarily well trained. It takes the average psychologist approximately 6 years of graduate training and supervision to become a professional psychologist. This represents more extensive and comprehensive training than that of our colleagues in nursing, social work, and marriage and family therapy (who, at the practice level, typically only possess master's degrees), and it compares favorably with our medical colleagues who possess 4 years of medical school education followed by an internship and probably (although not legally required) 3 years of residency training. Our clinical services are important in a wide range of arenas, including the entire physical health care system. Accordingly, we would rhetorically ask: Why are we consistently so reactive, rather than proactive? Why don't we collectively better control our own professional agenda?

In our judgment, there are a number of possible explanations, all of which go to the underlying issue of the relative maturation of our profession—and the slow but steady development of an appreciation that education, practice, and science are more intimately intertwined than many had suspected.

From an educational perspective, perhaps the lack of concerted direction is due to the fact that within our nation's educational institutions psychology has traditionally been considered one of the social sciences, rather than one of the health professions. As a direct consequence, psychology is usually accorded departmental status rather than school status. The individual "in charge" of psychology training programs is rarely a dean, and often not even a departmental chair. Our historical lack of aggressive leadership around professional issues is also undoubtedly related to the fact that few psychology training programs actually operate large-scale health programs with direct clinical responsibility for inpatient and outpatient care. Thus, few clinical psychologists ever really learn to grapple on a day-to-day basis with the intricacies of managing their own clinical programs or with the realities of constantly having to generate significant financial support.

From a professional practice perspective, psychology practitioners are traditionally employed in either small "cottage industry" private practices or in staff roles in large institutions or organized care systems. Historically, it has been the exception for one of our colleagues to be selected to head a treatment institution or state department of health (or mental health). As a direct consequence of these interrelated factors, few of our training and service delivery systems have established the type of truly collaborative contractual agreements that are so common within medicine and under which service delivery resources become readily available for programmatic training purposes (e.g., teaching hospital or teaching nursing home).

From a research perspective, we would note that service delivery institutions provide excellent opportunities for psychology to develop "state-of-the-art" health and mental health research projects (and often sites for basic research). It is noteworthy that there has been a "split" in the employment sites of research psychologists and professional psychologists. Most basic psychological research is done in academic psychology departments, often lacking a clinical services program. Most psychological services are provided in clinics and practices, often lacking a research program. It has been professional psychologists in medical schools and Veterans Administration hospitals who have most often been in settings that supported both service delivery and research (and provided access to research subjects). However, we are pleased to have observed recently that this historical separation between research and training and service delivery is gradually changing, as our field matures.

It has also become less remarkable for a psychologist to be appointed to a high-level federal administrative position or to serve as the chief mental health officer of a state—as has now been the case in such states as California, Colorado, Florida, Hawaii, Massachusetts, New York, Vermont, and Virginia. With such positions of responsibility and institutional "power," over time may also come programmatic vision, including an appreciation for the innate interrelationship between training/research and service delivery capacity.

Further, we must ensure that those psychologists experienced in high-level federal and state administration participate in the governance of APA. We must also involve such highly placed psychologists in our training institutions and other professional societies, so as to accord sufficient attention in our training programs to systematic exposure to broad public policy agendas, achieving a broader public health orientation within psychology, and understanding the business expertise that is so crucial in today's health care environment. With this change slowly evolving, we do expect programmatic modifications.

It has been only quite recently that psychology has even begun to conceptualize itself as one of the "health professions," rather than as exclusively a research discipline or only emphasizing mental health practice. Nevertheless, we can see that psychology is maturing as a profession. And, having done so, psychology must continue to develop a clearer vision of our potential contributions to society, a development that has caused consternation in our "natural competitors" within organized medicine. For, in our judgment, psychology must focus on society's real and perceived needs, if the survival of our profession is to be ensured.

THE EVOLUTIONARY BACKGROUND OF PROFESSIONAL RECOGNITION

The Vision of Federal Psychologists

World War II was to the psychotherapeutic training of psychologists what World War I was to the development of psychological assessment (VandenBos, Cummings, & DeLeon, 1992). Indeed, after World War II the federal government, particularly through the Veterans Administration (VA) psychology training programs, was more forward-thinking about psychological practice than was most of the field of psychology. It is a sign of psychology's professional youth that very few of today's psychologists have any idea who were the visionary leaders within our federal psychology corps at that time. The movement of psychologists from "assessment only" to "psychological intervention" was not uniformly viewed positively by the leaders of our own profession. In fact, this post-war clinical practice initiative was seen by some psychologists as a dangerous divergence from traditional psychology—a view that was naturally encouraged by other disciplines, particularly psychiatry (Cummings & VandenBos, 1983).

Of historical interest, Adelphi University and its post-doctoral program in psychotherapy were actually sued, in the early 1950s, by the Nassau County Neuropsychiatric Society for allegedly "practicing medicine without a license" and "establishing a medical school without a license," solely because the program was teaching psychologists to do psychotherapy. One can find numerous examples over the years of organized medicine's persistent refusal to recognize psychologists' professional expertise and competence. The essence of organized medicine's arguments against psychology's autonomous functioning have focused on the so-called inadequate training of psychologists. Physicians claimed psychologists allegedly were not skilled in physical diagnosis and therefore would miss important symptoms, ultimately leading to severe injury or even the death of patients. Organized medicine has promoted the belief that psychotherapy would naively be applied to organically based diseases, while simultaneously ignoring the growing clinical literature that stresses the important psychosocial aspects of physical health care. Simply stated, organized medicine has argued that psychology represents a significant "public health hazard" and should only be allowed to function under direct physician supervision (i.e., as a paraprofessional or physician extender). In medicine's judgment, if one did not attend medical (or, strangely, dental) school, one simply can not be a competent therapist—and certainly, cannot exercise independent clinical judgment. In sharp contrast, it has been extremely rare for the psychological profession to challenge the training (or clinical competence) of our medical colleagues—thereby, perhaps, actually giving credence to their allegations.

However, professional psychology overcame the roadblocks of organized medicine, and the expansion of professional training of clinical psychologists continued through the late 1940s and the 1950s. By the late 1950s a small but courageous number of psychologists were moving into independent practice. Today the APA Division of Psychologists in Independent Practice (Division 42) reports in excess of 7,800 members. It is thus the largest "interest group" within the association. This is an interesting development, given that initially the discipline of psychology itself was unsure about the appropriateness of this bold clinical training initiative or the need to be credentialed at an autonomous practice level.

Developing State Recognition

The first formal movement toward becoming an independent profession began on July 19, 1945 with the legal *certification* (statutory protection of title) of school psychologists in the State of Connecticut. To appreciate the policy significance of this movement one need only realize that for any other profession (e.g., law or medicine), being recognized by the state regulatory board is a *sine qua non* of professional identity. The first state psychology *licensure* act (i.e., protecting professional activities, rather than just professional title) was enacted into public law by the Commonwealth of Virginia a year later. It is interesting to note that concerns over what actually constituted the "practice of psychology" resulted in the creation of the American Board of Examiners in Professional Psychology (now the American Board of Professional Psychology [ABPP]) in 1946 by the APA, with a grant of $2,000 and the clear charge to "protect the public" from unqualified service providers.

Over the years, state regulation of the practice of psychology moved forward at an uneven pace, but in 1977 Missouri became the fiftieth state, along with the District of Columbia, to credential and regulate the practice of psychology (Cummings & VandenBos, 1983; VandenBos, Cummings, & DeLeon, 1992). Not surprisingly, along the way the practice of psychology has constantly been beset by obstacles placed in its path by organized medicine (and in particular, by psychiatry) in an attempt to impose various degrees of medical control over the psychology profession. In some states, licensure initially could be gained only by compromising and permitting medical boards to become involved in the licensing of psychologists. The process of clarifying and strengthening psychology practice acts continues even today, as we grapple at the state level with such policy issues as the locus of practice (e.g., hospital privileges), the exclusiveness of psychological testing, and the expansion of appropriate clinical responsibilities (e.g., prescription privileges).

Having successfully started on the path to achieving licensure (or "legal status"), the next confrontation for the fledgling profession might be considered the "recognition wars" (or the "I don't get no respect" battles). That is, in order for psychology to economically survive, there needed to be systematic recognition of its practitioners as autonomous providers under the various public and private health insurance programs. Although once again some national leaders of the profession actively decried such recognition, psychologists at the state level began to seek the enactment of what has come to be known collectively as "freedom of choice" acts, whereby the public is free to select practitioners of their choice, as long as the service is reimbursable and the individual practitioner is licensed and/or credentialed to provide that service (Dörken, 1976). Not surprisingly, as such statutes were proposed at the state and national level, physicians (and particularly psychiatrists) strenuously objected.

Athough there is some debate about which state actually signed the first freedom of choice act, it is generally agreed that the first laws were passed in 1968 in the states of New Jersey and Michigan. By 1995 forty-three states had enacted such "freedom of choice" statutes. At the federal level similar statutory progress has been made. In 1974 the Congress enacted a comparable provision for the Federal Employees' Health Benefit Program (FEHBP) [PL 93-363] and subsequently has also similarly modified most other federal reimbursement statutes (e.g., CHAMPUS and Medicare).

Although the issue of patient choice of provider and provider type may seem to have been resolved, as the Congress began to deliberate various proposed national health insurance reform (NHI) bills in the 102nd and 103rd Congresses, very serious consideration was given at the federal level to expressly preempting a wide range of state mandates, including the freedom of choice acts, under the guise of either ensuring uniformity of health benefits or curtailing ever escalating costs. The underlying policy notion is that if a particular health service is truly necessary, "market forces" will ensure its availability. Similar policy views also exist in the underlying conceptualizations of those advocating various "managed care" approaches (i.e., health maintenance organizations [HMOs]).

Judicial Recognition of Psychology

A pivotal event in the recognition of psychology as an autonomous profession occurred in Virginia in the mid-1970s (Resnick, 1985). The Virginia legislature enacted freedom of choice legislation in 1973. However, the dominant insurance carrier in the state, Blue Cross/Blue Shield ("the Blues"), simply refused to obey the law and reimburse beneficiaries for psychological services. The Blues denied such reimbursement over a 4-year period, unless specific criteria (which they had arbitrarily proposed) were satisfied. Initially, the psychologist's work had to be supervised by a physician—any physician, regardless of whether the physician possessed any mental health (psychiatric) training—and the required supervision did not even have to be face-to-face. Subsequently the Blues added another requirement: that the psychologist's patient had to be seen by the physician every 30 days. Not only was this an affront to psychology's autonomy, but it clearly also artificially inflated the cost of psychological care.

The "Virginia Blues" suit, as the litigation ultimately became known, was actually two legal initiatives. Psychologists in Virginia, under the leadership of the senior author, worked with the state's Office of the Attorney General to enforce the freedom of choice provisions within the state judicial system. Ultimately the Commonwealth of Virginia prevailed in a unanimous opinion by the State Supreme Court that, indeed, the act was constitutional and should be upheld. A separate action, initiated by the senior author and the Virginia Academy of Clinical Psychologists, alleged restraint of trade under the federal antitrust statute. For 3 years this latter suit was bitterly litigated through the federal courts, with the pro-psychology decision, expressly proclaiming that psychology and psychiatry were indeed competitors, ultimately being upheld by the U.S. Supreme Court. The Virginia Blues litigation is considered by many within professional psychology to be the cornerstone of what later was to become proactive advocacy on behalf of autonomous practice, as well as the establishment of clear legal precedent identifying psychologists as autonomous providers (Resnick, 1985).

The Federal Government as a "Purchaser" of Health Care

There are four major programs under which the federal government functions primarily as a "purchaser of health care" for identified beneficiary populations: the Federal Employees' Health Benefit Program (FEHBP), the Department of Defense (DoD) CHAMPUS program, Medicare, and Medicaid (DeLeon & VandenBos, 1980). As indicated earlier, in 1974 the Congress enacted a freedom of choice provision for the FEHBA, and since the enactment of the Fiscal Year 1976 Department of Defense Appropriations Act (PL 94-212), psychology has been recognized as a fully autonomous provider under CHAMPUS, essentially being treated in the same manner as physicians on both an inpatient and outpatient basis. Indeed, today psychology is the preminent provider of outpatient psychotherapeutic services under CHAMPUS. Psychology's efforts to be appropriately recognized under Medicare and Medicaid, however, took considerably longer.

Medicare and Medicaid were enacted by the Congress in 1965 (the Social Security Amendments of 1965) with an express "medical" orientation. Medicare is a federally administered program targeted toward senior citizens and those with certain definable chronic disabilities; the federal government alone determines the benefits and conditions under which they will be provided. Given the history of the federal government's role under Medicare, it is not surprising that over the years nearly every national health insurance (NHI) proposal has incorporated many of its basic provisions. And, in stark contrast, it is of considerable policy interest that every one of the major NHI proposals considered by the Congress in the 102nd and 103rd Congresses would have totally eliminated Medicaid.

Psychology's inclusion under Medicare (Title XVIII) represents over 20 years of struggle (Welch, 1990), beginning with a formal legislatively mandated study, acceptance under the HMO provision, development of a new mental health center provision, and finally obtaining direct recognition under the generic statute, as well as an express inpatient provision during the closing hours of the 103rd Congress (PL 103-432). With the complexity of the Medicare statute there will undoubtedly be further Medicare legislative agendas. Nevertheless, psychology would now seem to have finally obtained autonomous recognition under this, the largest federal health care program.

Medicaid, however, represents an entirely different situation (DeLeon et al., 1992; Resnick, 1983). Under this program (Title XIX) the federal government joins with the various states in a partnership to provide necessary health services for a subsection of the population that, simplistically stated, is economically disadvantaged (i.e., the poor). The federal statute provides for a basic benefit (interestingly, including mandatory access to the services of nurse midwives and certain categories of nurse practitioners). The states are authorized to enhance the benefit, with the federal government paying a significant share of the costs involved. Currently twenty-six states permit psychologists to be reimbursed directly for some services in certain settings, with eight states requiring physician referral. It is definitely a valid policy question to ask why nurses are so generously recognized under the federal Medicaid statute but not psychology. However, as we have indicated, Medicaid may soon be undergoing considerable federal modification, either outright elimination or the development of a substantial managed care orientation.

THE EXPANDING LOCUS OF PRACTICE

As professional psychology has matured into a clearly visible and effective health care profession, the need to expand our practice boundaries beyond traditional assessment and psychotherapy with identified mental health patients has become even clearer. Once again, however, the challenge to the profession initially came from outside of psychology, with the demand for "continuity of care" by recipients of psychological services.

The first step in this continuity of care paradigm could be considered a geographical one, addressing the locus of service delivery, that is, the expansion of psychological practice from outpatient to inpatient care, including within various partial hospitalization and nursing home and/or day care programs (Dörken, Webb, & Zaro, 1982). In many ways this expansion in locus of practice became a "scope of practice" issue for our colleagues in medicine and, as a direct result, evolved into a major underlying theme in psychology's quest for independent recognition under Medicare.

The APA developed a special task force that proposed specific credentialing guidelines so that psychologists might more effectively utilize all of their skills in organized health care delivery system settings. Psychology presently has acquired full hospital privileges by statute (or regulation) in eleven states, and, by virtue of "silent codes" (that is, where there is nothing expressly prohibiting psychologists from practicing in hospitals), are actively applying skills in hospitals all over the country. The Joint Commission on Accreditation of Health Care Organizations (JCAHO) standards formally recognize psychology's inpatient status. And we must not forget that psychologists hold faculty, staff training, and clinical positions in every medical school in the United States, as well as being active providers of psychological services within the various state and federal facilities where clinical restrictions are the exception, rather than a difficulty to be overcome (Thompson & Matarazzo, 1984).

PRESCRIPTION PRIVILEGES FOR PSYCHOLOGISTS?

As one becomes increasingly involved in providing "hands on" clinical services, the issue of psychology's role in ensuring the appropriate use of psychotropic medications readily surfaces. For the aspiring psychologist the multitude of contradictory treatment (and status or power relationship) messages surrounding prescription privileges are strikingly evident. On the one hand, there are patients who seem to need and demonstrably benefit from being "on meds." Conversely, there can be no question that there are significant clinical risks involved, including both unpleasant physiological side effects (immediate and perhaps long-term), as well as adverse psychological sequela (e.g., fostering dependency). At the same time, however, treatment team discussions regarding whether (and how) to medicate individual patients often seem to purposely exclude psychological input.

As psychologists we are led to "understand" that there are important (i.e., complex) physiological factors that must be considered. And, even though the psychological and behavioral aspects of the medication process are undoubtedly equally critical for successful treatment, we instinctively sense that there is very little interest in systematically considering them. Routinely, treatment staff with considerably less education and professional training than psychologists are accorded "correct judgment" and/or the assertion is flatly made that the residents' medication protocol is only to be discussed with the supervising psychiatrist. No other aspect of clinical diagnosis or treatment is so carefully guarded from scrutiny or objectivity. Simply stated, the psychotropic medication decision-making process is fundamentally flawed.

In talking with psychologists across the nation, it soon becomes clear that there is an almost universal institutional mythology that psychologists in particular, of all the mental health disciplines, are simply not to receive in-depth training about psychoactive medication. Accordingly, it does not take long for even the most naive therapist to appreciate that the prescription privilege agenda is, in fact, predominately driven by political and/or "turf" issues that have very little (if anything) to do with medicine's proffered concerns about providing "high quality" patient care. Those who possess this clinical responsibility (or power) simply do not want any other discipline to have it, no matter how competently trained these other practitioners might be.

Historical Perspectives

Few psychologists appreciate that in early Western history, pharmacy and medicine were so inextricably intertwined that, in effect, they were virtually one and the same profession. In fact, it was not until the twentieth century that pharmacists in the United States lost the right to prescribe—a clinical responsibility that, interestingly, they are just now beginning to reassert. In 1951 the federal government enacted legislation (the Durham-Humphrey amendments to the Food, Drug, and Cosmetic Act [PL 82-215]) that established the process for determining whether a particular drug was to be made available over the counter or by prescription only. Additionally, this federal regulatory schema relies exclusively upon the state authorities to determine which categories of health care providers are to be accorded the clinical responsibility for prescribing diagnostic or therapeutic pharmacological agents. We would clarify, however, that under our constitutional system of federal–state relationships the various federal agencies—including, for example, the VA, the Department of Justice, and the DoD—retain the exclusive authority to determine the "scope of practice" of their employees, notwithstanding state laws.

Generic State Prescription Models

In fulfilling their regulatory responsibilities, the various states have generally established a binary statutory schema for enumerating prescriptive authority. Each state's pharmacy act lists those professions that are authorized to prescribe medications, while the individual practice acts of the various health professions (e.g., nursing, optometry, and psychology) detail the specific legal parameters for their practitioners. Typically, the enabling statute is broad in nature, with the relevant professional regulatory board delegated to detail the specific conditions under which their practitioners can prescribe diagnostic or therapeutic medications.

In addressing the conditions under which nonphysician health care providers are authorized to prescribe, the states have generally structured their statutes along two conceptual classification models: (1) dependent versus independent and (2) limited versus unlimited. The former classification addresses the issue of whether there is to be mandatory physician involvement (i.e., supervision or consultation). The latter classification addresses the range or categories of medications that the nonphysician will be able to prescribe. And, not surprisingly, a state's medical practice act may include additional restrictions on prescriptive authority, even as this applies to other professions.

Unlike the very broad scope of practice authority of physicians (who are typically limited in their prescription practice by only their own individual clinical judgment), dentists, optometrists, and podiatrists are generally deemed to be "limited practitioners". That is, their interventions are restricted to specific body parts or conditions affecting those body parts. These professions are generally provided independent status, that is, requiring no physician involvement. On the other hand, nurse practitioners, physician assistants, and clinical pharmacists are usually considered to be "physician extenders," that is, practitioners who exercise limited independent clinical judgment. Accordingly, their regulatory statutes frequently require direct physician involvement through predetermined arrangements with medicine, such as requiring either: (1) a prearranged protocol or agreement between the nonphysician provider and a supervising physician or (2) a drug formulary established by the state's drug formulary commission, which determines a list of authorized drugs and provides specific guidelines for their use. Those nonphysician providers who prescribe by formulary are considered to be "limited but independent providers." Those who use protocols are considered to be "dependent providers," since they can prescribe only under the supervision of an attending physician.

Interestingly, professional nursing has recently begun moving toward the enactment of prescription legislation that expressly recognizes their independent clinical judgment, thus moving away from the physician extender model. What approach psychology will ultimately take in drafting its prescription statutes is still to be determined. To date, with the exception of Indiana (which will be discussed later), whenever this issue has been expressly addressed in the psychology statute, there has been a clear prohibition. Again, we want to emphasize that it is the various states, and not the federal government, that have the responsibility for determining under what conditions, if any, nonfederal employees can prescribe. (See Figure 14-1 for a summary of prescriptive authorities.)

A Beginning Step within Psychology

In 1984 U.S. Senator Daniel K. Inouye addressed the annual meeting of the Hawaii Psychological Association (HPA) and suggested that prescription privileges are

> . . . an entirely new legislative agenda which I think fits very nicely into the theme of your convention: Psychology in the 80s—Transcending Traditional Boundaries. As a United States Senator, I have also been working closely during the past decade with a number of your "natural allies." I am particularly thinking of our nation's nurse practitioners, nurse midwives, and optometrists. The members of these

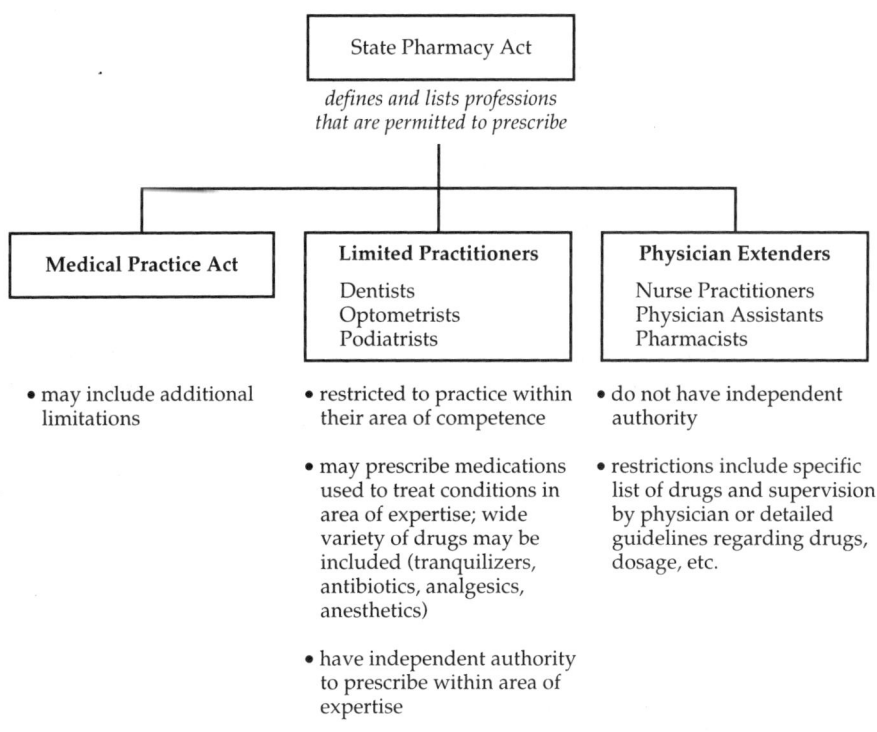

FIGURE 14-1 **Prescriptive Authority**

professions have been successful to differing degrees in amending their state practice acts to allow them to independently utilize drugs where appropriate. For example, presently 39 states allow optometrists to utilize diagnostic drugs and 4 states allow them to utilize therapeutic drugs. Eighteen states allow nurse practitioners to prescribe medications. . . . In my judgment, when you have obtained this statutory authority, you will have really made the big time. Then, you will be an autonomous profession and your clients will be well-served.

In 1985 the President of the APA Division of Psychologists in Independent Practice issued a similar challenge (Samuels, 1985). We would note that during the subsequent decade the various nonphysician health care providers have made considerable progress in the prescription privilege arena. As of this writing, nurse practitioners are recognized in all but three states, and optometrists possess diagnostic authority in all states and therapeutic privileges in forty states.

In reflecting upon the evolution toward prescription privileges within psychology, one must appreciate that it took our colleagues in organized optometry slightly more than 50 years to obtain diagnostic authority in all fifty states. We must also appreciate the policy significance of the fact that it was only back in 1977 that psychology became licensed/certified as an autonomous profession in each of the states—a journey that began 32 years earlier in Connecticut. At the same time, however, our numbers are dramatically increasing, as are the boundaries of our practice.

Developments within the State of Hawaii

Without question, the psychologists in Hawaii have from the beginning been in the forefront of the prescription privilege debate. Under the leadership of several of past-HPA presidents, relevant legislation was introduced twice in the late 1980s. Following extensive testimony (both pro and con), a House resolution was enacted in 1990 that requested the establishment by the Hawaii Center for Alternative Dispute Resolution, an agency of the state's Supreme Court, of an interdisciplinary roundtable to explore various alternatives. This body met over a period of 6 months, and a wide range of opposing views was discussed. It soon became evident that there was *no* condition under which organized psychiatry would ever support psychology obtaining this clinical responsibility. It also became clear that the essence of psychiatry's concerns centered around the alleged potential "public health hazard" that psychology's practitioners would represent if they had prescription privileges. That is, psychiatry claimed that psychologists would not responsibly utilize this clinical treatment modality and would instead intentionally harm their patients. A small but quite vocal subset of psychologists joined with medicine in expressing opposition to their own field becoming involved the prescription of medications.

The legislation proposed by Hawaii's psychologists called for 60 semester hours of targeted didactic training and no less than 400 hours of relevant supervised clinical (hands-on) experience. It was hoped that this level of intensive training would adequately address medicine's concerns. Subsequent research and discussions with educators from the other prescribing professions (and, in particular, with professional nursing), however, suggested that 100 *contact* hours (rather than 60 semester hours) of didactic training would be sufficient. Accordingly, a multi-weekend training module is being developed by faculty at the local professional psychology and nursing schools. This four-part training module will include: Psychopharmacology I, Pathophysiology, Health Assessment, and Psychopharmacology II. After completing the training, the participants will be deemed to have completed the equivalent of similar training provided to Hawaii's nurse practitioners, who since 1994 are legislatively authorized to prescribe. Compatibility of training will become a particularly important educational policy issue when Hawaii's psychologists again address the local legislature.

National Developments at the State Level

By 1995 more than twenty-five states had established prescription privilege task forces. The primary initial emphasis of almost all of these task forces has been on educating their state psychological association membership on the clinical, educational, and policy issues involved. It has generally been found that when the discussions first begin, approximately one-third of the membership is supportive, with another third somewhat oppositional. After extensive debate and exploration of relevant data—for example, that of the 135.8 million psychotherapeutic scripts written in 1991, only 17.3% were actually written by psychiatrists per se—the percentage expressing support rises to nearly 80% (DeLeon, Sammons, & Sexton, 1995).

To date, only Hawaii (and in a most unusual manner, Indiana) has actually had relevant legislation introduced into the state legislature. However, several of the task forces in other states are very close to having bills drafted in final form. Indiana represents an unusual situation in which during floor deliberations in 1993 on modifications to their Psychology Practice Act, language was adopted that would, on face value, seem to allow Indiana psychologists to prescribe under federal demonstration authority. Unfortunately, the psychology language was in direct conflict with other provisions of the Indiana health code, and an informal ruling by the state's Office of the Attorney General suggests that further modification is necessary.

In the long run, although seeming to be quite prolonged to some advocates, this evolutionary approach has probably worked out best for psychology. It has not only resulted in extensive policy discussions leading to significant involvement by the leadership of both the local and national psychological associations, but has furthermore highlighted the extent to which the prescription privilege agenda possesses both significant practice and educational components. We would further note that as a result of these extensive discussions, considerable technical and financial assistance has been forthcoming from APA to those states that have expressed serious interest in pursuing the agenda.

Federal Developments

During the Congressional deliberations on the Fiscal Year 1989 Appropriations Bill for the Department of Defense [PL 100-463] the conferees directed the DoD to establish a "demonstration pilot training project under which military psychologists may be trained and authorized to issue appropriate psychotropic medications under certain circumstances." DoD possesses an outstanding track record of training a wide range of health care professionals and in particular, of establishing focused mission-oriented modules. Further, numerous discussions with federal psychologists throughout the government have indicated that there has been a long history of individual psychologists competently prescribing under various federal programs, with this, for example, having been formally recognized in Indian Health Service (IHS) hospital bylaws. However, there has never been a formal training program, and there has been little formal recognition of psychology's psychopharmacology expertise.

Since the DoD psychopharmacology training program's inception, organized psychiatry has vigorously undertaken various administrative and legislative efforts to terminate it. Nevertheless, under considerable Congressional scrutiny, the program has survived and, in the process, undergone numerous substantive modifications in its training curricula based primarily on the recommendations of the participating psychology psychopharmacology Fellows. The didactic portion of the program has been shortened in length from 2 years to 1, and the training program has now become the responsibility of the recently established DoD school of nursing rather than consisting primarily of "off the shelf" medical school courses. The clinical hands-on component remains a full year in length, consisting of providing supervised clinical care at the Walter Reed Army Medical Center. Now, however, it includes both inpatient and outpatient exposure. Essentially, little by little the program has been custom-tailored to take into account the psychopharmacology Fellows' prior academic training and clinical expertise.

In January 1995 five psychopharmacology Fellows were enrolled in the first year of the program, with the expectation that in subsequent years there would be a minimum of six Fellows, two from each of the military services. It is hoped that eventually the VA, the IHS, and other federal agencies will decide to detail their own "students" to the program. This decision, however, is ultimately the responsibility of the various chief psychologists in their respective federal services, and, if it evolves, it will reflect a significant maturation of the federal service.

In retrospect, it is truly unfortunate that, of the first six Fellows enrolled in this ground-breaking DoD program, it was expected that only three would ultimately graduate. Although the initial "success rate" of the program was admittedly low, it is reassuring, and of considerable interest, that none of the Fellows who left the program did so for academic reasons. We would surmise that, in more ways than was ever anticipated, this initiative has indeed been on the "cutting edge" of psychology's maturation. Those who participated in the program have reported that their newly acquired in-depth knowledge of psychopharmacology resulted in a different conceptual appreciation of psychology's strengths and contributions to patient well-being. They have not found themselves, as some had feared, "medicalizing psychology," but, instead, have found that their psychological background and behavioral science expertise have allowed them to ensure that the psychological aspects of the medication decision making process are finally given appropriate weight. They report that they remain, above all else, psychologists!

Reflections on Psychology's Efforts

The prescription privilege agenda simultaneously contains both a significant clinical practice component and a significant educational component. Over the years a wide range of nonphysician health care providers have modified their state scope of practice acts to include this clinical responsibility. During the past decade a growing number of psychologists have expressed a similar interest. For the vast majority of practicing psychologists the decision as to when, and under what conditions, they will be authorized to prescribe psychotropic medications will ultimately be made by their state legislature and local psychology regulatory board.

Psychologists have been competently prescribing within the federal system (most extensively within the IHS) for years, with no demonstrable "quality of care" problems. Nevertheless, we must never expect overt support from organized medicine, no matter how rigorous our training programs may become. The Congressionally mandated psychopharmacology training program within the DoD is unique, although efforts are underway to develop similar but less-intensive training modules in the civilian sector. One might reasonably conceptualize the 2-year DoD program as "training the future trainers," while appreciating that 100 clinical hours of didactic exposure (plus an additional, yet to be determined, period of hands-on supervision) would be quite sufficient for those already practicing in the field. For psychology the prescription privilege agenda is above all else an evolutionary one, and we still have a substantial distance to travel (DeLeon, Fox, & Graham, 1991).

NATIONAL HEALTH INSURANCE

Beginning as far back as President Truman's administration, and perhaps reaching its zenith during the Clinton administration, there has been a concerted push toward the enactment of comprehensive national health care reform legislation. Throughout, there have been two underlying principles—improving access and curtailing ever escalating costs—although which is to receive priority has changed over time.

In the late 1960s and early 1970s the policy discussions (and resulting federal legislative proposals) dealt primarily with improving access to health care services and the issue of provider shortages. Although serious efforts were made, comprehensive legislation was not enacted. However, one example of legislation that was enacted during this period (and which has had a profound long term impact) was the Nixon administration's health maintenance organization (HMO) legislation, with its emphasis on controlling costs by actively administering and managing care.

Over the years, health care costs in the United States have continued to escalate significantly faster than any other segment of our economy (Dörken & DeLeon, 1986). As this spiral has continued and as health care has consumed an increasingly larger percentage of our gross domestic product, the need to control health care costs in some meaningful way has became ever more evident. Within the private sector the insurance industry, apparently recognizing the need to initiate changes, began offering a more extensive form of control over health care delivery. An increasing number of companies developed self-insured approaches, thus benefiting from federal preemption legislation (ERISA) and avoiding various state benefit mandates (including freedom of choice requirements). And there has been a steady increase in the number of governors and state legislatures who have seriously begun exploring ways to stretch their state's health care dollars, such as the program that exists in the State of Hawaii (VandenBos, 1993).

Managed Care

For psychologists the notion of purchasers of care actively "managing care" has became a cause of great concern. Major employers and governmental entities are "carving out" mental health services and, through a case manager or other intermediary, all psychological services. From its inception, "managed care" was met with great anxiety by the majority of health care providers. However, in 1943 the U.S. Supreme Court made it clear to the American Medical Association (AMA) that managed care was here to stay [*American Medical Association v. United States*, 130 F.2d 233 (D.C. Cir. 1942), *aff'd* 317 U.S. 519, 1943].

In our judgment as health care professionals, it is fair to state that some of the concerns raised by our psychology colleagues are clearly justified, while others are not. There are those providers who argue that all managed care is "bad," and there are those who argue just the opposite. Not surprisingly, neither extreme seems to be correct. There are some very significant problems with some managed care companies, particularly in the way they permit (or prevent) ready access to psychological services, and there are other managed care entities that are quite liberal with their benefits. The empirical evidence is quite clear that having an economic interest in providing (or in limiting access to) care does inappropriately influence one's perception of patient "need"; this applies to both providers and "payors." The key question is not whether managed care is good or bad, but whether or not the ultimate decision maker truly appreciates the clinical importance of *quality* psychological care.

A related policy question is whether psychologists have obtained appropriate training and experience to work in these environments, if they choose to do so. Given the emotional rhetoric currently surrounding managed care within organized psychology this is a significant matter. In our judgment, there clearly is a need, in addition to whatever clinical training new psychologists receive, for ensuring that they will be facile in working in a managed care environment and knowledgeable about the types of services that this particular health service environment will require (such as short-term, problem-oriented psychotherapy, pre-certification processes, case management, interdisciplinary collaboration, and so forth). It is becoming increasingly clear that fewer and fewer reimbursement programs will cover multi-year individual therapy, consciously preferring a problem-focused model. At the same time, Sigmund Freud never took an insurance card in his entire practice! What is evident, as well, is that managed care companies are becoming major players in the delivery of health care services and that psychologists must be prepared to be competitive in this particular market.

Health and Consultative Psychology

With the continuing evolution of psychological practice it is critical that psychologists broaden their training and market penetration and not be solely identified with, or conceptualize themselves as, "merely mental health care" providers. There is growing clinical and scientific evidence that behavioral and/or psychological health care services are extraordinarily important and highly cost-effective. These should be an integral component of the services that practicing psychologists proudly offer. Broadening and expanding our scope of practice will continue to make our profession dynamic and exciting, not to mention marketable.

As we have indicated, our field is not only pushing the boundaries by altering the site of practice (inpatient versus outpatient), but we are also adding additional competence to the services we provide. Psychologists today are providing rehabilitative services, consultation services, second opinion services, liaison services to other training and health care delivery programs, biofeedback, neuropsychology, geropsychology, organ transplantation evaluation, prevention services, "wellness" services, and employee assistance plans.

All these services are different from the traditional base of the "one-on-one psychotherapy" and psychological assessment that is our heritage. These traditional services will always be part of the core services the psychologist offers, but the profession must continue to broaden its horizons and its fundamental scope of practice to meet evolving health care needs (DeLeon & VandenBos, 1983).

Perhaps one of the most challenging and satisfying roles that a psychologist can undertake is that of a consultant in a variety of health care settings. It is important to note that these consultative services often run the complete range of integrated services and care and, accordingly, must be viewed in the broadest of possible perspectives. Thus, "points of service" can be found in traditional hospital-based practice; transitional programs such as partial hospitalization, residential treatment care, and hospices; day care programs and schools, and even practice within the patient's home or place of work. Consultation can focus around the patient, the family, or the system that is delivering services. Consultation can even occur with another provider of health services without direct contact with an identified patient, that is, by helping the provider understand the psychological component of the patient's functioning.

It becomes increasingly important for psychologists to recognize and understand that the nature of our training is such that our profession is simply not bound by setting, because psychological interventions and strategies are appropriate and necessary in all settings. More so than many appreciate, we are limited only by the myopia of our collective vision. It is an unfortunate reality that some of the service categories listed here may sound foreign to the reader, but they are among the most exciting services that psychology has to offer.

Additionally, psychology's ability to impact on the biological *and* psychological components of an individual's functioning has obtained increasing recognition within traditional medical care systems. Helping patients to adjust to a medical regime or to having diabetes, helping a youngster through prosthetic surgery, helping a young child to have a tooth extracted or to grieve over the loss of a relative, the development of employee assistance plans to prevent excessive loss of work, consultations to courts and police departments, the development of prevention programs as well as wellness programs—all of these are arenas in which psychologists can and do make significant contributions.

Our profession cannot survive if it stagnates; an appreciation for expansion and maturation will bring professional psychology into the twenty-first century. We would caution, however, that even today some of our national leaders openly decry our increasing numbers and expanding marketplace efforts. The past does, too often, accurately predict the future!

CONCLUDING OBSERVATIONS

During the two decades that we have been active in the governance of organized psychology our profession has matured considerably. Not only have our absolute numbers increased dramatically, but, equally importantly, the substance of "psychological care" has been significantly refined to reflect the growing awareness within our nation's health (and medical) delivery system of the fundamental importance of behavioral health. Above all else, we have gradually become sensitive to the crucial innate interrelationship between training, practice, and research endeavors.

Consistent with the theme of being responsive to evolving changes, the diversification of psychological services has been, for the most part, the result of change in health care delivery and the crisis in health care economics. New treatment modalities have developed, and the importance of outcome measures and accountability for what practitioners provide have moved psychology away from the traditional practice of outpatient psychotherapy and individual assessment to broad diversification in virtually every aspect of the delivery of health care.

Most importantly, no longer do psychologists see themselves as "merely mental health" specialists, but instead as psychological health care providers, or, simply stated, health care providers in psychology. This diversification of services will likely have a pivotal role in maintaining the marketability and attractiveness of psychological practice and services. Nontraditional services as well as service sites (both internal and external to the practitioner's office) will become the standard of psychological practice.

Although we have a long history of some national leaders in psychology decrying change, it is now, more than ever, incumbent upon us to obtain the nontraditional competence needed for continued market viability, through pre-doctoral training programs, post-doctoral training, and continuing education programs. What the First World War was to assessment, and the Second World War was to psychotherapy, the health care reform movement is, and will be, to the diversification of psychological practice.

REFERENCES

American Psychological Association (1945). *American Psychological Association Yearbook, 1945.* Washington, DC: Author.

American Psychological Association (1994). APA-accredited doctoral programs in professional psychology: 1994. *American Psychologist, 49,* 1056–1067

Cummings, N. A., & VandenBos, G. R. (1983). Relations with other professions. In C. E. Walker (Ed.), *The handbook of clinical psychology: Theory, research, and practice* (Vol. 2) (pp. 1301–1327). Homewood, IL: Dow Jones-Irwin.

DeLeon, P. H., & VandenBos, G. R. (1980). Psychotherapy reimbursement in federal programs: Political factors. In G. R. VandenBos (Ed.), *Psychotherapy: Practice, research, policy* (pp. 247–285). Beverly Hills, CA: Sage.

DeLeon, P. H., & VandenBos, G. R. (1983). The new federal health care frontiers—cost containment and "wellness." *Psychotherapy in Private Practice, 1*(2), 17–32.

DeLeon, P. H., Fox, R. E., & Graham, S. R. (1991). Prescription privileges: Psychology's next frontier? *American Psychologist, 46,* 384–393.

DeLeon, P. H., Sammons, M. T., & Sexton, J. L. (1995). Focusing on society's real needs: Responsibility and prescription privileges? *American Psychologist, 50*(12), 1022–1032.

DeLeon, P. H., Wedding, D., Wakefield, M. K., & VandenBos, G. R. (1992). Medicaid policy: Psychology's overlooked agenda. *Professional Psychology: Research and Practice, 23,* 96–107

Dörken, H. (1976). Laws, regulations, and psychological practice. In H. Dörken & Associates, *The Professional psychologist today: New developments in law, health insurance, and health practice* (pp. 33–58). San Francisco: Jossey-Bass.

Dörken, H., & DeLeon, P. H. (1986). Cost as the driving force in health care reform. In H. Dörken et al. (Eds.), *Professional psychology in transition: Meeting today's challenges* (pp. 313–349). San Francisco: Jossey-Bass.

Dörken, H., Webb, J. T., & Zaro, J. S. (1982). Hospital practice of psychology resurveyed: 1980. *Professional Psychology, 13,* 814–829.

Marquis, D. G. (1944). The mobilization of psychologists for war service. *Psychological Bulletin, 41,* 469–473.

Resnick, R. J. (1983). Medicaid: Direct provider recognition. *Professional Psychology: Research and Practice, 14,* 368–373.

Resnick, R. J. (1985). A case against the Blues: The Virginia challenge. *American Psychologist, 39,* 988–995.

Rodgers, D. A. (1980). The status of psychologists in hospitals: Technicians or professionals. *The Clinical Psychologist, 33*(4), 5–7.

Samuels, R. M. (1985). A prescription for psychologists. *The Independent Practitioner, 5*(3), 2–3.

Thompson, R. J., & Matarazzo, J. D. (1984). Psychology in United States medical schools: 1983. *American Psychologist, 39,* 988–995.

VandenBos, G. R. (1993). U.S. mental health policy: Proactive evolution in the midst of health care reform. *American Psychologist, 48,* 283–290.

VandenBos, G. R., Cummings, N. A., & DeLeon, P. H. (1992). A century of psychotherapy: Economic and environmental influences. In D. K. Freedheim (Ed.), *His-

tory of psychotherapy: A century of change (pp. 65–103). Washington, DC: American Psychological Association.

Welch, B. (1990). Medicare win demonstrates bill's strength in Congress. *APA Monitor, 21,* 18.

▶ 15

Professional
Associations

JANET R. MATTHEWS   C. EUGENE WALKER

Practicing psychologists, as well as students of psychology, often join professional associations. Questions that might be asked about this behavior include why they do so and how they select the organizations they join. This chapter presents information about a sampling of organizations to which practicing psychologists and students of psychology may belong. It is not a complete list of these organizations but rather is intended to illustrate the range of interests of practitioners as well as to discuss the reasons for the existence of these groups. There are many other organizations of interest to practicing psychologists. One source of information about associations is the list of professional meetings published monthly in the *American Psychologist*. Another source of information is the library because many of these associations publish professional journals. Reading journals in one's area of interest can lead to information about specialty organizations in that field.

One reason for joining professional organizations is the increased opportunity to meet others with similar interests. This factor is often called "networking." "Networks" are informal linkages among psychologists with common interests. Communication among these colleagues may be through such traditional means as letter or telephone or such newer methods as electronic mail (e-mail) via computer. The development of E-mail has allowed groups of psychologists to communicate quickly and efficiently. In addition to communication with specific individuals, E-mail allows for the development of group forms of communication in which one psychologist may ask for input from anyone else on that particular network or send such information to a large group of individuals.

Involvement in professional organizations may place the member on committees with people with whom the member would otherwise have no contact. Such organizations also have their own publications. Although many of these publications are in journal form and available on a subscription basis, newsletters and other less formal means of communication to the membership may provide a different level of information about the discipline from that obtained in journals. These less formal resources are also a source of information about current professional issues that may be quite important to the daily functioning of the individual practitioner.

Most professional organizations have regularly scheduled conventions, which are another setting for meeting peers with similar interests. These meetings also provide an opportunity for the practitioner to share what he or she is doing or current concerns about the discipline through program participation as well as less formal discussions. Data presented at such meetings may not appear for a year or more in the professional journals due to the publication lag for that particular journal. Thus, individuals who attend such sessions have the opportunity to hear about recent work or sometimes work in progress. Conventions also provide the possibility of discussing the research with the presenter. Although psychologists are expected to provide additional information about their published work to those who write to request it, the opportunity for a give-and-take discussion may lead to the raising of different questions than occur from just reading the material. This type of interaction may also lead to collaborative projects between individuals with similar interests but located geographically apart.

For many practitioners another reason for involvement in one or more professional organizations is the fact that they provide a group forum for action on issues affecting the discipline. Professional organizations may provide experts who talk to members of Congress regarding funding for research, training, and practice. Although legislators may listen to the concerns of an individual constituent, they may be more impressed by an individual who can legitimately indicate that she or he is speaking for a large number of professionals with similar interests. Such a central organization is also helpful when there is a need to assemble a group of professionals quickly, such as assisting with the psychological aftermath of a natural disaster like a hurricane or flood. National organizations have lists of professionals by geographic area and specialty and can thus more quickly reach individuals who may provide the needed services.

AMERICAN PSYCHOLOGICAL ASSOCIATION

For many psychologists the major generic organization with which they affiliate is the American Psychological Association (APA). This organization was founded in 1892 and incorporated in 1925. This corporation is chartered in the District of Columbia which is also the site of its Central Office. According to their 1995 membership statistics, the total of their fellows, members, and associate members was 81,000. These numbers do not include their growing list of special membership individuals listed under the headings of international affiliates, high school teacher affiliates and student affiliates, who may be either undergraduates or enrolled in a graduate program. Although individuals in these special membership categories cannot vote or hold office in APA, they do receive many benefits such as APA publications and discounts for convention registration. In 1995 there were 3,000 foreign and international affiliates, 1,500 high school teacher affiliates, and 46,500 student affiliates of APA. In order to better meet the needs of the large group of student affiliates, APA worked with these students to form the American Psychological Association of Graduate Students (APAGS), which reports to the APA Board of Directors. All graduate student affiliates of APA are automatically also members of APAGS and receive its newsletter. The leaders of APAGS attend relevant APA board and committee meetings as liaisons and have their own buttons and other paraphernalia, which are available through the APA bookstore.

As psychologists increase their interaction with their colleagues in other countries, it is not surprising that formal relations between their professional organizations would occur. The one country, other than the United States, in which the APA has periodically held its annual convention is Canada. The first time the convention was held in Canada was 1931, when the meeting was in Toronto. Starting in the 1970s, Canadian meeting sites became more common, with the 1973 meeting being in Montreal and 1978 in Toronto. Montreal was the site of the 1980 convention and Toronto for 1984. During the 1990s Canada had two APA conventions, with Toronto being selected for both the 1993 and 1996 meetings. A joint dues agreement was established between APA and the Canadian Psychological Association (CPA) whereby individuals who belong to both organizations pay the full dues to their parent association and 50% dues to the other association. At the 1993 APA convention, APA President Frank Farley announced a trilateral initiative with CPA and the Mexican Psychological Society. These initiatives, combined with APA's ongoing activities of its Committee on International Relations in Psychology (CIRP) are indicative of the interest of psychologists on an international level in interacting with each other.

When the APA reorganized its structure in 1945, one of the changes was the development of Divisions. Divisions are subgroups of the APA in which the members have special interests in common. Many of the APA divisions have their own journals focusing on their special interest areas, and some divisions even hold their own annual conventions to focus on their specialty. A list of the Division leaders is published annually in the July issue of the *American Psychologist*. Members of APA may join as many divisions as they choose. Each division has its own criteria for membership as well as an individual fee structure. Divisions of APA may also choose to include among their membership individuals who are not members of APA but have interests in common with that Division. These non-APA division members may participate actively in the business of the Division but cannot represent the Division on the APA Council of Representatives. In 1945 there were 17 divisions of APA. Since 1945 the number of divisions has increased as members developed diverse interests.

TABLE 15-1   Divisions of the American Psychological Association

 1. Division of General Psychology
 2. Division on the Teaching of Psychology
 3. Division of Experimental Psychology
 5. Division on Evaluation, Measurement and Statistics
 6. Division of Physiological and Comparative Psychology
 7. Division on Developmental Psychology
 8. The Society of Personality and Social Psychology -A Division of the APA
 9. The Society for the Psychological Study of Social Issues—A Division of the APA
10. Division of Psychology and the Arts
12. Division of Clinical Psychology
13. Division of Consulting Psychology
14. The Society for Industrial and Organizational Psychology—A Division of the APA
15. Division of Educational Psychology
16. Division of School Psychology
17. Division of Counseling Psychology
18. Division of Psychologists in Public Service
19. Division of Military Psychology
20. Division of Adult Development and Aging
21. Division of Applied Experimental and Engineering Psychology
22. Division of Rehabilitation Psychology
23. Division of Consumer Psychology
24. Division of Theoretical and Philosophical Psychology
25. Division for the Experimental Analysis of Behavior
26. Division of the History of Psychology
27. Division of Community Psychology
28. Division of Psychopharmacology
29. Division of Psychotherapy
30. Division of Psychological Hypnosis
31. Division of State Psychological Association Affairs
32. Division of Humanistic Psychology
33. Division on Mental Retardation and Developmental Disabilities
34. Division of Population and Environmental Psychology
35. Division of the Psychology of Women
36. Psychologists Interested in Religious Issues (PIRI)—A Division of the APA
37. Division of Child, Youth, and Family Services
38. Division of Health Psychology

(continued)

TABLE 15-1 *(Continued)*

39. Division of Psychoanalysis
40. Division of Clinical Neuropsychology
41. American Psychology-Law Society—A Division of the APA
42. Division of Psychologists in Independent Practice
43. Division of Family Psychology
44. The Society for the Psychological Study of Lesbian and Gay Issues—A Division of the APA
45. Society for the Psychological Study of Ethnic Minority Issues—A Division of the APA
46. Division of Media Psychology
47. Division of Exercise and Sport Psychology
48. Division of Peace Psychology
49. Division of Group Psychology and Group Psychotherapy
50. Division of Psychology of Addictive Behaviors
51. Society for the Psychological Study of Men and Masculinity

How are Divisions formed? When a group of APA members feel they have scientific and professional interests in common that are not represented by a current APA division, they may choose to circulate a petition to other APA members suggesting a new division. If at least 1% of the current APA membership signs that they are willing to join the new division if it is formed, that petition is then sent to the APA Council of Representatives for consideration. When the Council of Representatives considers this petition, they decide whether it represents an active and individual interest group whose objectives fall within the objectives of APA without having restrictive aspects to membership or being harmful to the welfare of any current APA division. If the petitioning group meets these criteria, it is likely to obtain the positive vote of two-thirds of the Council of Representatives that is needed for the formation of a new division. If accepted, the division holds the status of "candidate" 2 years in order to demonstrate the ongoing interest of the petitioners. During this intervening period, however, the division is given the same privileges as the fully established divisions. Table 15-1 provides a list of the APA divisions in existence in 1995. There are, however, a few numbers that are missing. When a division no longer includes at least one-half of 1% of the current APA membership, it may be dissolved. Divisions may also decide that they no longer have an interest in existing. Once a number is given to designate a particular interest area, however, it is not reissued.

Because APA is such a large organization, its administrative structure is somewhat complex. Much of the work of APA is conducted by a series of boards and committees. Members of these groups are typically elected by the Council of Representatives. In order to handle the regular business aspects of the corporation, however, the APA Central Office is run by a Chief

Executive Officer (CEO) who is responsible for its management and staffing. The APA Central Office has more than 400 employees and is located in a building in Washington, DC owned by APA.

Because the APA Central Office is so large, it is subdivided into four major units called Directorates. Each directorate addresses issues of specific interest to its area within psychology. The Directorates are Education, Practice, Public Interest, and Science. The Education Directorate is concerned with educational institutions and programs at all levels from pre-college through post-doctoral. Among the activities of this Directorate are the accreditation of graduate programs and internships in the applied areas of psychology and the approval of groups that provide continuing education credits for practicing psychologists. The Practice Directorate is concerned with the practice of psychology and the availability of psychological services to the public. Among their functions is the promotion of these activities through legislative and judicial advocacy. The focus of the Public Interest Directorate is the application of psychological principles to human welfare. Among the groups under this Directorate are Women's Programs and Ethnic Minority Affairs. The Science Directorate was formed to coordinate member activities related to the needs of the scientific and academic members of APA. During the APA Centennial and for a period thereafter, the Science Directorate coordinated the placement of APA's Traveling Psychology Exhibit which moved among many major cities and gave the general public an opportunity to learn more about scientific psychology. During the APA Centennial Celebration in 1992 this exhibit was housed at the Smithsonian Institution in Washington, DC. The exhibit continued to tour the country at various museums under a contract through 1997 after which it was leased to the Arizona Science Center in Phoenix for an additional 5 years. In order to maintain the continued high standards of the exhibit and to be able to update it, APA chose to lease it rather than to sell it. Given the overlapping nature of their areas of interest, the four Directorates must also work together on issues of common concern.

In addition to the major programs of the APA, the Central Office organizational structure includes full-time legal counsel, a financial services branch, and a communications office. This latter office's activities include the publication of APA's 27 different journals and newsletters, which are listed in Table 15-2.

The major legislative body of the APA is the Council of Representatives (Council). The Council meets during the annual convention as well as having a second meeting approximately 6 months after the convention to address additional business. Members of the Council are elected from Divisions as well as from State and Provincial Psychological Associations. In order to have a voice within this legislative body, the group must have the vote of at least one-half of 1% of the APA voting membership during the annual allocation balloting. Thus, some groups have several representatives on the Council while other groups do not have a voting member. Sometimes groups

TABLE 15-2 Journals Published by the American Psychological Association

American Psychologist
Behavioral Neuroscience
Clinician's Research Digest
Contemporary Psychology
Developmental Psychology
Experimental and Clinical Psychopharmacology
Health Psychology
Journal of Abnormal Psychology
Journal of Applied Psychology
Journal of Comparative Psychology
Journal of Consulting and Clinical Psychology
Journal of Counseling Psychology
Journal of Educational Psychology
Journal of Experimental Psychology: Animal Behavior Processes
Journal of Experimental Psychology: Applied
Journal of Experimental Psychology: General
Journal of Experimental Psychology: Human Perception and Performance
Journal of Experimental Psychology: Learning, Memory, and Cognition
Journal of Family Psychology
Journal of Personality and Social Psychology
Neuropsychology
Professional Psychology: Research and Practice
Psychological Abstracts
Psychological Assessment
Psychological Bulletin
Psychological Review
Psychology and Aging
Psychology, Public Policy, and Law
PsycSCAN: Applied Experimental and Engineering Psychology
PsycSCAN: Applied Psychology
PsycSCAN: Behavior Analysis & Therapy
PsycSCAN: Clinical Psychology
PsycSCAN: Developmental Psychology
PsycSCAN: LD/MR
PsycSCAN: Neuropsychology
PsycSCAN: Psychoanalytic Abstracts

who do not achieve the desired number of votes form a coalition and combine their votes in order to have a voting seat on the Council. Among the annual activities of the Council is review and approval of the APA's annual budget of over $50 million. About 25% of that money comes from member dues. The remainder of the organization's revenue comes from a range of activities including investments, publications, and real estate.

The Council elects six of its members to serve in at-large positions on the APA Board of Directors along with six elected officers. The elected officers are the president, past-president, president-elect, treasurer, recording secretary, and CEO. The first three of these elected officers are elected by the entire membership of APA by a mail ballot while the latter three are elected by the Council. The twelve-member Board of Directors is described in the APA bylaws as the administrative agent of the Council of Representatives. The Board of Directors reports to the Council. Between the meetings of Council the Board of Directors supervises the overall affairs of APA and has the power to take actions on behalf of the Council if a majority of the members of the Board of Directors declares the situation to be an emergency. The Board of Directors meets on a regular basis and sends liaisons to the meetings of each of the major boards and committees of APA. Members of the Board of Directors are often asked to represent the APA in such public settings as Congressional committees that are considering business related to psychology.

In order to conduct specific work for APA, volunteer services by the members are also needed. A major source of such volunteering is service on APA's boards, committees, and special task forces. Members of the standing boards and committees are elected by members of the Council of Representatives. The major standing boards and committees specified in the APA bylaws are given in Table 15-3. The specific composition and duties of each of these boards and committees are provided in the bylaws. Task forces are created as needed to address specific needs or concerns. The existence of these groups is time limited. There are also committees that deal with some of the work of the Directorates or the major standing boards or committees.

TABLE 15-3   Standing Boards and Committees of the American Psychological Association

Board for the Advancement of Psychology in the Public Interest
Board of Convention Affairs
Board of Educational Affairs
Board of Professional Affairs
Board of Scientific Affairs
Election Committee
Ethics Committee
Finance Committee
Membership Committee
Policy and Planning Board
Publications and Communication Board

AMERICAN PSYCHOLOGICAL SOCIETY

A second national association of psychologists is the American Psychological Society (APS). The APS was founded in August 1988 by a vote of the Assembly for Scientific and Applied Psychology (ASAP), which was a year old at that time. The ASAP was founded in 1987 as a society within the APA. The purpose of ASAP was to advocate for the interests of members of APA who identified themselves primarily as scientists in contrast to practitioners. The leaders of this group felt that they were underrepresented within the legislative structure of the organization and felt that the process of doing business was inordinately slow due to the procedures mandated by APA's bylaws and association rules. Thus a plan for reorganizing the structure of the legislative process was proposed. A major shift in the proposed plan was to move to a bicameral legislature rather than a unicameral system. One body would represent science and academic concerns while the other body would represent the practice and health care concerns. Members would be expected to identify with one of these two bodies; therefore the bodies would be directed by different individuals rather than having members who paid extra be able to have a greater voice based on finances. Members who viewed themselves as scientist-practitioners, trained in the Boulder model, voiced concerns about such a separation and suggested a third legislative body be formed to meet their needs. Numerous other issues were raised by groups of psychologists who felt strongly in favor of this proposed new system and those who opposed it. Factions developed and tensions were high among APA members who were actively involved in the proposed change process. The Council of Representatives voted to send the proposed bylaws change to the membership for a vote. Because of the divided opinion about the change among Council members, pro and con statements about the change accompanied the ballot. This proposed change in the bylaws was rejected by the APA membership in August 1988. Some advocates of this reorganization decided it was best to develop a separate organization from the APA. When the ASAP was formed, its bylaws had specified that if the then developing plan for APA reorganization were defeated, its members would form a separate society devoted to the science of psychology. This new organization was approved by the membership of the ASAP and named the American Psychological Society (APS).

The APS maintains a headquarters office in Washington, DC. In contrast to the large central office previously described for the APA, the APS specifically tried to keep its number of employees small. As of 1994, the APS had eleven paid staff members running its headquarters.

The stated purposes of the APS are to "promote, protect, and advance the interests of scientifically oriented psychology in research, application, teaching, and in the improvement of human welfare" (APS, 1994). By 1994 the APS included over 15,000 members and student affiliates. When APS members indicate their primary interest area within psychology, the largest percentage of them respond "general psychology." The second largest interest group is "clinical/counseling/school."

The APS maintains an active publication program. They publish two bimonthly journals. *Psychological Science* is a research journal that attempts to promote interdisciplinary knowledge among its readers. *Current Directions in Psychological Science* publishes invited mini-review articles spanning a range of current psychological research and theory. The APS also publishes a newsletter, "APS Observer," which includes news, research, announcements, and employment listings.

The APS holds an annual convention that includes invited addresses, research presentations, and poster presentations. During this convention they present achievement awards for exceptional contributions to the discipline. Although the APS was originally founded as a scientific society, over the years they have increased their activities related to the practice of psychology due to member interest in these domains.

OTHER PROFESSIONAL ORGANIZATIONS

Some professional organizations have been developed to focus on the ethnic heritage of the practitioner. The Council of National Psychological Associations for the Advancement of Ethnic Minority Interests was formed as a networking source where such groups have a regular opportunity to exchange information. This Council meets at least twice each year. The five organizations that make up this Council are the American Psychological Association, the Asian American Psychological Association, the Association of Black Psychologists, the National Association of Hispanic Psychologists, and the Society of Native American Psychologists. To illustrate the activities of these specialty organizations, information is provided about two of them, the Association of Black Psychologists and the Asian American Psychological Association. Information about the Council or addresses for any of its member groups is available from the APA's Committee on Ethnic Minority Affairs.

The Asian American Psychological Association (AAPA) was founded in 1974. The purpose of this organization is to provide a setting for sharing information about Asian American psychology. In 1994 this organization had 400 members. Student membership exists and students are encouraged to establish collegiate chapters of the AAPA. AAPA members have expertise in mental health services, education, violence, and related areas. Among the activities of the AAPA are a national convention, publication of a newsletter, student mentoring programs, networking services, and a range of community-based programs. Although a journal has been published, in 1994 it was not a regular activity of the organization. Illustrative of the service activities of AAPA was the provision of counseling services in Los Angeles following a civil disturbance in 1992.

The Association of Black Psychologists (ABPsi) was formed in 1968. The purpose of this organization is to address the needs of Black professionals and to have a positive impact on the mental health of the Black community on a national basis. In 1994 this organization had over 1,900 members including both professionals and students. Each member received the organization's journal, *Journal of Black Psychology*, plus a monthly news journal, "Psych Discourse." Other publications of the ABPsi include a sourcebook for teaching Black Psychology, a resource manual for Black psychology students, and a publication manual. With the assistance of a grant from The Centers for Disease Control and Prevention, they publish a technical assistance newsletter about issues related to work with HIV/STD. They hold an annual national convention and also have local chapters to further the interchange of information on a community level.

Other professional associations are formed based on specialty interests of the members. Some of these organizations are interdisciplinary while others are basically for psychologists. Some associations that fit this category are the American Association for Marriage and Family Therapy, American Group Psychotherapy Association, Association for the Advancement of Behavior Therapy, Association for the Care of Children's Health, National Academy of Neuropsychology, Society of Behavioral Medicine, and The Society for Research in Child Development. There are too many such groups to cover all of them here. These organizations were selected because they represent a range of specialty interests and were known to the chapter authors.

The American Association for Marriage and Family Therapy (AAMFT) was founded in 1942. The AAMFT is a professional association of more than 22,000 members, affiliates, and students in the United States and Canada. It was developed to provide a network representing both clinical and research interests of marriage and family therapists. Since its founding, the AAMFT has developed a set of training guidelines for the practice of marriage and family therapy as well as a Code of Ethics for such practice. Each Fall the AAMFT holds a national conference for the exchange of information, professional presentations, and networking. Formal training is offered each summer through a week-long series of institutes. The focus taught at these institutes is brief, solution-focused treatment. The major publications of the AAMFT are its journal, *Journal of Marriage and Family Therapy*, and its newsletter, "Family Therapy News." They also publish a variety of brochures and pamphlets that are intended for the general public to give them more information about issues related to marriage and family therapy. The AAMFT's Research and Education Foundation has developed a range of programs to advocate for the profession and assist the general public. Their briefing program, Family Impact Seminar, is a monthly offering for staff members of the U.S. Congress and federal agencies to address questions of family policy. With funding from the U.S. Department of Education, the AAMFT developed a series of videotapes titled "Listening to Families." These videotapes demonstrate family-centered approaches for human service providers.

The American Group Psychotherapy Association (AGPA) was founded in 1942 in New York City. The AGPA is interdisciplinary and open to mental health professionals and students who have an interest in the practice of group psychotherapy. Their stated purpose is to advance "knowledge, research, and training in Group Psychotherapy for professional and public benefit." In 1994 the AGPA included 4,000 members and thirty-one Affiliate Societies located throughout the United States. Their publications include a quarterly journal, *International Journal of Group Psychotherapy*, and a newsletter, "The Group Circle." They hold an annual convention that includes continuing education workshops. Their public service contributions include a consumer's guide to group psychotherapy ,which is written for individuals who may have questions about the process of group psychotherapy as well as the training of group psychotherapists.

The Association for the Advancement of Behavior Therapy (AABT) was founded in 1966 as an organization for mental health professionals and students who are interested in "behavior therapy, cognitive behavior therapy, behavioral assessment, and applied behavior analysis." In 1994 the AABT had 4,300 members. Membership categories are full, associate, and student. They have both state and city chapter affiliates in addition to their national organization. Their special-interest groups reflect the range of topics addressed by the AABT. Some of these groups focus on addictive behavior, disaster and trauma, insomnia, mental retardation, schizophrenia, and spiritual and religious issues. The AABT holds an annual convention at which both research and clinical findings are presented. Their publications include a newsletter, "The Behavior Therapist," and directories of both graduate programs and internships that offer training in behavior therapy. AABT members also qualify for reduced rate subscriptions to the research journal, *Behavior Therapy*.

The Association for the Care of Children's Health (ACCH) was founded in 1965. In 1994 the ACCH had 4,500 members. Members may be individuals, hospitals and other health care facilities, specialized departments within hospitals, and organizations committed to issues relevant to children and families. The 1994 Membership Directory of ACCH listed thirty-one different discipline abbreviations. In addition to psychologists the ACCH includes practitioners from such diverse specialties as chaplain, music therapist, and volunteer. The ACCH defines itself as "an international nonprofit advocacy and educational organization of multidisciplinary professionals and family members working together to promote family-centered, psychosocially supportive, and developmentally appropriate health care for children." Among ACCH's activities is serving as a clearinghouse for professionals and families of infants who have disabilities or life-threatening diseases. They hold an annual convention at which participants share knowledge, skills, and experiences. Their publications include a quarterly research-based journal, *Children's Health Care,* and two newsletters, "ACCH News" and "Child Health Design."

The National Academy of Neuropsychology (NAN) was founded in 1975 and held its first annual convention in 1981. By 1994, NAN had grown to an organization of approximately 2,400 individuals. Its membership materials indicate that it is a professional society that includes both clinicians and researchers who are interested in neuropsychology. NAN has varying levels of membership depending on the individual's educational background as well as experience in neuropsychology. There is a student membership category for individuals who are enrolled in graduate school. According to NAN's 1994 membership information brochure, "The Academy is dedicated to the advancement of knowledge in the understanding, assessment, and remediation of brain dysfunction." NAN holds an annual convention in which professional continuing education workshops in neuropsychology are offered in addition to general workshops and poster presentations of research. NAN's publications include a research journal, *Archives of Clinical Neuropsychology,* and a newsletter, "Bulletin."

The Society of Behavioral Medicine (SBM) was founded in 1978 as a multidisciplinary, nonprofit organization for health professionals. By 1994, SBM had grown to an organization of over 3,000 members. The major focus of SBM is to integrate behavioral and biomedical methods and data that relate to issues of both health and illness. In addition to "psychologist," the SBM membership application form lists such diverse professions as anthropologist, geneticist, and social worker. They also have a category for "in training/student." SBM holds an annual scientific meeting for the exchange of research and professional information. The overall meeting has a different theme each year. For example, in 1995 the theme was "Stress-Diathesis: Behavioral Medicine and the Biological Predisposition to Disease." Their publications include a research journal, *Annals of Behavioral Medicine,* the "Annual Meeting Proceedings," and a directory of training opportunities.

The Society for Research in Child Development (SRCD) was founded in 1933. The purpose of SRCD is to provide an "informational network for scholars and professionals studying the development of children." In 1994 the organization had almost 5,000 members, including professionals and students. SRCD publishes three journals. *Child Development* is a bi-monthly publication containing original research and theory articles. *Child Development Abstracts & Bibliography* is a tri-annual publication containing both abstracts of research articles and book reviews related to child development. *Monographs of the Society for Research in Child Development* are published whenever there is a research report that is considered too extensive for the regular journal or a series of reports that is best presented as a unit rather than in separate issues of a journal. To foster face-to-face interchanges of information, SRCD sponsors conferences and a biannual convention. To facilitate the implementation of findings of child development research, SRCD maintains ten committees which address such topics as public policy and ethical conduct of research.

STATE, PROVINCIAL, AND TERRITORIAL ASSOCIATIONS

For many practicing psychologists a primary source of professional support is the state, provincial, or territorial psychological association for the distinct in which they reside. These organizations typically hold an annual convention that offers both research and professional presentations. Such meetings often include workshops offered for continuing education credit as well. Many of these associations also serve practitioners as a monitor of activities within the area impacting the practice of psychology. As the practice of psychology has become more political over its history, such groups have hired lobbyists who assaist them in dealing with the state legislature on issues such as licensing laws and other items that impact the practice of psychology within its borders. As these associations have increased their functions, some have hired professional administrators rather than being run solely by professional psychologists.

These associations may, based on a vote of the APA Council of Representatives, become affiliated with the APA. These affiliated groups are listed on the annual apportionment ballot sent to APA members when selecting the groups to have seats on the Council of Representatives. A list of the leaders of these groups with addresses and phone numbers of the executive office are published annually in the *American Psychologist*. In order to facilitate interaction among these affiliated groups as well as to discuss issues that are of mutual concern to them and to the APA, the APA holds an annual state leadership conference to which they are invited. The APA also maintains close contact with these leaders as a grass roots network for issues within the U.S. Congress that impact the practice of psychology.

REGIONAL ASSOCIATIONS

The United States is geographically divided into overlapping regions that have psychological associations. Some states are included in more than one region and psychologists may choose to be members not only of regional associations in which they maintain residence but in any of the other regional associations as well. These organizations have as their main function an annual convention at which both scientific and professional presentations occur. Because the distance is often less than to national meetings, the cost of attendance may be less. Also, with their more limited scope of activities the regional associations often have a dues structure and convention cost that is less than most national groups. Regional psychological associations can, by vote of the APA Council of Representatives, affiliate with the APA. As of the 1994 APA bylaws, however, these groups do not appear on the annual apportionment ballot. The affiliated regional associations in 1994 were Eastern Psychological Association, Midwestern Psychological Association, New England Psychological Association, Rocky Mountain Psychological Association, Southeastern Psychological Association, Southwestern Psychological Association, and Western Psychological Association.

SUMMARY

This chapter has provided general information about a sample of professional organizations with which practicing psychologists may choose to affiliate. Some of these organizations are broad-based while others have a more specific focus. There is no mandate for psychologists to join these organizations and some psychologists do not choose to do so. This chapter has provided not only a description of some professional organizations, but also reasons for choosing to affiliate and become active in them.

FURTHER INFORMATION

Professional organizations are very willing to provide students and professionals with information about membership and services. Listed here are addresses for many of the organizations discussed in this chapter.

AMERICAN ASSOCIATION FOR
MARRIAGE AND FAMILY
THERAPY
1100 17th Street, NW
10th Floor
Washington, DC 20036-4601
(202) 452-0109

AMERICAN GROUP PSYCHO-
THERAPY ASSOCIATION

25 East 21st Street
6th Floor
New York, NY 10010
(212) 477-2677

AMERICAN PSYCHOLOGICAL
ASSOCIATION
705 First Street, NE
Washington, DC 20002-4242
(202) 336-5500

AMERICAN PSYCHOLOGICAL
  SOCIETY
1010 Vermont Avenue, NW
Suite 1100
Washington, DC 20005-4907
(202) 783-2077

ASIAN AMERICAN PSYCHO-
  LOGICAL ASSOCIATION
Contact American Psychological
  Association
Office of Ethnic Minority Affairs for
  address of current president of
  AAPA

ASSOCIATION FOR ADVANCE-
  MENT OF BEHAVIOR THERAPY
305 Seventh Avenue
New York, NY 10001
(800) 685-AABT

THE ASSOCIATION OF BLACK
  PSYCHOLOGISTS
P.O. Box 55999
Washington, DC 20040-5999
(202) 722-0808

ASSOCIATION FOR THE CARE
  OF CHILDREN'S HEALTH
7910 Woodmont Avenue, Suite 300
Bethesda, MD 20814
(301) 654-6549

ASSOCIATION FOR THE CARE
  OF CHILDREN'S HEALTH
7910 Woodmont Avenue, Suite 300
Bethesda, MD 20814
(301) 654-6549

NATIONAL ACADEMY OF
  NEUROPSYCHOLOGY
c/o Executive Secretary
C. Munro Cullum, Ph.D.
University of Colorado Health
  Sciences Center
University North Pavilion
4455 E. 12th Avenue, Suite 129
Denver, CO 80220
(303) 372-3123

THE SOCIETY OF BEHAVIORAL
  MEDICINE
103 South Adams Street
Rockville, MD 20850
(301) 251-2790

SOCIETY FOR RESEARCH IN
  CHILD DEVELOPMENT
Executive Offices
University of Michigan
300 N. Ingalls
10th Floor
Ann Arbor, MI 48109-0406

CLOSING COMMENTS

We developed this book because we felt there was a need for it. It is our hope that you have found the material provided by our colleagues useful not only for your practicum experience but also as you conceptualize your role as a practicing psychologist. As we noted in the Preface, this book is really a chance for you to have individual lectures from specialists in a range of domains related to clinical practice. As with any lecture, some were probably more interesting to you than others. Some topics may not be as relevant to you at this moment as they may be in the future.

One reader of the original manuscript for this book suggested that our final chapter should include comments about the future of clinical practice.

We are not visionaries and cannot predict the direction of clinical practice. As students of the history of our profession we have noted shifts in focus from psychological testing to psychotherapy. With the rise of such specialties as clinical neuropsychology, psychological testing has had a resurgence of popularity. Both individual and group psychotherapy continue to be popular activities for practitioners.

Many issues continue to be raised that may influence the shape of clinical practice in the future. As an increasing number of individuals become part of managed care health plans, will these plans rather than the practitioner dictate the length and form of treatment? We have seen the average length of stay in inpatient facilities decrease as a direct result of these fiscal changes. Entire treatment programs are restructured to meet the changing reimbursement policies. These plans typically include qualifications about the number of hospitalization days or outpatient sessions that can be reimbursed depending upon the diagnosis and provider. Will long-term therapy be reserved for those who can afford to pay for it with their personal resources? At this time that seems likely. Over the years there have been periodic attempts by psychologists to obtain prescription privileges. With an increasing number of psychologists obtaining medical staff privileges, the prescriptive option has once again become a major one. Both the general topic and Hawaii's example are covered in our book. The Department of Defense developed a test program to train psychologists to prescribe, and some psychologists have completed that program successfully at the time of this writing. The American Psychological Association has developed recommended courses of study for psychologists who are interested in obtaining such privileges. Bills to allow prescriptive privileges for psychologists continue to be introduced in various state legislatures. At this writing the outcome of these efforts is unknown. The impact on the role of the clinical psychologist if such legislation is passed is also unknown.

What will a "typical" practitioner's day be like in the future? We question whether there will be a "typical" or "average" practitioner. For us, versatility becomes a key attribute. Future practitioners will continue to have basic skills that are common to us all. What may be different is that practitioners will need to be more open to applying these skills in a range of markets. They will also need to learn how to market themselves. We do not mean to imply that high-pressure advertising will be the rule. On the other hand, clinicians of the future will not be likely to just place an ad in the yellow pages of their local phone directory and then expect to have a full practice. They will have to explain what they have to offer and negotiate fees with prospective health carrier consumers.

Future practitioners will also benefit from a strong support system. That support system includes a network of peers with whom to discuss professional issues, active use of continuing education to further develop skills and learn new ways to apply them, and participation in relevant professional associations. These associations provide not only a source for networking and learning but also a public education platform that needs to be shaped to meet the changing needs of the practitioner. Professional associations are becoming more actively involved in speaking for the profession with members of the government as well as providing lists of interviewees for network news programs. These sites can be effective venues for educating the public about the varied roles of professional psychologists.

Both of us were trained in traditional scientist-practitioner Ph.D. clinical psychology programs. Over our careers we have been fortunate to be able to teach as well as engage in clinical practice. Each of us has been involved in professional association activities and leadership positions. We have seen changes in our activities that have been related to the demands of our employment sites, shifts in the marketplace, and our personal development. We have come to appreciate the rich diversity of our discipline. It is our belief that only through the excitement of new members of the profession can clinical psychology continue to thrive and reach the potential we continue to believe it has. We hope some of our enthusiasm for the profession has reached you as a reader and that you will nurture this spirit not only in yourself but also in your peers and future students.

Ethical Principles of Psychologists and Code of Conduct

CONTENTS

December 1992 • American Psychologist
Copyright 1992 by the American Psychological Association, Inc.
Vol. 47, No. 12, 1597–1611.

This vesion of the APA Ethics Code was adopted by the American Psychological Association's Council of Representatives during its meeting, August 13 and 16, 1992, and is effective beginning December 1, 1992. Inquiries concerning the substance or interpretation of the APA Ethics Code should be addressed to the Director, Office of Ethics, American Psychological Association, 750 First Street, NE, Washington, DC 20002-4242.

This Code will be used to adjudicate complaints brought concerning alleged conduct occurring on or after the effective date. Complaints regarding conduct occurring prior to the effective date will be adjudicated on the basis of the version of the Code that was in effect at the time the conduct occurred, except that no provisions repealed in June 1989, will be enforced even if an earlier version contains the provision. The Ethics Code will undergo continuing review and study for future revisions; comments on the Code may be sent to the above address.

The APA has previously published its Ethical Standards as follows:

American Psychological Association. (1953) *Ethical standards of psychologists.* Washington, DC: Author.

American Psychological Association. (1958). Standards of ethical behavior for psychologists. *American Psychologist, 13,* 268–271.

American Psychological Association. (1963). Ethical standards of psychologists. *American Psychologist, 18,* 56–60.

American Psychological Association. (1968). Ethical standards of psychologists. *American Psychologist, 23,* 357–361.

American Psychological Association. (1977, March). Ethical standards of psychologists. *APA Monitor,* pp. 22–23.

American Psychological Association. (1979). *Ethical standards of psychologists.* Washington, DC: Author.

American Psychological Association. (1981). Ethical principles of psychologists. *American Psychologist, 36,* 633–638.

American Psychological Association. (1990). Ethical principles of psychologists (Amended June 2, 1989). *American Psychologist, 45,* 390–395.

Request copies of the APA's Ethical Principles of Psychologists and Code of Conduct from the APA Order Department, 750 First Street, NE, Washington, DC 20002-4242, or phone (202) 336-5510.

INTRODUCTION

The American Psychological Association's (APA's) Ethical Principles of Psychologists and Code of Conduct (hereinafter referred to as the Ethics Code) consists of an Introduction, a Preamble, six General Principles (A–F), and specific Ethical Standards. The Introduction discusses the intent, organization, procedural considerations, and scope of application of the Ethics Code. The Preamble and General Principles are *aspirational* goals to guide psychologists toward the highest ideals of psychology. Although the Preamble and General Principles are not themselves enforceable rules, they should be considered by psychologists in arriving at an ethical course of action and may be considered by ethics bodies in interpreting the Ethical Standards. The Ethical Standards set forth *enforceable* rules for conduct as psychologists. Most of the Ethical Standards are written broadly, in order to apply to psychologists in varied roles, although the application of an Ethical Standard may vary depending on the context. The Ethical Standards are not exhaustive. The fact that a given conduct is not specifically addressed by the Ethics Code does not mean that it is necessarily either ethical or unethical.

Membership in the APA commits members to adhere to the APA Ethics Code and to the rules and procedures used to implement it. Psychologists and students, whether or not they are APA members, should be aware that the Ethics Code may be applied to them by state psychology boards, courts, or other public bodies.

This Ethics Code applies only to psychogists' work-related activities, that is, activities that are part of the psychologists' scientific and professional functions or that are psychological in nature. It includes the clinical or counseling practice of psychology, research, teaching, supervision of trainees, development of assessment instruments, conducting assessments, educational counseling, organizational consulting, social intervention, administration, and other activities as well. These work-related activities can be distinguished from the purely private conduct of a psychologist, which ordinarily is not within the purview of the Ethics Code.

The Ethics Code is intended to provide standards of professional conduct that can be applied by the APA and by other bodies that choose to adopt them. Whether or not a psychologist has violated the Ethics Code does not by itself determine whether he or she is legally liable in a court action, whether a contract is enforceable, or whether other legal consequences occur. These results are based on legal rather than ethical rules. However, compliance with or violation of the Ethics Code may be admissible as evidence in some legal proceedings, depending on the circumstances.

In the process of making decisions regarding their professional behavior, psychologists must consider this Ethics Code, in addition to applicable laws and psychology board regulations. If the Ethics Code establishes a higher standard of conduct than is required by law, psychologists must meet the higher ethical standard. If the Ethics Code standard appears to conflict with the requirements of law, then psychologists make known their commitment to the Ethics Code and take steps to resolve the conflict in a responsible manner. If neither law nor the Ethics Code resolves an issue, psychologists should consider other professional materials[1] and the dictates of their own conscience, as well as seek consultation with others within the field when this is practical.

The procedures for filing, investigating, and resolving complaints of unethical conduct are describ ed in the current Rules and Procedures of the APA Ethics Committee. The actions that APA may take for violations of the Ethics Code include actions such as reprimand, censure, termination of APA membership, and referral of the matter to other bodies. Complaints who seek remedies such as monetary damages in alleging ethical violations by a psychologist must resort to private negotiation, administrative bodies, or the courts. Actions that violate the Ethics Code may lead to the imposition of sanctions on a psychologist by bodies other than APA, including state psychological associations, other professional groups, psychology boards, other state or federal agencies, and payors for health services. In addition to actions for violation of the Ethics Code, the APA Bylaws provide that APA may take action against a member after his or her conviction of a felony, expulsion or suspension from an affiliated state psychological association, or suspension or loss of licensure.

PREAMBLE

Psychologists work to develop a valid and reliable body of scientific knowledge based on research. They may apply that knowledge to human behavior in a variety of contexts. In doing so, they perform many roles, such as researcher, educator, diagnostician, therapist, supervisor, consultant, adminis-

---

[1] Professional materials that are most helpful in this regard are guidelines and standards that have been adopted or endorsed by professional psychological organizations. Such guidelines and standards, whether adopted by the American Psychological Association (APA) or its Divisions, are not enforceable as such by this Ethics Code, but are of educative value to psychologists, courts, and professional bodies. Such materials include, but are not limited to, the APA's *General Guidelines for Providers of Psychological Services* (1987), *Specialty Guidelines for the Delivery of Services by Clinical Psychologists, Counseling Psychologists, Industrial/Organizational Psychologists, and School Psychologists* (1981), *Guidelines for Computer Based Tests and Interpretations* (1987), *Standards for Educational and Psychological Testing* (1985), *Ethical Principles in the Conduct of Research With Human Participants* (1982), *Guidelines for Ethical Conduct in the Care and Use of Animals* (1986), *Guidelines for Providers of Psychological Services to Ethnic, Linguistic, and Culturally Diverse Populations* (1990), and *Publication Manual of the American Psychological Association* (3rd ed., 1983). Materials not adopted by APA as a whole include the APA Division 41 (Forensic Psychology)/American Psychology—Law Society's *Specialty Guidelines for Forensic Psychologists* (1991).

trator, social interventionist, and expert witness. Their goal is to broaden knowledge of behavior and, where appropriate, to apply it pragmatically to improve the condition of both the individual and society. Psychologists respect the central importance of freedom of inquiry and expression in research, teaching, and publication. They also strive to help the public in developing informed judgments and choices concerning human behavior. This Ethics Code provides a common set of values upon which psychologists build their professional and scientific work.

This Code is intended to provide both the general principles and the decision rules to cover most situations encountered by psychologists. It has as its primary goal the welfare and protection of the individuals and groups with whom psychologists work. It is the individual responsibility of each psychologist to aspire to the highest possible standards of conduct. Psychologists respect and protect human and civil rights, and do not knowingly participate in or condone unfair discriminatory practices.

The development of adynamic set of ethical standards for a psychologist's work-related conduct requires a personal commitment to a lifelong effort to act ethically; to encourage ethical behavior by students, supervisees, employees, and colleagues, as appropriate; and to consult with others, as needed, concerning ethical problems. Each psychologist supplements, but does not violate, the Ethics Code's values and rules on the basis of guidance drawn from personate, values, culture, and experience.

GENERAL PRINCIPLES

Principle A: Competence

Psychologists strive to maintain high standards of competence in their work. They recognize the boundaries of their particular competencies and the limitations of their expertise. They provide only those services and use only those techniques for which they are qualified by education, training, or experience. Psychologists are cognizant of the fact that the competencies required in serving, teaching, and/or studying groups of people vary with the distinctive characteristics of those groups. In those areas in which recognized professional standards do not yet exist, psychologists exercise careful judgment and take appropriate precautions to protect the welfare of those with whom they work. They maintain knowledge of relevant scientific and professional information related to the services they render, and they recognize the need for ongoing education. Psychologists make appropriate use of scientific, professional, technical, and administrative resources.

Principle B: Integrity

Psychologists seek to promote integrity in the science, teaching, and practice of psychology. In these activities psychologists are honest, fair, and respectful of others. In describing or reporting their qualifications, services, products, fees, research, or teaching, they do not make statements that are false, misleading, or deceptive. Psychologists strive to be aware of their own belief systems, values, needs, and limitations and the effect of these on their work. To the extent feasible, they attempt to clarify for relevant parties the roles they are performing and to function appropriately in accordance with those roles. Psychologists avoid improper and potentially harmful dual relationships.

Principle C: Professional and Scientific Responsibility

Psychologists uphold professional standards of conduct, clarify their professional roles and obligations, accept appropriate responsibility for their behavior, and adapt their methods to the needs of different populations. Psychologists consult with, refer to, or cooperate with other professionals and institutions to the extent needed to serve the best interests of their patients, clients, or other recipients of their services. Psychologists' moral standards and conduct are personal matters to the same degree as is true for any other person, except as psychologists' conduct may compromise their professional responsibilities or reduce the public's trust in psychology and psychologists. Psychologists are concerned about the ethical compliance of their colleagues' scientific and professional conduct. When appropriate, they consult with colleagues in order to prevent or avoid unethical conduct.

Principle D: Respect for People's Rights and Dignity

Psychologists accord appropriate respect to the fundamental rights, dignity, and worth of all people. They respect the rights of individuals to privacy, confidentiality, self-determination, and autonomy, mindful that legal and other obligations may lead to inconsistency and conflict with the exercise of these rights. Psychologists are aware of cultural, individual, and role differences, including those due to age, gender, race, ethnicity, national origin, religion, sexual orientation, disability, language, and socioeconomic status.

Psychologists try to eliminate the effect on their work of biases based on those factors, and they do not knowingly participate in or condone unfair discriminatory practices.

Principle E: Concern for Others' Welfare

Psychologists seek to contribute to the welfare of those with whom they interact professionally. In their professional actions, psychologists weigh the welfare and rights of their patients or clients, students, supervisees, human research participants, and other affected persons, and the welfare of animal subjects of research. When conflicts occur among psychologists' obligations or concerns, they attempt to resolve these conflicts and to perform their roles in a responsible fashion that avoids or minimizes harm. Psychologists are sensitive to real and ascribed differences in power between themselves and others, and they do not exploit or mislead other people during or after professional relationships.

Principle F: Social Responsibility

Psychologists are aware of their professional and scientific responsibilities to the community and the society in which they work and live. They apply and make public their knowledge of psychology in order to contribute to human welfare. Psychologists are concerned about and work to mitigate the causes of human suffering. When undertaking research, they strive to advance human welfare and the science of psychology. Psychologists try to avoid misuse of their work. Psychologists comply with the law and encourage the development of law and social policy that serve the interests of their patients and clients and the public. They are encouraged to contribute a portion of their professional time for little or no personal advantage.

ETHICAL STANDARDS

1. General Standards

These General Standards are potentially applicable to the professional and scientific activities of all psychologists.

1.01 Applicability of the Ethics Code

The activity of a psychologist is suspect cholo ist subject to the Ethics Code may be reviewed under these Ethical Standards only if the activity is part of his or her work-related functions or the activity is psychological in nature. Personal activities having no connection to or effect on psychological roles are not subject to the Ethics Code.

1.02 Relationship of Ethics and Law

If psychologists' ethical responsibilities conflict with law, psychologists make known their commitment to the Ethics Code and take steps to resolve the conflict in a responsible manner.

1.03   Professional and Scientific Relationship

Psychologists provide diagnostic, therapeutic, teaching, research, supervisory, consultative, or other psychological services only in the context of a defined professional or scientific relationship or role. (See also Standards 2.01, Evaluation, Diagnosis, and Interventions in Professional Context, and 7.02, Forensic Assessments.)

1.04   Boundaries of Competence

(a) Psychologists provide services, teach, and conduct research only within the boundaries of their competence, based on their education, training, supervised experience, or appropriate professional experience.

   (b) Psychologists provide services, teach, or conduct research in new areas or involving new techniques only after first undertaking appropriate study, training, supervision, and/or consultation from persons who are competent in those areas or techniques.

   (c) In those emerging areas in which generally recognized standards for preparatory training do not yet exist, psychologists nevertheless take reasonable steps to ensure the competence of their work and to protect patients, clients, students. research participants, and others from harm.

1.05   Maintaining Expertise

Psychologists who engage in assessment, therapy, teaching, research, organizational consulting, or other professional activities maintain a reasonable level of awareness of current scientific and professional information in their fields of activity, and undertake ongoing efforts to maintain competence in the skills they use.

1.06   Basis for Scientific and Professional Judgments

Psychologists rely on scientifically and professionally derived knowledge when making scientific or professional judgments or when engaging in scholarly or professional endeavors.

1.07   Describing the Nature and Results of Psychological Services

(a) When psychologists provide assessment, evaluation, treatment, counseling, supervision, teaching, consultation, research, or other psychological services to an individual, a group, or an organization, they provide, using language that is reasonably understandable to the recipient of those services, appropriate information beforehand about the nature of such services and appropriate information later about results and conclusions. (See also Standard 2.09, Explaining Assessment Results.)

   (b) If psychologists will be precluded by law or by organizational roles from providing such information to particular individuals or groups, they so inform those individuals or groups at the outset of the service.

1.08 Human Differences

Where differences of age, gender, race, ethnicity, national origin, religion, sexual orientation, disability, language, or socioeconomic status significantly affect psychologists' work concerning particular individuals or groups, psychologists obtain the training, experience, consultation, or supervision necessary to ensure the competence of their services, or they make appropriate referrals.

1.09 Respecting Others

In their work-related activities, psychologists respect the rights of others to hold values, attitudes, and opinions that differ from their own.

1.10 Nondiscrimination

In their work-related activities, psychologists do not engage in unfair discrimination based on age, gender, race, ethnicity, national origin, religion, sexual orientation, disability, socioeconomic status, or any basis proscribed by law.

1.11 Sexual Harassment

(a) Psychologists do not engage in sexual harassment. Sexual harassment is sexual solicitation, physical advances, or verbal or nonverbal conduct that is sexual in nature, that occurs in connection with the psychologist's activities or roles as a psychologist, and that either (1) is unwelcome, is offensive, or creates a hostile workplace environment, and the psychologist knows or is told this; or (2) is sufficiently severe or intense to be abusive to a reasonable person in the context. Sexual harassment can consist of a single intense or severe act or of multiple persistent or pervasive acts.

(b) Psychologists accord sexual-harassment complainants and respondents dignity and respect. Psychologists do not participate in denying a person academic admittance or advancement, employment, tenure, or promotion, based solely upon their having made, or their being the subject of, sexual harassment charges. This does not preclude taking action based upon the outcome of such proceedings or consideration of other appropriate infor-mation.

1.12 Other Harassment

Psychologists do not knowingly engage in behavior that is harassing or demeaning to persons with whom they interact in their work based on factors such as those persons' age, gender, race, ethnicity, national origin, religion, sexual orientation, disability, language, or socioeconomic status.

1.13 Personal Problems and Conflicts

(a) Psychologists recognize that their personal problems and conflicts may interfere with their effectiveness. Accordingly, they refrain from undertaking an activity when they know or should know that their personal problems are likely to lead to harm to a patient, client, colleague, student, research participant, or other person to whom they may owe a professional or scientific obligation.

(b) In addition, psychologists have an obligation to be alert to signs of, and to obtain assistance for, their personal problems at an early stage, in order to prevent significantly impaired performance.

(c) When psychologists become aware of personal problems that may interfere with their performing work related duties adequately, they take appropriate measures, such as obtaining professional consultation or assistance, and determine whether they should limit, suspend, or terminate their work-related duties.

1.14 Avoiding Harm
Psychologists take reasonable steps to avoid harming their patients or clients, research participants, students, and others with whom they work, and to minimize harm where it is foreseeable and unavoidable.

1.15 Misuse of Psychologists' Influence
Because psychologists' scientific and professional judgments and actions may affect the lives of others, they are alert to and guard against personal, financial, social, organizational, or political factors that might lead to misuse of their influence.

1.16 Misuse of Psychologists' Work
(a) Psychologists do not participate in activities in which it appears likely that their skills or data will be misused by others, unless corrective mechanisms are available. (See also Standard 7.04, Truthfulness and Candor.)

(b) If psychologists learn of misuse or misrepresentation of their work, they take reasonable steps to correct or minimize the misuse or misrepresentation.

1.17 Multiple Relationships
(a) In many communities and situations, it may not be feasible or reasonable for psychologists to avoid social or other nonprofessional contacts with persons such as patients, clients, students, supervisees, or research participants. Psychologists must always be sensitive to the potential harmful effects of other contacts on their work and on those persons with whom they deal. A psychologist refrains from entering into or promising another personal, scientific, professional, financial, or other relationship with such persons if it appears likely that such a relationship reasonably might impair the psychologist's objectivity or otherwise interfere with the psychologist's effectively performing his or her functions as a psychologist, or might harm or exploit the other party.

(b) Likewise, whenever feasible, a psychologist refrains from taking on professional or scientific obligations when preexisting relationships would create a risk of such harm..

(c) If a psychologist finds that, due to unforeseen factors, a potentially harmful multiple relationship has arisen, the psychologist attempts to resolve it with due regard for the best interests of the affected person and maximal compliance with the Ethics Code.

1.18 Barter (With Patients or Clients)
Psychologists ordinarily refrain from accepting goods, services, or other nonmonetary remuneration from patients or clients in return for psychological services because such arrangements create inherent potential for conflicts, exploitation, and distortion of the professional relationship. A psychologist may participate in bartering *only* if (1) it is not clinically contraindicated, *and* (2) the relationship is not exploitative. (See also Standards 1.17, Multiple Relationships, and 1.25, Fees and Financial Arrangements.)

1.19 Exploitative Relationships
(a) Psychologists do not exploit persons over whom they have supervisory, evaluative, or other authority such as students, supervisees, employees, research participants, and clients or patients. (See also Standards 4.05-4.07 regarding sexual involvement with clients or patients.)

(b) Psychologists do not engage in sexual relationships with students or supervisees in training over whom the psychologist has evaluative or direct authority, because such relationships are so likely to impair judgment or be exploitative.

1.20 Consultations and Referrals
(a) Psychologists arrange for appropriate consultations and referrals based principally on the best interests of their patients or clients, with appropriate consent, and subject to other relevant considerations, including applicable law and contractual obligations. (See also Standards 5.01, Discussing the Limits of Confidentiality, and 5.06, Consultations.)

(b) When indicated and professionally psychologists cooperate with other professionals in order to serve their patients or clients effectively and appropriately.

(c) Psychologists' referral practices are consistent with law.

1.21 Third-Party Requests for Services
(a) When a psychologist agrees to provide services to a person or entity at the request of a third party, the psychologist clarifies to the extent feasible, at the outset of the service, the nature of the relationship with each party. This clarification includes the role of the psychologist (such as therapist, organi-

zational consultant, diagnostician, or expert witness), the probable uses of the services provided or the information obtained, and the fact that there may be limits to confidentiality.

(b) If there is a foreseeable risk of the psychologist's being called upon to perform conflicting roles because of the involvement of a third party, the psychologist clarifies the nature and direction of his or her responsibilities, keeps all parties appropriately informed as matters develop, and resolves the situation in accordance with this Ethics Code.

1.22 Delegation to and Supervision of Subordinates

(a) Psychologists delegate to their employees, supervisees, and research assistants only those responsibilities that such persons can reasonably be expected to perform competently, on the basis of their education, training, or experience, either independently or with the level of supervision being provided.

(b) Psychologists provide proper training and supervision to their employees or supervisees and take reasonable steps to see that such persons perform services responsibly, competently, and ethically.

(c) If institutional policies, procedures, or practices prevent fulfillment of this obligation, psychologists attempt to modify their role or to correct the situation to the extent feasible.

1.23 Documentation of Professional and Scientific Work

(a) Psychologists appropriately document their professional and scientific work in order to facilitate provision of services later by them or by other professionals, to ensure accountability. and to meet other requirements of institutions or the law.

(b) When psychologists have reason to believe that records of their professional services will be used in legal proceedings involving recipients of or participants in their work, they have a responsibility to create and maintain documentation in the kind of detail and quality that would be consistent with reasonable scrutiny in an adjudicative forum. (See also Standard 7.01, Professionalism, under Forensic Activities.)

1.24 Records and Data

Psychologists create, maintain, disseminate, store, retain, and dispose of records and data relating to their research, practice, and other work in accordance with law and in a manner that permits compiliance with the requirements of this Ethics Code. (See also Standard 5.04, Maintenance of Records.)

1.25 Fees and Financial Arrangements

(a) As early as is feasible in a professional or scientific relationship, the psychologist and the patient, client, or other appropriate recipient of psychological services reach an agreement specifying the compensation and the billing arrangements.

(b) Psychologists do not exploit recipients of services or payors with respect to fees.

(c) Psychologists' fee practices are consistent with law.

(d) Psychologists do not misrepresent their fees.

(e) If limitations to services can be anticipated because of limitations in financing, this is discussed with the patient, client, or other appropriate recipient of services as early as is feasible. (See also Standard 4.08, Interruption of Services.)

(f) If the patient, client, or other recipient of services does not pay for services as agreed, and if the psychologist wishes to use collection agencies or legal measures to collect the fees, the psychologist first informs the person that such measures will be taken and provides that person an opportunity to make prompt payment (See also Standard 5.1 1, Withholding Records for Nonpayment.)

1.26   Accuracy in Reports to Payors and Funding Sources
In their reports to payors for services or sources of research funding, psychologists accurately state the nature of the research or service provided, the fees or charges, and where applicable, the identity of the provider, the findings, and the diagnosis. (See also Standard 5.05, Disclosures.)

1.27   Referrals and Fees
When a psychologist pays, receives payment from, or divides fees with another professional other than in an employer-employee relationship, the payment to each is based on the services (clinical, consultative, administrative, or other) provided and is not based on the referral itself.

2.   Evaluation, Assessment, or Intervention

2.01   Evaluation, Diagnosis, and Interventions in Professional Context
(a) Psychologists perform evaluations, diagnostic services, or interventions only within the context of a defined professional relationship. (See also Standard 1.03, Professional and Scientific Relationship.)

(b) Psychologists' assessments, recommendations, reports, and psychological diagnostic or evaluative statements are based on information and techniques (including personal interviews of the individual when appropriate) sufficient to provide appropriate substantiation for their findings. (See also Standard 7.02, Forensic Assessments.)

2.02 Competence and Appropriate Use of Assessments and Interventions

(a) Psychologists who develop, administer, score, interpret, or use psychological assessment techniques, interviews, tests, or instruments do so in a manner and for purposes that are appropriate in light of the research on or evidence of the usefulness and proper application of the techniques.

(b) Psychologists refrain from misuse of assessment techniques, interventions, results, and interpretations and take reasonable steps to prevent others from misusing the information these techniques provide. This includes refraining from releasing raw test results or raw data to persons, other than to patients or clients as appropriate, who are not qualified to use such information. (See also Standards 1.02, Relationship of Ethics and Law, and 1.04. Boundaries of Competence.)

2.03 Test Construction

Psychologists who develop and conduct research with tests and other assessment techniques use scientific procedures and current professional knowledge for test design, standardization, validation, reduction or elimination of bias, and recommendations for use.

2.04 Use of Assessment in General and With Special Populations

(a) Psychologists who perform interventions or administer, score, interpret, or use assessment techniques are familiar with the reliability, validation, and related standardization or outcome studies of, and proper applications and uses of, the techniques they use.

(b) Psychologists recognize limits to the certainty with which diagnoses, judgments, or predictions can be made about individuals.

(c) Psychologists attempt to identify situations in which particular interventions or assessment techniques or norms may not be applicable or may require adjustment in administration or interpretation because of factors such as individuals' gender, age, race, ethnicity, national origin, religion, sexual orientation, disability. language, or socioeconomic status.

2.05 Interpreting Assessment Results

When interpreting assessment results, including automated interpretations, psychologists take into account the various test factors and characteristics of the person being assessed that might affect psychologists' judgments or reduce the accuracy of their interpretations. They indicate any significant reservations they have about the accuracy or limitations of their interpretations.

2.06   Unqualified Persons
Psychologists do not promote the use of psychological assessment techniques by unqualified persons. (See also Standard 1.22, Delegation to and Supervision of Subordinates.)

2.07   Obsolete Tests and Outdated Test Results
(a) Psychologists do not base their assessment or intervention decisions or recommendations on data or test results that are outdated for the current purpose.

(b) Similarly, psychologists do not base such decisions or recommendations on tests and measures that are obsolete and not useful for the current purpose.

2.08   Test Scoring and Interpretation Services
(a) Psychologists who offer assessment or scoring procedures to other professionals accurately describe the purpose, norms, validity, reliability, and applications of the procedures and any special qualifications applicable to their use.

(b) Psychologists select scoring and interpretation services (including automated services) on the basis of evidence of the validity of the program and procedures as well as on other appropriate considerations.

(c) Psychologists retain appropriate responsibility for the appropriate application, interpretation, and use of assessment instruments, whether they score and interpret such tests themselves or use automated or other services.

2.09   Explaining Assessment Results
Unless the nature of the relationship is clearly explained to the person being assessed in advance and precludes provision of an explanation of results (such as in some organizational consulting, preemployment or security screenings, and forensic evaluations), psychologists ensure that an explanation of the results is provided using language that is reasonably understandable to the person assessed or to another legally authorized person on behalf of the client. Regardless of whether the scoring and interpretation are done by the psychologist, by assistants, or by automated or other outside services, psychologists take reasonable steps to ensure that appropriate explanations of results are given.

2.10   Maintaining Test Security
Psychologists make reasonable efforts to maintain the integrity and security of tests and other assessment techniques consistent with law, contractual obligations, and in a manner that permits compliance with the requirements of this Ethics Code. (See also Standard 1.02, Relationship of Ethics and Law.)

3. *Advertising and Other Public Statements*

3.01 *Definition of Public Statements*
Psychologists comply with this Ethics Code in public statements relating to their professional services, products, or publications or to the field of psychology. Public statements include but are not limited to paid or unpaid advertising, brochures, printed matter, directory listings, personal resumes or curricula vitae, interviews or comments for use in media, statements in legal proceedings, lectures and public oral presentations, and published materials,

3.02 *Statements by Others*
(a) Psychologists who engage others to create or place public statements that promote their professional practice, products, or activities retain professional responsibility for such statements.

(b) In addition, psychologists make reasonable efforts to prevent others whom they do not control (such as employers, publishers, sponsors, organizational clients, and representatives of the print or broadcast media) from making deceptive statements concerning psychologists' practice or professional or scientific activities.

(c) If psychologists learn of deceptive statements about their work made by others, psychologists make reasonable efforts to correct such statements.

(d) Psychologists do not compensate employees of press, radio, television, or other communication media in return for publicity in a news item.

(e) A paid advertisement relating to the psychologist's activities must be identified as such, unless it is already apparent from the context.

3.03 *Avoidance of False or Deceptive Statements*
(a) Psychologists do not make public statements that are false, deceptive, misleading, or fraudulent, either because of what they state, convey, or suggest or because of what they omit, concerning their research, practice, or other work activities or those of persons or organizations with which they are affiliated. As examples (and not in limitation) of this standard, psychologists do not make false or deceptive statements concerning (1) their training, experience, or competence; (2) their academic degrees; (3) their credentials; (4) their institutional or association affiliations; (5) their services; (6) the scientific or clinical basis for, or results or degree of success of, their services; (7) their fees; or (8) their publications or research findings. (See also Standards 6.15, Deception in Research, and 6.18, Providing Participants With Information About the Study.)

(b) Psychologists claim as credentials for their psychological work, only degrees that (1) were earned from a regionally accredited educational institution or (2) were the basis for psychology licensure by the state in which they practice.

3.04   Media Presentations

When psychologists provide advice or comment by means of public lectures, demonstrations, radio or television programs, prerecorded tapes, printed articles, mailed material, or other media, they take reasonable precautions to ensure that (1) the statements are based on appropriate psychological literature and practice, (2) the statements are otherwise consistent with this Ethics Code, and (3) the recipients of the information are not encouraged to infer that a relationship has been established with them personally.

3.05   Testimonials

Psychologists do not solicit testimonials from current psychotherapy clients or patients or other persons who because of their particular circumstances are vulnerable to undue influence.

3.06   In-Person Solicitation

Psychologists do not engage, directly or through agents, in uninvited in-person solicitation of business from actual or potential psychotherapy patients or clients or other persons who because of their particular circumstances are vulnerable to undue influence. However, this does not preclude attempting to implement appropriate collateral contacts with significant others for the purpose of benefiting an already engaged therapy patient.

4.   Therapy

4.01   Structuring the Relationship

(a)   Psychologists discuss with clients or patients as early as is feasible in the therapeutic relationship appropriate issues, such as the nature and anticipated course of therapy, fees, and confidentiality. (See also Standards 1.25, Fees and Financial Arrangements, and 5.01, Discussing the Limits of Confidentiality.)

(b)   When the psychologist's work with clients or patients will be supervised, the above discussion includes that fact, and the name of the supervisor, when the supervisor has legal responsibility for the case.

(c)   When the therapist is a student intern, the client or patient is   informed of that fact.

(d)   Psychologists make reasonable efforts to answer patients' questions and to avoid apparent misunderstandings about therapy. Whenever possible, psychologists provide oral and/or written information, using language that is reasonably understandable to the patient or client.

4.02   Informed Consent to Therapy

(a)   Psychologists obtain appropriate informed consent to therapy or related procedures, using language that is reasonably understandable to participants.

The content of informed consent will vary depending on many circum stances; however, informed consent generally implies that the person (1) has the capacity to consent, (2) has been informed of significant information concerning the procedure, (3) has freely and without undue influence expressed consent, and (4) consent has been appropriately documented.

(b) When persons are legally incapable of giving informed consent, psychologists obtain informed permission from a legally authorized person, if such substitute consent is permitted by law.

(c) In addition, psychologists (1) inform those persons who are legally incapable of giving informed consent about the proposed interventions in a manner commensurate with the persons' psychological capacities, (2) seek their assent to those interventions, and (3) consider such persons' preferences and best interests.

4.03   Couple and Family Relationships

(a) When a psychologist agrees to provide services to several persons who have a relationship (such as husband and wife or parents and children), the psychologist attempts to clarify at the outset (1) which of the individuals are patients or clients and (2) the relationship the psychologist will have with each person. This clarification includes the role of the psychologist and the probable uses of the services provided or the information obtained. (See also Standard 5.01, Discussing the Limits of Confidentiality.)

(b) As soon as it becomes apparent that the psychologist may be called on to perform potentially conflicting roles (such as marital counselor to husband and wife, and then witness for one party in a divorce proceeding), the psychologist attempts to clarify and adjust, or withdraw from, roles appropriately. (See also Standard 7.03, Clarification of Role, under Forensic Activities.)

4.04   Providing Mental Health Services to Those Served by Others

In deciding whether to offer or provide services to those already receiving mental health services elsewhere, psychologists carefully consider the treatment issues and the potential patient's or client's welfare. The psychologist discusses these issues with the patient or client, or another legally authorized person on behalf of the client, in order to minimize the risk of confusion and conflict, consults with the other service providers when appropriate, and proceeds with caution and sensitivity to the therapeutic issues.

4.05   Sexual Intimacies With Current Patients or Clients

Psychologists do not engage in sexual intimacies with current patients or clients.

4.06   Therapy With Former Sexual Partners

Psychologists do not accept as therapy patients or clients persons with whom they have engaged in sexual intimacies.

4.07   Sexual Intimacies With Former Therapy Patients

(a) Psychologists do not engage in sexual intimacies with a former therapy patient or client for at least two years after cessation or termination of professional services.

(b) Because sexual intimacies with a former therapy patient or client are so frequently harmful to the patient or client, and because such intimacies undermine public confidence in the psychology profession and thereby deter the public's use of needed services, psychologists do not engage in sexual intimacies with former therapy patients and clients even after a two-year interval except in the most unusual circumstances. The psychologist who engages in such activity after the two years following cessation or termination of treatment bears the burden of demonstrating that there has been no exploitation, in light of all relevant factors, including (1) the amount of time that has passed since therapy terminated, (2) the nature and duration of the therapy, (3) the circumstances of termination, (4) the patient's or client's personal history, (5) the patient's or client's current mental status, (6) the likelihood of adverse impact on the patient or client and others, and (7) any statements or actions made by the therapist during the course of therapy suggesting or inviting the possibility of a posttermination sexual or romantic relationship with the patient or client. (See also Standard 1.17, Multiple Relationships.)

4.08   Interruption of Services

(a) Psychologists make reasonable efforts to plan for facilitating care in the event that psychological services are interrupted by factors such as the psychologist's illness, death, unavailability, or relocation or by the client's relocation or financial limitations. (See also Standard 5.09, Preserving Records and Data.)

(b) When entering into employment or contractual relationships, psychologists provide for orderly and appropriate resolution of responsibility for patient or client care in the event that the employment or contractual relationship ends, with paramount consideration given to the welfare of the patient or client

4.09   Terminating the Professional Relationship

(a) Psychologists do not abandon patients or clients. (See also Standard 1.25e, under Fees and Financial Arrangements.)

(b) Psychologists terminate a professional relationship when it becomes reasonably clear that the patient or client no longer needs the service, is not benefiting, or is being harmed by continued service.

(c) Prior to termination for whatever reason, except where precluded by the patient's or client's conduct, the psychologist discusses the patient's or client's views and needs, provides appropriate pretermination counseling, suggests alternative service providers as appropriate, and takes other reasonable steps to facilitate transfer of responsibility to another provider if the patient or client needs one immediately.

5. Privacy and Confidentiality

These Standards are potentially applicable to the professional and scientific activities of all psychologists.

5.01 Discussing the Limits of Confidentiality

(a) Psychologists discuss with persons and organizations with whom they establish a scientific or professional relationship (including, to the extent feasible, minors and their legal representatives) (1) the relevant limitations on confidentiality, including limitations where applicable in group, marital, and family therapy or in organizational consulting, and (2) the foreseeable uses of the information generated through their services.

(b) Unless it is not feasible or is contraindicated, the discussion of confidentiality occurs at the outset of the relationship and thereafter as new circumstances may warrant.

(c) Permission for electronic recording of interviews is secured from clients and patients.

5.02 Maintaining Confidentiality

Psychologists have a primary obligation and take reasonable precautions to respect the confidentiality rights of those with whom they work or consult, recognizing that confidentiality may be established by law, institutional rules, or professional or scientific relationships. (See also Standard 6.26, Professional Reviewers.)

5.03 Minimizing Intrusions on Privacy

(a) In order to minimize intrusions on privacy, psychologists include in written and oral reports, consultations, and the like, only information germane to the purpose for which the communication is made.

(b) Psychologists discuss confidential information obtained in clinical or consulting relationships, or evaluative data concerning patients, individual or organizational clients, students, research participants, supervisees, and employees, only for appropriate scientific or professional purposes and only with persons clearly concerned with such matters.

5.04 Maintenance of Records
Psychologists maintain appropriate confidentiality in creating, storing, accessing, transferring, and disposing of records under their control, whether these are written, automated, or in any other medium. Psychologists maintain and dispose of records in accordance with law and in a manner that permits compliance with the requirements of this Ethics Code.

5.05 Disclosures
(a) Psychologists disclose confidential information without the consent of the individual only as mandated by law, or where permitted by law for a valid purpose, such as (1) to provide needed professional services to the patient or the individual or organizational client, (2) to obtain appropriate professional consultations, (3) to protect the patient or client or others from harm, or (4) to obtain payment for services, in which instance disclosure is limited to the minimum that is necessary to achieve the purpose.

(b) Psychologists also may disclose confidential information with the appropriate consent of the patient or the individual or organizational client (or of another legally authorized person on behalf of the patient or client), unless prohibited by law.

5.06 Consultations
When consulting with colleagues, (1) psychologists do not share confidential information that reasonably could lead to the identification of a patient, client, research participant, or other person or organization with whom they have a confidential relationship unless they have obtained the prior consent of the person or organization or the disclosure cannot be avoided, and (2) they share information only to the extent necessary to achieve the purposes of the consultation. (See also Standard 5.02, Maintaining Confidentiality.)

5.07 Confidential Information in Databases
(a) If confidential information concerning recipients of psychological services is to be entered into databases or systems of records available to persons whose access has not been consented to by the recipient, then psychologists use coding or other techniques to avoid the inclusion of personal identifiers.

(b) If a research protocol approved by an institutional review board or similar body requires the inclusion of personal identifiers, such identifiers are deleted before the information is made accessible to persons other than those of whom the subject was advised.

(c) If such deletion is not feasible, then before psychologists transfer such data to others or review such data collected by others, they take reasonable steps to determine that appropriate consent of personally identifiable individuals has been obtained.

5.08   Use of Confidential Information for Didactic or Other Purposes

(a) Psychologists do not disclose in their writings, lectures, or other public media, confidential, personally identifiable information concerning their patients, individual or organizational clients, students, research participants, or other recipients of their services that they obtained during the course of their work, unless the person or organization has consented in writing or unless there is other ethical or legal authorization for doing so.

(b) Ordinarily, in such scientific and professional presentations, psychologists disguise confidential information concerning such persons or organizations so that they are not individually identifiable to others and so that discussions do not cause harm to subjects who might identify themselves.

5.09   Preserving Records and Data

A psychologist makes plans in advance so that confidentiality of records and data is protected in the event of the psychologist's death, incapacity, or withdrawal from the position or practice.

5.10   Ownership of Records and Data

Recognizing that ownership of records and data is governed by legal principles, psychologists take reasonable and lawful steps so that records and data remain available to the extent needed to serve the best interests of patients, individual or organizational clients, research participants, or appropriate others.

5.11   Withholding Records for Nonpayment

Psychologists may not withhold records under their ontrol that are requested and imminently needed for a patient's or client's treatment solely because payment has not been received, except as otherwise provided by law.

6.   Teaching, Training Supervision, Research, and Publishing

6.01 Design of Education and Training Programs

Psychologists who are responsible for education and training programs seek to ensure that the programs are competently designed, provide the proper experiences, and meet the requirements for licensure, certification, or other goals for which claims are made by the program.

6.02   Descriptions of Education and Training Programs

(a) Psychologists responsible for education and training programs seek to ensure that there is a current and accurate description of the program content, training goals and objectives, and requirements that must be met for satisfactory completion of the program. This information must be made readily available to all interested parties.

(b) Psychologists seek to ensure that statements concerning their course outlines are accurate and not misleading, particularly regarding the subject matter to be covered, bases for evaluating progress, and the nature of course experiences. (See also Standard 3.03, Avoidance of False or Deceptive Statements.)

(c) To the degree to which they exercise control, psychologists responsible for announcements, catalogs, brochures, or advertisements describing workshops, seminars, or other non-degree-granting educational programs ensure that they accurately describe the audience for which the program is intended, the educational objectives, the presenters, and the fees involved.

6.03   Accuracy and Objectivity in Teaching
(a) When engaged in teaching or training, psychologists present psychological information accurately and with a reasonable degree of objectivity.

(b) When engaged in teaching or training, psychologists recognize the power they hold over students or supervisees and therefore make reasonable efforts to avoid engaging in conduct that is personally demeaning to students or supervisees. (See also Standards 1.09, Respecting Others, and 1.12, Other Harassment.)

6.04   Limitation on Teaching
Psychologists do not teach the use of techniques or procedures that require specialized training, licensure, or expertise, including but not limited to hypnosis, biofeedback, and projective techniques, to individuals who lack the prerequisite training, legal scope of practice, or expertise.

6 .05   Assessing Student and Supervisee Performance
(a) In academic and supervisory relationships, psychologists establish an appropriate process for providing feedback to students and supervisees.

(b) Psychologists evaluate students and supervises on the basis of their actual performance on relevant and established program requirements.

6.06   Planning Research
(a) Psychologists design, conduct, and report research in accordance with recognized standards of scientific competence and ethical research.

(b) Psychologists plan their research so as to minimize the possibility that results will be misleading.

(c) In planning research, psychologists consider its ethical acceptability under the Ethics Code. If an ethical issue is unclear, psychologists seek to resolve the issue through consultation with institutional review boards, animal care and use committees, peer consultations. or other proper mechanisms.

(d) Psychologists take reasonable steps to implement appropriate protections for the rights and welfare of human participants, other persons affected by the research, and the welfare of animal subjects.

6.07 Responsibility

(a) Psychologists conduct research competently and with due concern for the dignity and welfare of the participants.

(b) Psychologists are responsible for the ethical conduct of research conducted by them or by others under their supervision or control.

(c) Researchers and assistants are permitted to perform only those tasks for which they are appropriately trained and prepared.

(d) As part of the process of development and implementation of research projects, psychologists consult those with expertise concerning any special population under investigation or most likely to be affected.

6.08 Compliance With Law and Standards

Psychologists plan and conduct research in a manner consistent with federal and state law and regulations, as well as professional standards governing the conduct of research, and particularly those standards governing research with human participants and animal subjects.

6.09 Institutional Approval

Psychologists obtain from host institutions or organizations appropriate approval prior to conducting research, and they provide accurate information about their research proposals. They conduct the research in accordance with the approved research protocol.

6.10 Research Responsibilities

Prior to conducting research (except research involving only anonymous surveys, naturalistic observations, or similar research), psychologists enter into an agreement with participants that clarifies the nature of the research and the responsibilities of each party.

6.11 Informed Consent to Research

(a) Psychologists use language that is reasonably understandable to research participants in obtaining their appropriate informed consent (except as provided in Standard 6.12, Dispensing With Informed Consent). Such informed consent is appropriately documented.

(b) Using language that is reasonably understandable to participants, psychologists inform participants of the nature of the research; they inform participants that they are free to participate or to decline to participate or to withdraw from the research; they explain the foreseeable consequences of declining or withdrawing; they inform participants of significant factors that may be expected to influence their willingness to participate (such as risks, discomfort, adverse effects, or limitations on confidentiality, except as provided in Standard 6.15, Deception in Research); and they explain other aspects about which the prospective participants inquire.

c) When psychologists conduct research with individuals such as students or subordinates, psychologists take special care to protect the prospective participants from adverse consequences of declining or withdrawing from participation.

(d) When research participation is a course requirement or opportunity for extra credit, the prospective participant is given the choice of equitable alternative activities.

(e) For persons who are legally incapable of giving informed consent, psychologists nevertheless (1) provide an appropriate explanation, (2) obtain the participant's assent, and (3) obtain appropriate permission from a legally authorized person, if such substitute consent is permitted by law.

6.12   Dispensing With Informed Consent
Before determining that planned research (such as research involving only anonymous questionnaires, naturalistic observations, or certain kinds of archival research) does not require the informed consent of research participants, psychologists consider applicable regulations and institutional review board requirements, and they consult with colleagues as appropriate.

6 .13   Informed Consent in Research Filming or Recording
Psychologists obtain informed consent from research participants prior to filming or recording them in any form, unless the research involves simply naturalistic observations in public places and it is not anticipated that the recording will be used in a manner that could cause personal identification or harm.

6.14   Offering Inducements for Research Participants
(a) In offering professional services as an inducement to obtain research participants, psychologists make clear the nature of the services, as well as the risks, obligations, and imitations. (See also Standard 1. 18, Barter [With Patients or Clients].)

(b) Psychologists do not offer excessive or inappropriate financial or other inducements to obtain research participants, particularly when it might tend to coerce participation.

6.15   Deception in Research
(a) Psychologists do not conduct a study involving deception unless they have determined that the use of deceptive techniques is justified by the study's

prospective scientific, educational, or applied value and that equally effective alternative procedures that do not use deception are not feasible.

(b) Psychologists never deceive research participants about significant aspects that would affect their willingness to participate, such as physical risks, discomfort, or unpleasant emotional experiences.

(c) Any other deception that is an integral feature of the design and conduct of an experiment must be explained to participants as early as is feasible, preferably at the conclusion of their participation, but no later than at the conclusion of the research. (See also Standard 6.18, Providing Participants With Information About the Study.)

6.16 Sharing and Utilizing Data

Psychologists inform research participants of their anticipated sharing or further use of personally identifiable research data and of the possibility of unanticipated future uses.

6.17 Minimizing Invasiveness

In conducting research, psychologists interfere with the participants or milieu from which data are collected only in a manner that is warranted by an appropriate research design and that is consistent with psychologists' roles as scientific investigators.

6.18 Providing Participants With Information About the Study

(a) Psychologists provide a prompt opportunity for ' participants to obtain appropriate information about the nature, results, and conclusions of the re search, and psychologists attempt to correct any misconceptions that participants may have.

(b) If scientific or humane values justify delaying or withholding this information, psychologists take reasonable measures to reduce the risk of harm.

6.19 Honoring Commitments

Psychologists take reasonable measures to honor all commitments they have made to research participants.

6.20 Care and Use of Animals in Research

(a) Psychologists who conduct research involv ing animals treat them humanely.

(b) Psychologists acquire, care for, use, and dispose of animals in compliance with current federal, state, and local laws and regulations, and with professional standards.

(c) Psychologists trained in research methods and experienced in the care of laboratory animals supervise all procedures involving animals and are responsible for ensuring appropriate consideration of their comfort, health, and humane treatment.

(d) Psychologists ensure that all individuals using animals under their supervision have received instruction in research methods and in the care, maintenance, and handling of the species being used, to the extent appropriate to their role.

(e) Responsibilities and activities of individuals assisting in a research project are consistent with their respective competencies.

(f) Psychologists make reasonable efforts to minimize the discomfort, infection, illness, and pain of animal subjects.

(g) A procedure subjecting animals to pain, stress, or privation is used only when an alternative procedure is unavailable and the goal is justified by its prospective scientific, educational, or applied value.

(h) Surgical procedures are performed under appropriate anesthesia; techniques to avoid infection and minimize pain are followed during and after surgery.

(i) When it is appropriate that the animal's life be terminated, it is done rapidly, with an effort to minimize pain, and in accordance with accepted procedures.

6.21   Reporting of Results

(a) Psychologists do not fabricate data or falsify results in their publications.

(b) If psychologists discover significant errors in their published data, they take reasonable steps to correct such errors in a correction, retraction, erratum, or other appropriate publication means.

6.22   Plagiarism

Psychologists do not present substantial portions or elements of another's work or data as their own, even if the other work or data source is cited occasionally.

6.23   Publication Credit

(a) Psychologists take responsibility and credit, including authorship credit, only for work they have actually performed or to which they have contributed.

(b) Principal authorship and other publication credits accurately reflect the relative scientific or professional contributions of the individuals involved, regardless of their relative status. Mere possession of an institutional position, such as Department Chair, does not justify authorship credit. Minor contributions to the research or to the writing for publications are appropriately acknowledged, such as in footnotes or in an introductory statement.

(c) A student is usually listed as principal author on any multiple-authored article that is substantially based on the student's dissertation or thesis.

6.24 Duplicate Publication of Data

Psychologists do not publish, as original data, data that have been previously published. This does not preclude republishing data when they are accompanied by proper acknowledgment.

6.25 Sharing Data

After research results are published, psychologists do not withhold the data on which their conclusions are based from other competent professionals who seek to verify the substantive claims through reanalysis and who intend to use such data only for that purpose, provided that the confidentiality of the participants can be protected and unless legal rights concerning proprietary data preclude their release.

6.26 Professional Reviewers

Psychologists who review material submitted for publication, grant, or other research proposal review respect the confidentiality of and the proprietary rights in such information of those who submitted it.

7. Forensic Activities

7.01 Professionalism

Psychologists who perform forensic functions, such as assessments, interviews, consultations, reports, or expert testimony, must comply with all other provisions of this Ethics Code to the extent that they apply to such activities. In addition, psychologists base their forensic work on appropriate knowledge of and competence in the areas underlying such work, including specialized knowledge concerning special populations. (See also Standards 1.06, Basis for Scientific and Professional Judgments; 1.08, Human Differences; 1.15, Misuse of Psychologists' Influence; and 1.23, Documentation of Professional and Scientific Work.)

7.02 Forensic Assessments

(a) Psychologists' forensic assessments, recommendations, and reports are based on information and techniques (including personal interviews of the individual, when appropriate) sufficient to provide appropriate substantiation for,, their findings. (See also Standards 1.03, Professional and Scientific Relationship; 1.23, Documentation of Professional and Scientific Work; 2.01, Evaluation, Diagnosis, and Interventions in Professional Context; and 2.05, Interpreting Assessment Results.)

(b) Except as noted in (c), below, psychologists provide written or oral forensic reports or testimony of the psychological characteristics of an individual only after they have conducted an examination of the individual adequate to support their statements or conclusions.

(c) When, despite reasonable efforts, such an examination is not feasible, psychologists clarify the impact of their limited information on the reliability and validity of their reports and testimony, and they appropriately limit the nature and extent of their conclusions or recommendations.

7.03   Clarification of Role
In most circumstances, psychologists avoid performing multiple and potentially conflicting roles in forensic matters. When psychologists may be called on to serve in more than one role in a legal proceeding—for example, as consultant or expert for one party or for the court and as a fact witness—they clarify role expectations and the extent of confidentiality in advance to the extent feasible, and thereafter as changes occur, in order to avoid compromising their professional judgment and objectivity and in order to avoid misleading others regarding their role.

7.04   Truthfulness and Candor
(a) In forensic testimony and reports, psychologists testify truthfully, honestly, and candidly and, consistent with applicable legal procedures, describe fairly the bases for their testimony and conclusions.

(b) Whenever necessary to avoid misleading, psychologists acknowledge the limits of their data or conclusions.

7.05   Prior Relationships
A prior professional relationship with a party does not preclude psychologists from testifying as fact witnesses or from testifying to their services to the extent permitted by applicable law. Psychologists appropriately take into account ways in which the prior relationship might affect their professional objectivity or opinions and disclose the potential conflict to the relevant parties.

7.06   Compliance With Law and Rules
In performing forensic roles, psychologists are reasonably familiar with the rules governing their roles. Psychologists are aware of the occasionally competing demands placed upon them by these principles and the requirements of the court system, and attempt to resolve these conflicts by making known their commitment to this Ethics Code and taking steps to resolve the conflict in a responsible manner. (See also Standard 1.02, Relationship of Ethics and Law.)

8.   Resolving Ethical Issues

8.01   Familiarity With Ethics Code
Psychologists have an obligation to be familiar with this Ethics Code, other applicable ethics codes, and their application to psychologists' work. Lack of

awareness or misunderstanding of an ethical standard is not itself a defense to a charge of unethical conduct.

8.02 Confronting Ethical Issues
When a psychologist is uncertain whether a particular situation or course of action would violate this Ethics Code, the psychologist ordinarily consults with other psychologists knowledgeable about ethical issues, with state or national psychology ethics committees, or with other appropriate authorities in order to choose a proper response.

8.03 Conflicts Between Ethics and Organizational Demands
If the demands of an organization with which psychologists are affiliated conflict with this Ethics Code, psychologists clarify the nature of the conflict, make known their commitment to the Ethics Code, and to the extent feasible, seek to resolve the conflict in a way that permits the fullest adherence to the Ethics Code.

8.04 Informal Resolution of Ethical Violations
When psychologists believe that there may have been an ethical violation by another psychologist, they attempt to resolve the issue by bringing it to the attention of that individual if an informal resolution appears appropriate and the intervention does not violate any confidentiality rights that may be involved.

8.05 Reporting Ethical Violations
If an apparent ethical violation is not appropriate for informal resolution under Standard 8.04 or is not resolved properly in that fashion, psychologists take further action appropriate to the situation, unless such action conflicts with confidentiality rights in ways that cannot be resolved. Such action might include referral to state or national committees on professional ethics or to state licensing boards.

8.06 Cooperating With Ethics Committees
Psychologists cooperate in ethics investigations, proceedings, and resulting requirements of the APA or any affiliated state psychological association to which they belong. In doing so, they make reasonable efforts to resolve any issues as to confidentiality. Failure to cooperate is itself an thics violation.

8.07 Improper Complaints
Psychologists do not file or encourage the filing of ethics complaints that are frivolous and are intended to harm the respondent rather than to protect the public.

▶ Index

355

This novel is inspired by a famous image called *Mixed Bathing in Aberystwyth* taken in 1911.

Whilst some events are from local historical accounts the story and all characters and modern events in the book are fictional.